A Handbook of
Appendix

A Handbook of
Appendix

Vinod Kumar Nigam MBBS MS FICS FIAGES
Associate Director, General and Minimal Access Surgery
Max Hospital
Gurugram, Haryana, India

Siddharth Nigam MBBS MS(General Surgery)
Senior Consultant, General and Minimal Access Surgery
Max Hospital
Gurugram, Haryana, India

Foreword

Pradeep Chowbey

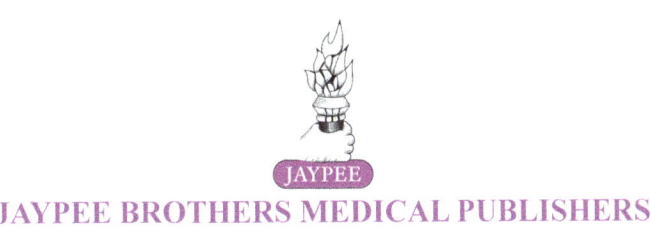

JAYPEE BROTHERS MEDICAL PUBLISHERS
The Health Sciences Publisher
New Delhi | London

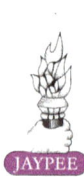 **Jaypee Brothers Medical Publishers (P) Ltd**

Headquarters
EMCA House
23/23-B, Ansari Road, Daryaganj
New Delhi 110 002, India
Landline: +91-11-23272143, +91-11-23272703
+91-11-23282021, +91-11-23245672
E-mail: jaypee@jaypeebrothers.com

Overseas Office
JP Medical Ltd.
83, Victoria Street, London
SW1H 0HW (UK)
Phone: +44-20 3170 8910
Fax: +44(0)20 3008 6180
E-mail: info@jpmedpub.com

Corporate Office
Jaypee Brothers Medical Publishers (P) Ltd.
4838/24, Ansari Road, Daryaganj
New Delhi 110 002, India
Phone: +91-11-43574357
Fax: +91-11-43574314
E-mail: jaypee@jaypeebrothers.com

EU GPSR Authorised Representative
LOGOS EUROPE, 9 rue Nicolas Poussin
17000, LA ROCHELLE, France
Phone: +33 (0) 6 67 93 73 78
Email: Contact@logos europe.eu

Website: www.jaypeebrothers.com
Website: www.jaypeedigital.com

© 2024, Jaypee Brothers Medical Publishers

The views and opinions expressed in this book are solely those of the original contributor(s)/author(s) and do not necessarily represent those of editor(s) or publisher of the book.

All rights reserved. No part of this publication may be reproduced, stored or transmitted in any form or by any means, electronic, mechanical, photocopying, recording or otherwise, without the prior permission in writing of the publishers.

All brand names and product names used in this book are trade names, service marks, trademarks or registered trademarks of their respective owners. The publisher is not associated with any product or vendor mentioned in this book.

Medical knowledge and practice change constantly. This book is designed to provide accurate, authoritative information about the subject matter in question. However, readers are advised to check the most current information available on procedures included and check information from the manufacturer of each product to be administered, to verify the recommended dose, formula, method and duration of administration, adverse effects and contraindications. It is the responsibility of the practitioner to take all appropriate safety precautions. Neither the publisher nor the author(s)/editor(s) assume any liability for any injury and/or damage to persons or property arising from or related to use of material in this book.

This book is sold on the understanding that the publisher is not engaged in providing professional medical services. If such advice or services are required, the services of a competent medical professional should be sought.

Every effort has been made where necessary to contact holders of copyright to obtain permission to reproduce copyright material. If any have been inadvertently overlooked, the publisher will be pleased to make the necessary arrangements at the first opportunity.

Inquiries for bulk sales may be solicited at: jaypee@jaypeebrothers.com

A Handbook of Appendix / Vinod Kumar Nigam, Siddharth Nigam

First Edition: **2024**

ISBN: 978-93-5696-446-4

DEDICATED TO

All our patients and surgical colleagues

Appendicitis can be fatal, even when treated by the most experienced surgeon.
— **Vinod Kumar Nigam**

Appendix is known more due to its misdeeds than to its deeds.
— **Vinod Kumar Nigam**

No one should die of appendicitis.
— **Paul Georges Dieulafoy**

Foreword

I was pleased to learn about the Handbook on Appendix written by my colleagues and friends Dr Vinod Kumar Nigam and Dr Siddharth Nigam. We are currently navigating unprecedented times in our existence. The practice of surgery is also subject to increased scrutiny, challenge, and validation. Ubiquitous social media has added to debate, controversy, and decision-making. The wide array of pathology, clinical presentation, and management options can make the subject more controversial and confusing, especially for our younger colleagues. This handbook provides a comprehensive, overarching, and holistic view of the appendix from the perspective of an experienced surgeon.

All practicing physicians and surgeons are destined to encounter the innocuous appendix with its varied presentations in their patients on some occasions. The introduction of this handbook is a testament to the possibilities that exist in the management of pathology of this innocuous organ. As such, this handbook shall prove to be a treatise not only to practicing surgeons but also to all clinicians dealing with patients.

The contents of this handbook are contemporary and have been provided in a lucid, easy-to-read format that is not stressful. The operative pictures are excellent and the live diagrams provide a clean and concise depiction that is easy to understand. I wish to congratulate the authors for their expertise and lucid presentation. This publication will provide a ready handbook for all references for the appendix as also technical details and handy tips for clinicians who manage patients with different pathologies and presentations related to the appendix.

I wish this handbook great success and popularity that it richly deserves.

Warm Regards,

Pradeep Chowbey
MS MNAMS FRCS(London) FIMSA FAIS FICS FACS FIAGES FALS FAMS
Padmashri Awarded by The President of India
Chairman, Max Institute of Minimal Access, Metabolic and Bariatric Surgery
Chairman, Surgery and Allied Surgical Specialities
Honorary Laparoscopic Surgeon to The President of India
Honorary Laparoscopic Surgeon to Armed Forces Medical Services (AFMS)
Doctor of Science (Honoris Causa)
Surgeon to His Holiness Dalai Lama

Preface

*'To acquire knowledge, one must study;
but to acquire wisdom, one must observe.'*
—Marilyn vos Savant

Medical understanding of diseases is fast improving. The surgical procedures are also developing at a high pace with the trend toward minimal invasive surgery. It is becoming difficult to accommodate all in one small and handy book which can be taken towards, to bedsides of patients, and to clinics for ready reference. That is why we thought of taking out one topic in one volume and include everything about that subject, from anatomy to recent advancements. The sole purpose of this book is to get everything about appendix in one short book. We hope that this will be helpful to the undergraduate and postgraduate students as well as to practicing surgeons and to those who are interested in acquiring knowledge about appendix and its diseases.

Appendicitis is one of the most important and common problems in the field of surgery. The book is primarily written for clinical students, surgeons, and higher surgical trainees. This book will be helpful to those who require an understanding of the basic science and essential principles of surgery while dealing with the diseases of appendix. This book is also designed to be a reference book for family practice doctors and for the doctors in other specialties who are interested to know about appendix and its diseases. We are sure that this book will have the greatest appeal among its readers who want to enhance their knowledge. There is a vast difference between this book and any other textbook of surgery having appendix and its diseases as a chapter. This is a book about appendix having an extensive description with a view to have the pathophysiology, anatomy, clinical problems, differential diagnosis, management, and operative details in simple language and manner. The book has simple, informative, and easy to practice line diagrams which will be very helpful to the students. Photographs of the patients, investigative procedures, and operations are chosen carefully to explain the salient points rather than just filling the space. Unnecessary text diagrams and photographs are avoided to remove confusion. The clinical material in this book is from our day to day clinical practice. QR codes are given at various sites in the book to confirm "seeing is believing".

Abbreviations given are the standard abbreviations used the world over. To avoid monotonous design and text, the book has many quotations. These quotations are to keep interest and enthusiasm of readers alive in reading the book. Care is taken to explain the operative procedures step-by-step to make it short, simple, easy to understand, and quick to refer.

"Controversies, Arguments and Discussions" are there to understand different views and to follow the overall accepted procedures and to know the pros and cons of various ways of dealing with a situation. Recent advancements and modern trends make the reader aware of what is recent and what is obsolete. Mnemonics, questions and answers, and MCQs are important for students and will also enhance the knowledge of a surgeon. The medicolegal aspect of management of appendicitis is important in today's time, so that you can avoid unnecessary medicolegal implications. QR Codes are there to explain the clinical features and procedures in a simple way and make a mental impact. At the end of each chapter, there is an exhaustive list of references which is important for a reader who wishes to know more.

Vinod Kumar Nigam
Siddharth Nigam

Acknowledgments

*'After all, he thinks conscience is a sort of vermiform appendix.
Chop it out and you'll feel all the better.'*
—**Dorothy L Sayers**

We are thankful to all our colleagues who helped us by providing valuable information, suggestions, and photographs used in this book. We are obliged to Late Mr Mukul Sharma, science writer and scientific editor of "Times of India", for important suggestions and editing the book without which the book would not have come to this shape. We thank Dr Kunal Nigam, for helping us out to write anatomy and other basic sciences. Dr Madhur Arora, helped us by drawing beautiful line diagrams and searching medical literature and bibliography. Dr Charvi Chawla, deserves thanks for proofreading and suggestions.

Mrs Kumud acted as the backbone for allowing me to take as much time as required from personal life to devote in writing this book without any complaints. She also did the excellent job of proof reading of the book. Mr Vipin Sharma earns my thanks and gratitude for typing and computer work. Ms Jasleen Kaur deserves credit for helping in preparing QR Codes for the book.

I am extremely thankful to Shri Jitendar P Vij (Group Chairman), Mr Ankit Vij (Managing Director), Mr MS Mani (Group President), Ms Chetna Malhotra (Senior Director—Professional Publishing, Marketing, and Business Development), Ms Pooja Bhandari [Director—Production (Books and Journals)], and Mr Akhilesh Saxena (Publishing Coordinator), M/s Jaypee Brothers Medical Publishers (P) Ltd, New Delhi, India, for constant encouragement.

Vinod Kumar Nigam
Siddharth Nigam

Abbreviations

AA	: Acute appendicitis	NPO	: Nil per oral
APUD	: Amine precursor uptake decarboxylase (cells)	NSAIDs	: Nonsteroidal anti-inflammatory drugs
ASIS	: Anterior superior iliac spine	OSR	: Ochsner–Sherren regimen
CBC	: Complete blood count	OT	: Operation theater
CHF	: Congestive heart failure	PAC	: Preanesthetic checkup
CT	: Computerized tomography	PID	: Pelvic inflammatory disease
DLC	: Differential leukocyte count	PPI	: Proton-pump inhibitor
DRE	: Digital rectal examination	QoL	: Quality of life
DVT	: Deep vein thrombosis	PR	: Per rectal
GA	: General anesthesia	RBC	: Red blood cell
GALT	: Gut-associated lymphoid tissue	RIF	: Right iliac fossa
GIT	: Gastrointestinal tract	RLQ	: Right lower quadrant
IV	: Intravenous	RT	: Ryle's tube
IVU	: Intravenous urogram	RUQ	: Right upper quadrant
LA	: Local anesthesia	SA	: Spinal anesthesia
LIF	: Left iliac fossa	TLC	: Total leukocyte count
LLQ	: Left lower quadrant	UTI	: Urinary tract infection
LUQ	: Left upper quadrant	USG	: Ultrasonogram
NCCT	: Noncontrast CT	WBC	: White blood cell

Contents

1. **Introduction**   1
2. **Historical Background—Milestones**   3
3. **Surgical Anatomy**   10
   - Development of Appendix   *10*
   - Surface Marking of Appendix   *12*
   - Position of Appendix   *12*
   - Subhepatic Appendix   *13*
   - Size of the Appendix   *15*
   - Appendicular Orifice   *15*
   - Lumen of the Appendix   *15*
   - Why Appendix is Prone to Infection   *15*
   - Mesoappendix or Mesentery of Appendix   *16*
   - Variations in Arterial Supply of Appendix   *17*
   - Venous Drainage of Appendix   *18*
   - Lymphatic Drainage of Appendix   *18*
   - Nerve Supply of Appendix   *20*
   - Folds and Recesses in Relation to the Appendix   *20*
   - Jackson's Membrane   *20*
4. **Histology of Appendix**   22
   - Serosa   *23*
   - Muscle Coat   *23*
   - Submucosa   *23*
   - Mucosa   *23*
5. **Functions of Appendix**   25
   - To Maintain Gut Flora   *25*
   - Immune Function   *26*
   - Vestigiality   *26*
6. **Diseases of Appendix**   28
   - Congenital Anomalies of Appendix   *28*
     - Agenesis of Appendix   *28*
     - Duplication of Appendix   *29*
   - Appendicitis   *30*
     - Types of Appendicitis   *30*

- Acute Appendicitis 33
  - Historical Background 33
  - Acute Catarrhal Appendicitis 34
  - Purulent Appendicitis 35
  - Gangrenous Appendicitis 36
  - Perforative Appendicitis 36
- Etiology of Acute Appendicitis 37
  - Diet 38
  - Familial Tendency 39
  - Hereditary Factor 39
  - Nationality 39
  - Viral Infection 39
  - Lumen of Appendix 40
  - Socioeconomic Status 40
  - Obstruction of the Lumen of the Appendix 40
  - Nonobstructive Theory 41
- Pathology of Acute Appendicitis 43
  - Bacteriology 43
  - Common Organisms Seen in Patients with Acute Appendicitis 44
  - Types of Acute Appendicitis 44
- Clinical Features of Acute Appendicitis 48
  - Incidence 48
  - Symptoms 50
  - Examination 52
  - Signs 53
  - Other Important Points in Clinical Features of Appendicitis 58
- Clinical Features According to the Type of Appendicitis 59
  - Obstructive Appendicitis 59
  - Nonobstructive Appendicitis 60
- Clinical Features According to the Position of the Appendix 61
  - Retrocecal Appendicitis 61
  - Pelvic Appendicitis 62
- Investigations for Appendicitis 62
  - Complete Blood Count 63
  - Urine Examination 63
  - Pregnancy Test 63
  - Blood Urea, Creatinine and Electrolytes (Sodium, Potassium, and Calcium) 64
  - C-reactive Protein 64
  - Radiography 64
  - Barium Meal or Enema 65
  - Ultrasound of Abdomen 65
  - Computed Tomography Scan of Abdomen 66
  - Diagnostic Laparoscopy 68

- Scoring Systems 68
- Nuclear Medicine Investigations 70
- Vaginal Examination 70
- Urinary 5-hydroxyindoleacetic Acid 70
- Diagnosis of Acute Appendicitis 70
  - Computer-assisted Diagnosis 72
  - Problems of Acute Appendicitis at Different Age and Stage 72
  - Appendicitis in Patients with Human Immunodeficiency Virus Infection 76
  - Stump Appendicitis 77
  - Asymptomatic Appendicolith 77
- Differential Diagnosis of Acute Appendicitis 78
  - In Children 78
  - In Adult Male 80
  - In Adult Female 82
  - In Elderly 84
  - Rare Differential Diagnosis 85
- Complications of Appendicitis 86
  - Perforation of Appendix 86
  - General Peritonitis 88
  - Appendicular Abscess 89
  - Appendicular Lump or Mass (Phlegmon) 91
  - Septicemia 95
  - Portal Pyaemia or Suppurative Pylephlebitis and Pyemic Abscesses 95
  - Infertility 96
  - Recurrent Appendicitis 96
  - Obliteration of the Appendix 96
  - Intestinal Obstruction 96
  - Appendicular Cysts 96
  - Vascular Infections as Complication of Appendicitis 96
- Treatment of Acute Appendicitis 97
  - General Principles 97
  - Prognosis of Acute Appendicitis 97
- Some Golden Rules in Acute Appendicitis 97
- Role of Antibiotics in Right Iliac Fossa Pain 98
- Some Important and Practical Hints to the Beginners 98
  - Solution 99
  - Other Conditions of Appendix 99
  - Mucocele of Appendix 99
  - Pyocele of Appendix or Empyema of Appendix 99
  - Intussusception of Appendix 100
- Tumors of Appendix 100
  - Benign Tumors of Appendix 101
  - Malignant Tumors of Appendix 101

Contents

7. **Operative Surgery of Appendix** 108
    - Anatomy of Right Iliac Fossa in Relation to Appendix Surgery *108*
    - Muscles of Anterior Abdominal Wall *109*
    - Inferior Epigastric Artery *111*
    - Preoperative Preparation for Appendicectomy *111*
    • Appendicectomy or Appendectomy *112*
        - Appendicectomy *112*
        - Definition *113*
        - Indications of Appendicectomy *113*
        - Open or Conventional Appendicectomy *113*
        - Operation Site Preparation *114*
        - Steps of Appendicectomy *114*
    • Incisions *114*
        - Gridiron Incision *115*
        - Lanz or Crease Incision *116*
        - Rutherford Morison's Muscle Cutting Incision *116*
        - Fowler–Weir Approach *117*
        - Battle's Pararectal Incision *118*
        - Rockey–Davis Incision *118*
        - Identification of Cecum *118*
        - Cutting of Mesoappendix *119*
        - Removal of Appendix *119*
        - Inspection of Operative Site, Terminal Ileum, and Pelvic Organs *121*
        - Closure of the Wound *122*
    • Laparoscopic Appendicectomy *122*
        - Historical Background *122*
        - Indications *123*
        - Preoperative Preparation *124*
        - Removal of Appendix *127*
        - Closure *128*
        - Interval Appendicectomy *129*
        - Incidental Appendicectomy *129*
        - Retrograde Appendicectomy *130*
        - Inversion Appendicectomy *130*
    • How to Deal with Special Circumstances during Appendicectomy? *130*
        - Postoperative Complications of Open Appendicectomy *131*
        - Postoperative Complications after Laparoscopic Appendicectomy *134*
    • Postoperative Care *135*
        - Follow-up of Appendicectomy Patient *136*
        - Things to Remember about Appendicitis *136*

8. **Recent Advancements and Modern Trends** 140
    - Immunity and Appendix *140*
    • Diminishing Incidence of Appendicitis *141*
    • Appendicostomy (Malone Procedure) *142*

9. Some Rituals and Thoughts that are Becoming Obsolete	143
10. Questions Patients may ask	145
11. Difficulties and Problems in Appendicectomy	148

- If the Cecum cannot be Found? *148*
- If Cecum is Found but cannot be Delivered in Wound? *148*
- If Appendix cannot be Found? *149*
- Cecum may not be Cecum but it is Sigmoid Colon or Transverse Colon *149*
- When Whole Appendix is not Removed? *149*
- When in Gangrenous Appendix the Discoloration has Reached up to Cecum? *149*
- When the Omentum is Adherent to the Appendix? *150*
- What if a Tumor is Found? *150*
- When a Stump after Appendicectomy Leaks? *150*
- When Hemorrhage Occurs from Appendicular Mesentery? *150*

12. Arguments, Controversies, and Discussions in Diseases of Appendix — **152**

- Whether Appendix is Vestigial Organ or Not *152*
- Open or Conventional versus Laparoscopic Appendicectomy *153*
- Disadvantages of Laparoscopic Appendicectomy *153*
- Debate I: Perforated Appendix—Open or Laparoscopic Appendicectomy *154*
- Debate II: Appendicectomy—Ligation or Stapling of Base of Appendix *154*
- Debate III: Normal Looking Appendix—Remove or Leave it? *155*
- Debate IV: Pregnancy—Open or Laparoscopic Appendicectomy? *156*

13. Pharmacology of Drugs Used in Diseases of Appendix — **157**

- Antibiotics *157*
- Analgesics *159*
- Antispasmodics *160*
- Antiemetics *160*
- H_2 Receptor Antagonists *160*
- Proton Pump Inhibitors *160*

14. Statistics about Appendix and its Diseases — **162**

15. Surgical Audit — **165**

- Audit *165*
- Register *165*
- Aims *166*

16. Medicolegal Aspects: Legal Eagle — **168**

17. Mnemonics — **170**

18.	Frequently Asked Questions	**173**
19.	Multiple Choice Questions	**180**

Further Readings **185**

Index **187**

Video Contents

CHAPTER 6

Video 1: Acute on Chronic Appendicitis—Spiral Appendix
Video 2: Adhesions due to Previous Attacks of Appendicitis
Video 3: Purulent Appendicitis with Perforation
Video 4: Acutely Inflamed Appendix
Video 5: Retrocaecal Appendicitis—Exploration
Video 6: Subcecal Appendicitis
Video 7: Appendicular Lump—Base of Appendix Detached
Video 8: Appendicular Lump—Exploration

CHAPTER 7

Video 9: Insertion of Trocar
Video 10: Cautery of Mesoappendix
Video 11: Exploration of Acutely Inflamed Appendix
Video 12: Cutting of Mesoappendix
Video 13: Extraction of Appendix
Video 14: Application of Clips on Mesoappendix
Video 15: Ligation of Base of Appendix
Video 16: Cutting of Base of Appendix
Video 17: Adhesiolysis

To access the videos contents, simply scan this QR code.

CHAPTER 1

Introduction

> *'To study the phenomenon of disease without books is to sail an uncharted sea, while to study books without patients is not to go to sea at all.'*
> —**Sir William Osler**

The word 'vermiform appendix' is derived from Latin words 'vermis' meaning 'worm' and 'forma' meaning 'shape' so shaped like a worm and 'appendere' means to 'hang upon'. The vermiform appendix is a worm-like tubular structure which hangs from cecum in abdominal cavity.

Morphologically appendix is an undeveloped distal end of large cecum found in many animals.

The appendix was considered as a vestigial organ, an organ which becomes rudimentary and functionless in the course of evolution.

Charles Darwin's theory: Appendix was merely a useless vestige of evolution, a small worm-like sac that was once a giant organ to aid the digestion of greens (Norman Swan, The Appendix—Darwin's Mistake).

The vermiform appendix is found in man, some apes, and wombat, (the nocturnal burrowing Australian marsupial) only.

> The vermiform appendix is found in certain herbivorous animals and not in most of the carnivorous animals. It indicates influence of vermiform appendix in digestion of plant foods.

In many herbivorous animals the appendix is replaced by a big diverticulum in cecum. This diverticulum breaks down the cellulose by bacteriolytic activity. The vermiform appendix differs from this diverticulum due to its rich collection of lymphoid follicles. The vermiform appendix is now considered a specialized part of gastrointestinal tract and not a vestigial organ. The notion that appendix is only a vestigial organ (a structure that has lost all or most of its original functions or that has evolved to take on a new function) has changed since the early 2000s.[1] It may be a reservoir for beneficial gut bacteria. William Parker, Randy Bollinger and colleagues at Duke University proposed in 2007 that the appendix serves as a haven for useful bacteria when illness flushes the bacteria from the rest of the intestines.[2,3] Parker explained that, 'Darwin simply did not have access to the information we have,... if Darwin had been aware of the species that have an appendix attached to a large cecum, and if he had known about the widespread nature of the appendix, he probably would not have thought of the appendix as a vestige of evolution'. This proposition is based on an understanding that emerged by the early 2000s of how the immune system supports the growth of beneficial intestinal bacteria,[4,5] in combination with many well-known features of the appendix, including its architecture, its location which is just below the normal one-way flow of food and germs in the large intestine and its association with copious amounts of immune tissue. The presence of abundant amount of lymphoid tissue and the present scenario of immunity-related sicknesses make us think that it is not a vestigial organ but a specialized one.

Appendicitis is an extraordinarily common disease, and can result in a great deal of difficulty for patient and surgeon alike.[6] Appendicitis is the main cause of pain in right side of lower abdomen.

> **Key Point**
>
> The vermiform appendix is now considered as a specialized part of gastrointestinal tract (GIT) and not a vestigial organ.

REFERENCES

1. Kooij IA, Sahani S, Meijer SL, Buskens CJ, Te Velde AA. The immunology of the vermiform appendix: a review of the literature. Clin Experiment Immunol. 2016;186(1):1-9.
2. Associated Press. Scientists may have Found Appendix's Purpose. NBC News; 2007.
3. Randal Bollinger R, Barbas AS, Bush EL, Lin SS, Parker W. Biofilms in the large bowel suggest an apparent function of the human vermiform appendix. J Theor Biol. 2007;249(4):826-31.
4. Sonnenburg JL, Angenent LT, Getting a grip on things: how do communities of bacterial symbionts become established in our intestine? Nat Immunol. 2004;5(6):569-73.
5. Evertt ML, Patestrant D, Miller SL, Bollinger RR, Parker W. Immune exclusion and immune inclusion: a new model of host-bacterial interactions on the gut. Clin App Immunol Rev. 2004;5(5):321-32.
6. Fischer JE. Appendicitis and appendiceal abscess. In: Bland KI, Callery MP, Clagett GP, Jones DB. Mastery of Surgery, 5th edition. Lippincott Williams and Wilkins; 2006. p. 1433.

CHAPTER 2
Historical Background—Milestones

'Those who cannot remember the past are condemned to repeat it.'
—**George Santayana**

Important Milestones

- In 1736 Claudius Amyand did first appendicectomy.
- In 1880 Lawson Tait did first appendicectomy but reported in 1890.
- In 1886 Reginald Heber Fitz, coined the term 'Appendicitis'.
- In 1886 Kronlein reported first appendicectomy.
- In 1889 McBurney described McBurney's point.
- In 1889 McBurney also described Gridiron incision.
- In 1902 Ochsner–Sherren Regimen was given by Ochsner and Sherren.
- In 1982 Kurt Semm performed first laparoscopic appendicectomy.
- In 2009: First transvaginal removal of the appendix by Santiago Horgan and Mark A. Talamini—a procedure called Natural Orifice Transluminal Endoscopic Surgery (NOTES).

INTRODUCTION

Vermiform appendix and appendicitis remained a mystery for centuries. Donald C Collins, The Mayo Foundation mentioned in his research paper, 'Historic Phases of Appendicitis' in 1931 that, "It seemed reasonable to believe that the presence of appendix was well known when the pyramids were built, because all the visera were removed from the body during the process of mummification and placed in four separate coptic jars. In fact, certain coptic jars in which the intestines were placed contained inscriptions on the exterior referring to the 'worm' of the bowel..... In 1543, The Fleming, Andreas Vesalius, Professor of Anatomy at Padua, accurately described and illustrated the normal appendix, with its relationship to other organs, in the magnificent, 'De fabrica humani corporis.' "

- Appendix was found preserved in the mummy of a young princess of Egypt as described by Arthur Morgan Spencer, Powick Hospital, England.[1]
- 2000 years back appendix was shown in some Greek drawings of human body. It was shown as a small tail-like structure attached to the intestine which indicates that this is wrongly called vestigial organ.

- In 1492 appendix was found sketched by Leonardo da Vinci in his notebook of anatomy.[2-5] It was called an ear (Orecchio).[6]
- In 1736 first appendicectomy was performed by Claudius Amyand,[7,8] (1685–1740) **(Fig. 1)**, who was a French born surgeon at St. George's Hospital London, England, who was Surgeon to King George-1st and 2nd and also was sergeant surgeon to Queen Ann. He was first principal surgeon to Westminster Hospital, and founder and first principal surgeon to St. George's Hospital.[8] This patient was an 11-year-old boy named Hanvil Anderson with right inguinal hernia. He developed a fecal fistula after a pin-prick of hernia leading to perforation of gut. The appendix was lying inside the hernial sac and the pin had perforated the appendix causing fecal fistula. The appendix and the culprit pin were removed during operation.[9] The patient improved and survived. He also repaired the hernia after removing the appendix.[10] The operation was performed without anesthesia. When the appendix is included in the hernia sac, it is known as Amyand's hernia. Amyand's hernia is very uncommon and characterized by the presence of the appendix in the hernia sac and it is 0.4–1% of all inguinal hernia cases, literature review also showed that incidence of Amyand's hernia is very rare, whereas only 0.1% of cases complicate into acute appendicitis due to late presentation and missed diagnosis **(Fig. 2)**.[11]
- In 1755 Lorenz Heister **(Fig. 3)**, German anatomist, surgeon, and botanist, reported the inflammation of appendix at an autopsy. Usually acute appendicitis was wrongly called as typhlitis or perityphlitis.[12]

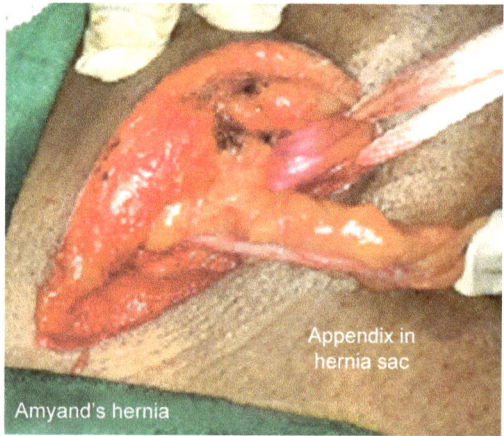

FIG. 2: Amyand's hernia—appendix present in a hernial sac.

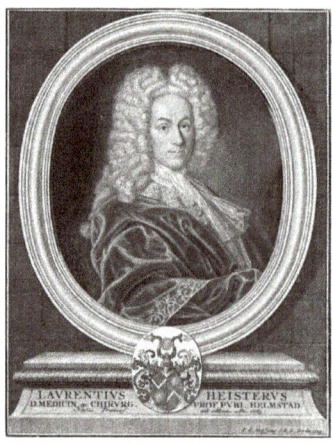

FIG. 1: Claudius Amyand.

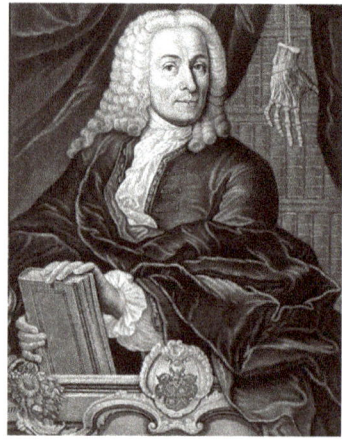

FIG. 3: Lorenz Heister.

- In 1824 Louyer-Villermay a French Surgeon reported two cases of appendicitis in two autopsies. In 1827 François Milior, a French physician, reported six autopsy cases of appendicitis and he was the first who suggested the recognition of appendicitis. In 1839 Bright and Addison described symptoms of appendicitis and identified it as the primary cause of inflammatory process of right lower quadrant in their book 'Elements of practical medicine'. [13,14]
- In 18th century right lower quadrant (RLQ) pain was called perityphlitis and paratyphlitis. In 1827 Milior described several autopsy cases of appendicitis and declared that appendix was the likely cause.
- Thomas Hodgkin (1798–1866), a British physician, considered one of the most prominent pathologists of his time and a pioneer in preventive medicine. He is best known for the first account of Hodgkin's disease, a form of lymphoma and blood disease. In 1836 opined that partial inflammation of the peritoneum in the right iliac fossa is sometimes set up by disease in the appendix caeci.
- In 1848 Henry Hancock (**Fig. 4**), Surgeon, Chairing Cross Hospital London, operated first reported case of appendicular abscess without removing the appendix. In those days the standard treatment was to drain RLQ after perforation of appendix.
- In 1880 Matterstock of Germany published papers writing that appendix was the cause of right iliac fossa inflammation.
- Reginald Heber Fitz (1843–1913) (**Fig. 5**), Professor of Pathology, Anatomy and Medicine at Harvard University, coined the term 'Appendicitis' in 1886. He published this study of 257 cases. For the first time, he described the clinical features, pathological changes in appendicitis and classified the pathology in appendicitis in 1886. He published 'Perforating Inflammation of the Vermiform Appendix: With Special Reference to its Early Diagnosis and Treatment'. He distinguished it from 'typhlitis.'[15] He advocated early appendicectomy but as he was not a surgeon so his advice was not taken seriously (**Fig. 6**).
- Rudolf Ulrich Kronlein (**Fig. 7**), a Swiss Surgeon, is the man in reality who reported first detail account of appendicectomy in 1886. He performed the first appendicectomy in 1884. The patient died on 3rd postoperative day. He was a 17-year-old boy with acute appendicitis. Kronlein operated another patient on the same day and this patient had

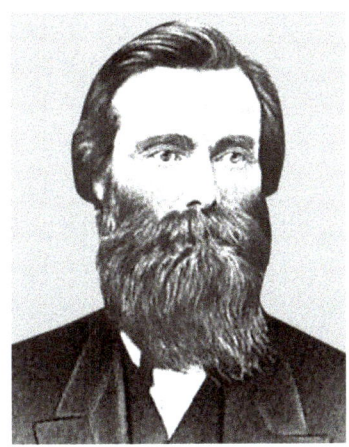

FIG. 4: Henry Hancock.

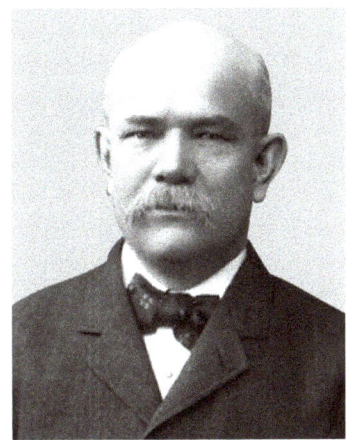

FIG. 5: Reginald Heber Fitz.

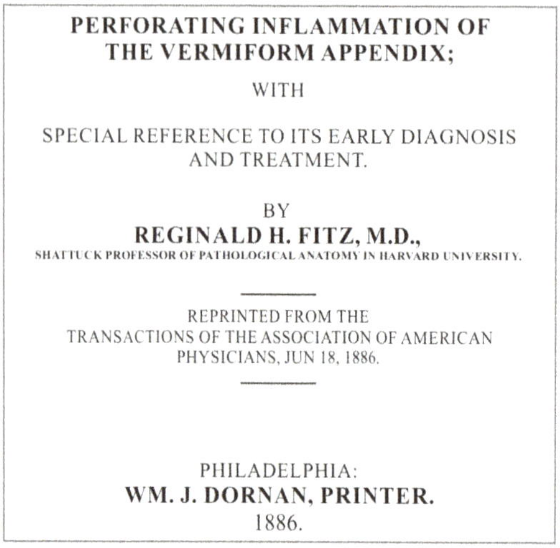

PERFORATING INFLAMMATION OF
THE VERMIFORM APPENDIX;

WITH

SPECIAL REFERENCE TO ITS EARLY DIAGNOSIS
AND TREATMENT.

BY
REGINALD H. FITZ, M.D.,
SHATTUCK PROFESSOR OF PATHOLOGICAL ANATOMY IN HARVARD UNIVERSITY.

REPRINTED FROM THE
TRANSACTIONS OF THE ASSOCIATION OF AMERICAN
PHYSICIANS, JUN 18, 1886.

PHILADELPHIA:
WM. J. DORNAN, PRINTER.
1886.

FIG. 6: Book on appendix by Reginald H Fitz.

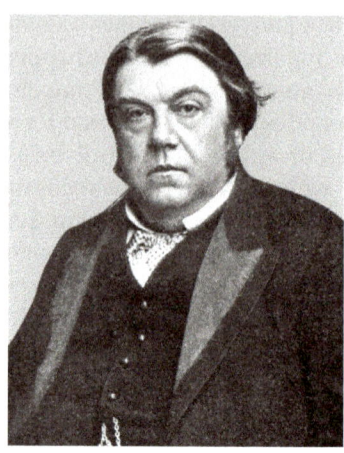

FIG. 8: Lawson Tait.

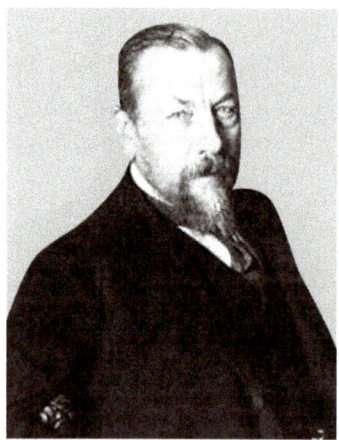

FIG. 7: Rudolf Ulrich Kronlein.

developed acute peritonitis probably due to perforation of appendix. He did not remove the appendix but only cleansed and lavaged the peritoneal cavity. This patient recovered and survived. He was a reputable Professor of Surgery at Zurich University and was nominated for Nobel Prize in 1902.[16]

- Lawson Tait **(Fig. 8)**, Surgeon, Hospital for Diseases of Women, Birmingham, England[17] did first appendectomy in 1880 but he published his account after 10 years in 1890 so Kronlein was credited with first appendicectomy.
- In 1887, Thomas Morton, Philadelphia, USA, diagnosed correctly a case of appendicitis and operated successfully a perforated appendix and saved the patient.
- In 1889 Charles McBurney, Professor of Surgery **(Fig. 9)**, Columbia, College of Physician and Surgeons, New York, USA, described 'McBurney's Point'. He became Surgeon-in-Chief of the Roosevelt Hospital in 1888. Here he did his most famous work on appendicitis, presenting his report on operative management to the New York Surgical Society in 1889. He published his famous landmark paper in New York Medical Journal.
- McBurney's Point is the point of maximum tenderness in acute appendicitis. It is the meeting pint of lateral 1/3rd and medial 2/3rd of a line drawn from umbilicus to right anterior superior iliac spine. In his own words 'Very exactly between an inch and a half and two inches from the anterior superior process of ileum on a straight line drawn from that process to the umbilicus'.[18]
- McBurney incorrectly stated that this was an almost constant finding in patients with appendicitis. McBurney used to keep

CHAPTER 2 Historical Background—Milestones

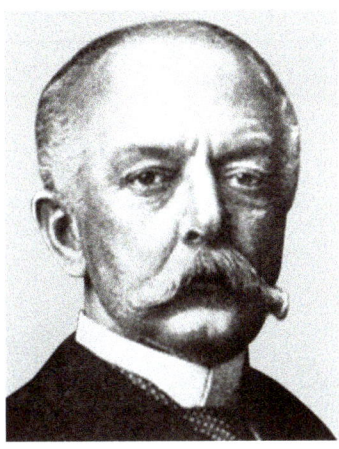

FIG. 9: Charles Mc Burney.

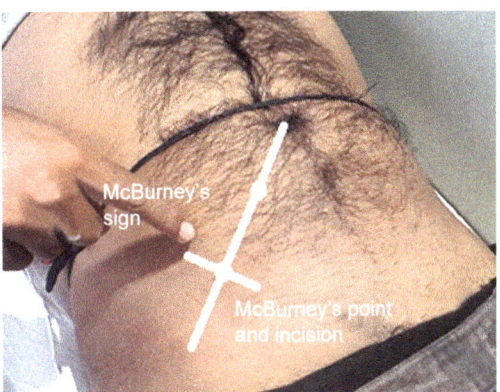

FIG. 10: McBurney's point of maximum tenderness and McBurney's incision.

his patients for at least 4 weeks on bed rest after surgery.[19]
- McBurney's incision, a muscle splitting incision for appendectomies, also called gridiron incision. In 1894, McBurney described 'Gridiron incision or McBurney's incision' **(Fig. 10)**.[20]
- McBurney's operation, operation for inguinal hernia.
- McBurney's sign, tenderness at McBurney's point in acute appendicitis.
- Albert John Ochsner, Professor of Clinical Surgery, University of Illinois, Chicago, and James Sherren, Surgeon. The London Hospital, London, advised a conservative management for late presentation of appendicitis with a lump. It is called 'Ochsner-Sherren Regimen'.
- In 1920, Sir Fredrick Treves **(Fig. 11)**, Surgeon, London Hospital, London, England[21] drained the appendicular abscess and removed the appendix of King Edward VII two days before his intended coronation. He performed the first appendicectomy in England, on 29 June 1888. King Edward was diagnosed with appendicitis. The King had opposed surgery because of upcoming coronation and Treves insisted, stating that if he was not permitted to operate, there would instead be a funeral.[22] The next day, Edward was sitting up in bed, smoking

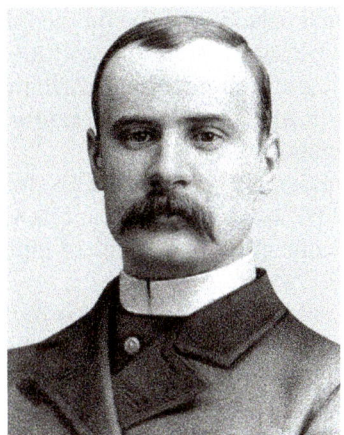

FIG. 11: Sir Fredrick Treves.

a cigar. He was applauded and earned a big name and fame as the man who saved the king. This incidence increased the confidence of public in surgery. By 1901, Treves had removed a thousand appendices.[23]
- In 1905 John Benjamin Murphy **(Fig. 12)**, Professor of Surgery, Northwestern University, Chicago, USA described sequence of symptoms of pain followed by nausea and vomiting with fever and tenderness in the position occupied by appendix[24] Murphy described this syndrome in 1903. In 1896, he was the first person to successfully suture a severed femoral artery; in 1898, he was

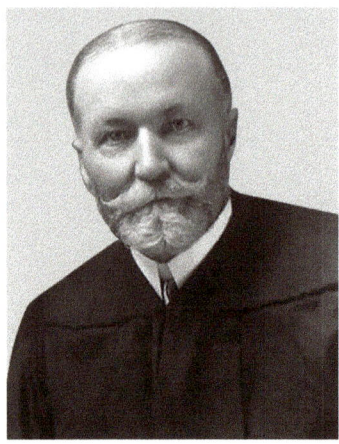

FIG. 12: John Benjamin Murphy.

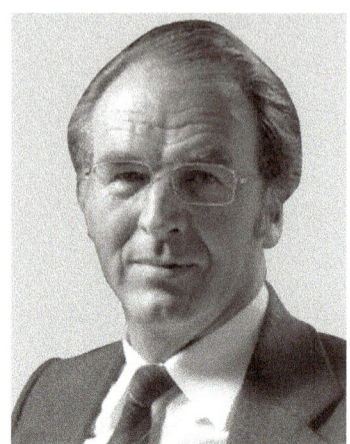

FIG. 13: Kurt Semm.

the first person to do the thoracoplasty for pulmonary tuberculosis and pioneered bone grafting technique. William Mayo said of him 'The surgical genius of our generation'.[25]

- The mortality by appendicitis decreased to 20% by 1945 with availability of penicillin. The current rate of mortality is 0.25%.[26,27]
- In 1982 Kurt Semm **(Fig. 13)** performed successfully the first laparoscopic appendicectomy much before the first laparoscopic cholecystectomy[28] as a prophylactic measure during an ancillary procedure to a gynecologic operation.[29-33]
- The first reported case of appendicitis appeared in 1554, when Jean Fernel noted at autopsy the luminal obstruction, necrosis, and perforation of the appendix and cecum.[34-36]

It was not properly documented but some writings indicate that Indian ancestors of today's physicians and surgeons probably knew about appendix and appendicitis. As per Ayurveda Unduka is derived from Shonitakittabhaga.[37] Therefore Undukapuccha is also derived from it because Unduka is a terminology used both for Unduka and Undukapuccha (i.e., cecum and appendix).[37]

Key Point
Charles Darwin's Theory of Appendix, a vestigial organ is proved wrong.

REFERENCES

1. Mann CV, Russell RCG, Williams NS. Bailey and Love's Short Practice of Surgery, 22nd edition. Chapman and Hall; 1995. p. 829.
2. Gough DB, Donohue JH, Schutt AJ, Gonchoroff N, Goellner JR, Wilson TO, et al. Pseudomyxoma peritonei. Long-term patient survival with an aggressive regional approach. Ann Surg. 1994;219(2):112-9.
3. Finaly DJ, Doherty GM. Acute Abdominal pain and appendicitis, The Washington Manual of Surgery. Lippincott Williams and Wilkins; 2002. p. 258.
4. Doherty GM, Lewis FR Jr. Appendicitis: continuing diagnostic challenge. Emerg Med Clin North Am. 1989;7:537.
5. Finaly DJ, Doherty GM. Suit Abdominal Pain and appendicitis, The Washington Manual of Surgery, Lippincott Williams and Wilkins; 2002. p. 26.
6. Soybel DI. Appendix. In: Norton JA, Bollinger RR, Chang AE, Lowry SF, Mulvihill SJ, Pass HI (Eds). Surgery: Basic Science and Clinical Evidence. Springer, Berlin, Heidelberg; 2001.

7. Chumber S. Appendix. In: Essentials of Surgery. New Delhi: Jaypee Brothers Pvt. Ltd. 2005. p. 833.
8. Mohamed AAR. Amyand: A Forgotten Surgeon and Hernia Case presentation and Literature Review. J Urol. 2009;7(1).
9. Amyand C. of an inguinal rupture, with a pin in the appendix Caeci, incrusted with stone; and some observations on wounds in the gut. Philos. Trans R Soc Lond B Biol Sci. 1735;39:329-36.
10. Ellis H. Appendix. In: Schwartz SI (Ed). Maingot's Abdominal Operations. 8th edition. Volume 2. Norwalk: Appleton-Century-Crofts; 1985. p 1255.
11. Khalid H, Khan NA, Aziz MA. Amyand's Hernia a case report. Int J Surg Case Rep. 2021;86:106332.
12. The Royal Society. Fellows. [online] Available from https://royalsociety.org/fellows/ [Last accessed December, 2023].
13. Lewis F. Appendix. In: Davis JH (Ed). Clinical Surgery. 1st edition. Volume 1. St. Louis: Mosby; 1987. p. 1581.
14. Addison T. An Essay on the Operation of Poisonous Agents upon the Living Body. Leopold Classic Library; 2015.
15. Fitz RH. Perforating inflammation of the vermiform appendix: with special reference to its early diagnosis and treatment. Trans Assoc Am Physicians. 1886;1:107.
16. Laios K. Rudolf Ulrich Kronlein (1847-1910): An Innovative General, Thoracic, Neuro, and Ocular Surgeon. Surg Innov. 2017;24(6):627-9.
17. Meade RH. An Introduction to the History of General Surgery. Philadelphia PA: Saunders; 1968.
18. McBurney C. Experience with early operative interference in cases of disease of the vermiform appendix. NY State Med J. 1889;50:676.
19. Lally KP, Cox CS, Androssy RJ. Appendix. In: Townsend CM, Beauchamp RD, Evers BM, Mattex KL (Eds). Sabiston Textbook of Surgery. 17th ed. Philadelphia: Elsevier Saunders; 2004. p. 1382.
20. McBurney C. The incision made in the abdominal wall in cases of appendicitis. Ann Surg. 1994;20:38.
21. Richardson RG. The Surgeon's Tale. New York, NY: Scribner's; 1958.
22. Treves SF. An account of the illness of King Edward VII in June 1902. Royal Archive Victoria. p. 9.
23. Ramchandran M, Aronson JK. Frederick Treves first surgical operation for appendicitis. JR Soc Med. 2011;104(5):191-7.
24. Murphy JB. Appendicitis with original report histories and analysis of one hundred and forty one laparotomies for that disease under personal observation. JAMA. 1984;22:302-4.
25. Williams SN, Bulstrode CJK, O'Connell PR. The Vermiform Appendix, Bailey and Love's, Short Practice of Surgery. 26th edition; 2013. p. 1203.
26. Blomqvist PG, Andersson RE, Granath F, Lambe MP, Ekbom AR. Mortality after appendectomy in Sweden, 1987-1996. Ann Surg. 2001;233(4):455-60.
27. Hale DA, Molloy M, Pearl RH, Schutt DC, Jaques DP. Appendectomy: a contemporary appraisal. Ann Surg. 1997;225(3):252-61.
28. Semm K. Endoscopic appendectomy. Endoscopy. 1983;15:59-64.
29. Cameron JL. Current Surgical Therapy. St Louis: Mosby; 1995. pp. 1025-8.
30. Gotz F, Pier A, Bacher C. Modified laparoscopic appendectomy in surgery: a report on 388 operations. Surg Endosc. 1990;4:6-9.
31. Valla JS, Limonne B, Valla V, Montupet P, Daoud N, Grinda A, et al. Laparoscopic appendectomy in children: report of 465 cases. Surg Laparosc Endosc. 1990;1:166-172.
32. Pier A, Cotz F, Bacher: Laparscopic appendectomy in 625 cases: from innovation to routine. Surg Laparosc Endosc. 1991;1(3):8-13.
33. Neugebauer E, Troidl H, Kum CK, Eypasch E, Miserez M, Paul A. The EAES consensus development on laparoscopic cholecystectomy. Appendectomy, and hernia repair. Surg Endosc. 1995;9(5):550-63.
34. Fernel J. Universa medicina. In: Major RH. Classic Description of Disease. 3rd edition. Springfield, IL: CC Thomas; 1945. pp, 646-8.
35. Graffeo CS, Counselman FL. Appendicitis. Emerg Med Clin North Am. 1996;14:653-71.
36. Gallos G, Cosgrove JM. Laparoscopic Appendicectomy. In; Brooks DC. Current View of Minimally Invasive Surgery, Springer; 1998. p. 53.
37. Reshma M, Shubha Devi V, Thyagarju K, Azaruddin MD. Morphological features and morphometric parameters of human fetal vermiform appendix at different gesetatoinal ages. J Anat. 2013;2: 18-25.

CHAPTER
3

Surgical Anatomy

*'Remember that your patient is a human
being like yourself..........
Your knowledge of anatomy may save his or her life.'*
—Richard S Snell

INTRODUCTION

The vermiform appendix is an important organ in the abdominal cavity. Anatomy of the appendix must be clear in the mind of the operating surgeon. As we all know the appendix is more known for its nuisance than its functions. It was considered as a vestigial organ earlier, but now the recent researches have confirmed it having immunological functions.

The appendix is called 'vermiform appendix' **(Fig. 1)** due to its worm-like shape. Morphologically it is the undeveloped distal part of cecum. The appendix is attached at the posteromedial aspect of cecum, due to uneven growth of walls of cecum, which pushes it medially and posteriorly. It arises about 2.5 cm below the ileocecal valve from the point where three taenia coli of colon merge.

The base of appendix is fixed but its tip lies free in the pelvis and can point to any direction. The appendix hangs freely in peritoneal cavity.

In very rare cases, the appendix may not be present at all (laparotomies for suspected appendicitis have given a frequency of one in 1,00,000)[1].

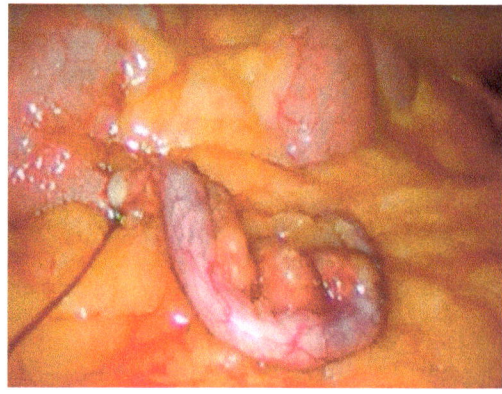

FIG. 1: Vermiform appendix.

DEVELOPMENT OF APPENDIX

The appendix develops as a diverticulum from the wall of cecum. The appendix appears first as a prominence in the terminal part of cecum in 8th week of intrauterine life, it attains the shape of tubular structure by about the age of 2 years.[2] In an early embryonic age appendix has the same diameter as the cecum and it lies in the line of cecum. The excessive growth of the right and anterior walls of cecum pushes the appendix to medial side and posteriorly. In later stages of development, the lumen disparity between cecum and appendix develops. The lumen of cecum goes on enlarging and developing fast but the lumen of appendix enlarges much slowly and the disparity develops. By 5th month of intrauterine life appendix elongates and becomes vermiform in shape. At birth, the appendix is broad and short then gradually around 2 years of age it acquires tubular shape. The position of appendix in relation to cecum varies greatly but the relation between the attachment of base of appendix and cecum is always constant. The base of appendix is always attached at same spot with cecum in relation to the ileocecal valve **(Figs. 2 to 4)**. The location of appendix is determined by the location of the cecum.[3]

Appendix is devoid of lymphoid tissue before birth and it appears only after 2 weeks of birth. The lymphoid tissue increases in amount continuously from birth to puberty, then its amount becomes stationary for 10–12 years then it starts regressing with age and by the age of 60 years again appendix becomes almost devoid of lymphoid tissue.

The excessive growth of the right and anterior walls of cecum pushes the appendix to medial side and posteriorly.

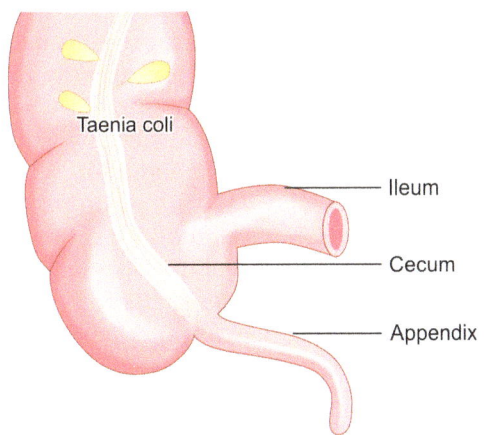

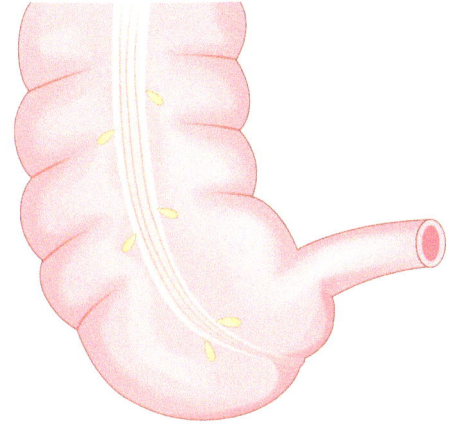

FIG. 3: Agenesis of appendix.

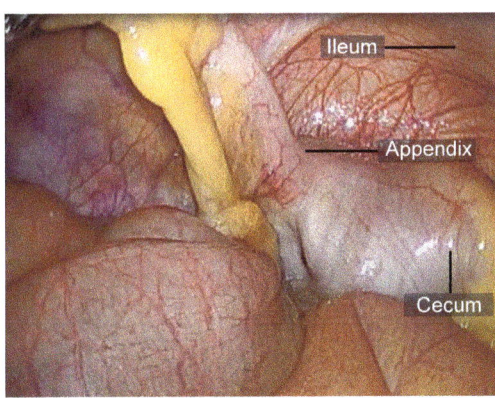

FIG. 2: Vermiform appendix, cecum and ileum.

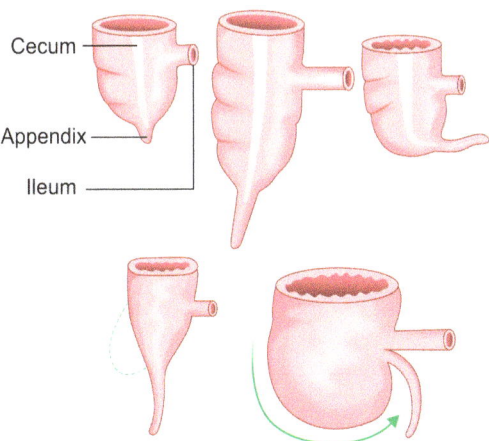

FIG. 4: Development of appendix.

SURFACE MARKING OF APPENDIX

Base of the appendix can be marked on anterior abdominal wall at a point 2 cm below the point where transtubercular plane crosses vertical right lateral plane. McBurney's point is the site of maximum tenderness in acute appendicitis. McBurney's point is situated at the junction of medial 2/3rd and lateral 1/3rd of the imaginary line joining umbilicus and anterior superior iliac spine **(Fig. 5)**. Position of appendix can be marked in relation to the face of a clock (for example, pelvic position of appendix is mentioned as 4 o'clock position). The base of the appendix is fixed as it is attached to the cecum so is marked as the center of clock where hands of the clock meet. The appendix is marked as hand of a clock.

POSITION OF APPENDIX

The appendix is situated in right iliac fossa (RIF) **(Fig. 6)**. The anatomical position of appendix in the peritoneal cavity is inconstant. The position of the base of the appendix is always constant in relation to cecum. However, true but, Howard Atwood Kelly, mentioned in his book, *'Appendicitis and Other Diseases of the Vermiform Appendix'*, that the location of the point of origin depends, entirely upon the topography of the cecum. According to whether the cecal pouch is directed upward or downward, outward or inward, forward or backward or whether colon and cecum have rotated insufficiently or too much around their long axis, the point of origin of the appendix varies in position. It may be found at almost any point of the cecal pouch. The base of appendix during operation is traced by identifying and following the 3 taenia coli, specially the anterior taenia coli. The position of the appendix is extremely variable, more than that of any other organ. As the appendix is attached to cecum so its position depends upon position of cecum. Usually it is in RIF but due to incomplete descent of cecum it may be subhepatic. Cecum may be in pelvis or even on left side due to malrotation of gut or arrest in rotation of gut. Appendix usually hangs and floats free in peritoneal cavity and is fixed only in retrocecal position or when it is inflamed. Appendix can take any of the following positions **(Figs. 7 A and B)**:

- *Retrocecal (12 o'clock) position (in 70% persons)*: The normal location of appendix is retrocecal. The appendix lies behind the cecum. It may be embedded in cecal wall. It is intraperitoneal but sometimes extraperitoneal also. It may

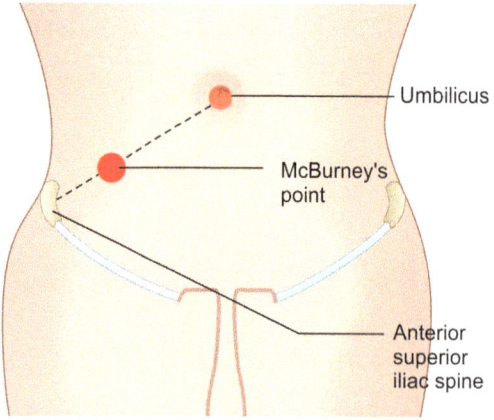

FIG. 5: McBurney's point.

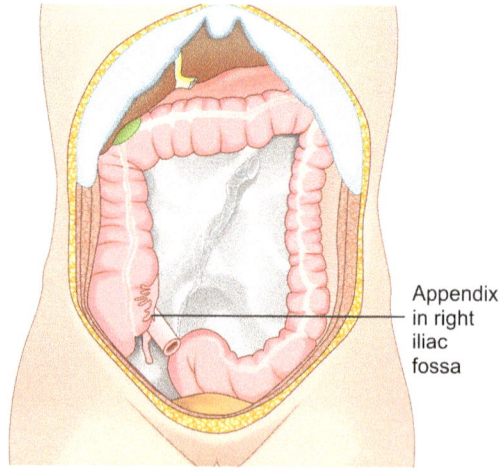

FIG. 6: Location of appendix.
Source: Kelly HA. Appendicitis and Others Diseases of the Vermiform Appendix. Philadelphia: JB Lippincott Company; 1905.

CHAPTER 3 Surgical Anatomy

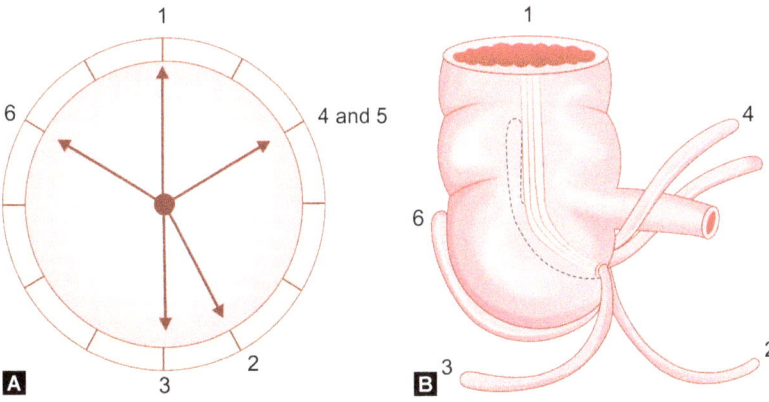

FIGS. 7A AND B: Positions of appendix.

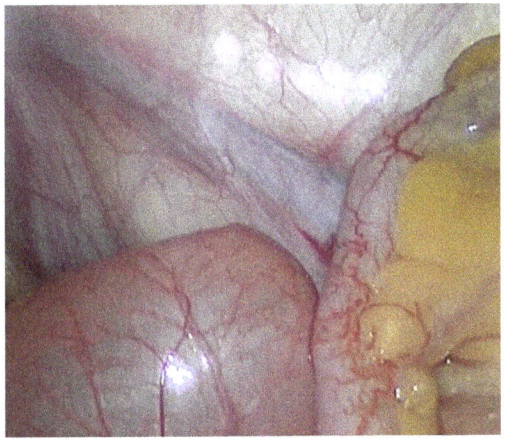

FIG. 8: Retrocecal appendix.

be sometime difficult to elicit tenderness in RIF, as inflamed appendix is lying behind cecum, which is distended with gas. Long retrocecal appendix can mimic cholecystitis if only the tip is inflamed or it can mimic ureteric colic if it touches the ureter **(Fig. 8)**.

- *Pelvic (4 o'clock) position (in 25% persons)*: The appendix hangs down in pelvis. There may be no tenderness in RIF as the inflamed appendix lies in pelvis but deep tenderness may be elicited on digital rectal examination. The tip of the appendix if touches ureter or bladder patient will have urinary symptoms. When the tip of appendix touches rectum patient will have rectal symptoms.

- *Subcecal (3 o'clock) position (in 2% of population)*: The appendix lies just below the cecum.
- *Preileal (2 o'clock) position (in 1% of population)*: The appendix lies in front of terminal part of ileum.
- *Postileal (2 o'clock) position (in 1% of population)*: The appendix lies behind the terminal part of ileum.
- *Paracolic (6 o'clock) position (in 1% of population)*: It lies just along lateral wall of cecum.

The location of the place of origin of the appendix from cecum does not vary whether the cecum is directed toward upward, downward, right or left.

Though retrocecal position of appendix is commonest but in some countries it is different as in Iran and Bosnia, pelvic position is most common, with 55.8% and 57.7% occurrence respectively.[4,5]

SUBHEPATIC APPENDIX

Malrotation of gut puts cecum with appendix below the liver. It is a very rare incidence. It gives great challenge to diagnosis. It can mimic cholecystitis and liver abscess, may lead to delayed diagnosis and increases the chances of appendicular rupture **(Figs. 9A and B)**.[6,7]

CHAPTER 3 Surgical Anatomy

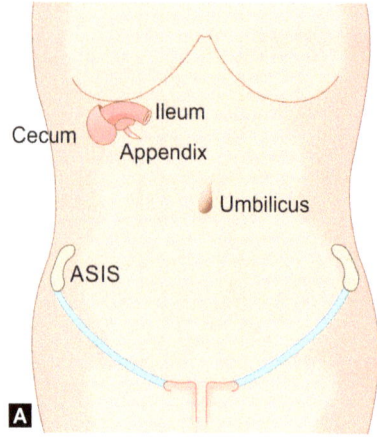 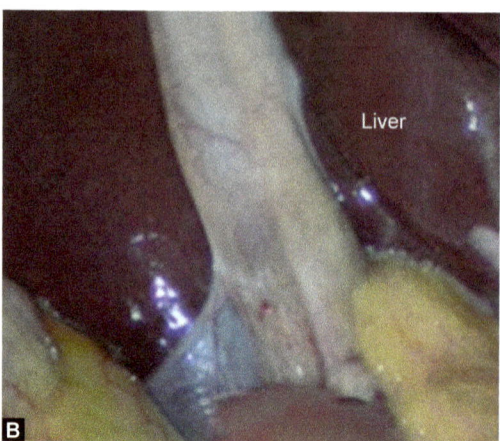

FIGS. 9A AND B: Subhepatic appendix.

Subserous appendix
Sometimes appendix is found buried in the wall of cecum under the serosa which causes difficulty in dissecting out the appendix while performing appendicectomy, especially laparoscopic.

Dissection for subserous appendix can cause damage to the wall of cecum which can be dangerous if deep and can lead to fecal fistula so all precautions must be taken while dealing with appendicectomy for subserous appendix **(Fig. 10)**.

Amyand's hernia is the presence of a vermiform appendix in an inguinal hernia sac, the appendix may be normal or inflamed. It is named after Claudius Amyand (1685–1740), who was surgeon at St. George's Hospital, London. He removed successfully an inflamed appendix from hernia sac of an 11-year-old boy in 1736. Amyand's hernia is a rare and difficult to diagnose preoperatively **(Fig. 11)**.

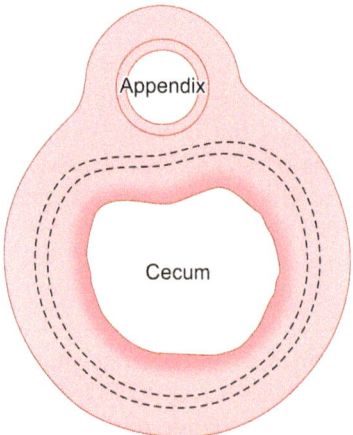 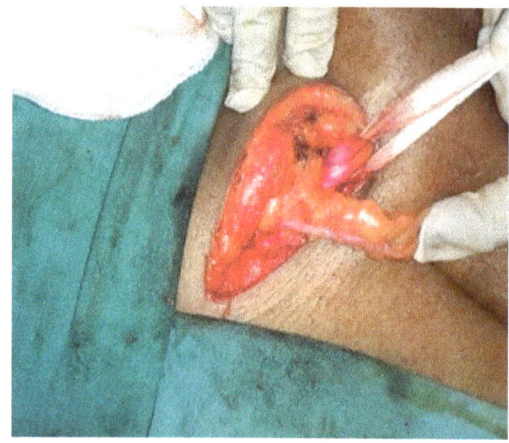

FIG. 10: Subserous appendix.

FIG. 11: Amyand's hernia, appendix in hernial sac.

SIZE OF THE APPENDIX

The size of appendix varies from person to person. Some studies have indicated a relation of length of appendix with height of a person but it is not confirmed. The usual length of the appendix is approximately 7.5 cm but it may vary from 2 to 20 cm. It is longer in children and may atrophy after mid-adult life. The longest appendix ever removed was 26 cm long.[8]

The average length of the appendix is about 8.3 cm, or between 3 and 3.5 inches. Extremely shorts appendices have been described by Bryant, 6 mm; Huntington 5 mm, and HT Marshall 2 mm. Authentic cases of complete absence of the appendix have been described by Zuckerkandl, Bryant, and Huntington. From the minimum of 2 mm appendices range in length up to 24 cm (9.5 inches) or more. The longest appendix on record, to our knowledge, is one presented by F Grauer, of New York, to the Northwestern Medical and Surgical Society in 1890. It measured $12^{7/8}$ inches in length (33 cm). The width of appendix varies from 3 to 8 mm with 6 mm as the normal.[9]

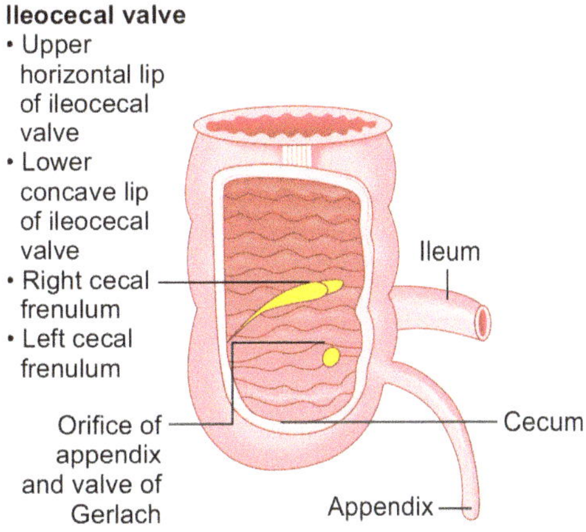

APPENDICULAR ORIFICE

It is situated 2 cm below and lateral to the ileocecal orifice at posteromedial aspect of cecum. It approximately corresponds to McBurney's point. Often it lies to a point below it **(Fig. 12)**. The appendicular orifice is sometimes, not always, having a semilunar fold of mucus membrane, which acts as a valve and is called 'valve of Gerlach' **(Figs. 9A and B)**.

LUMEN OF THE APPENDIX

The lumen of appendix is approximately 2 mm wide just sufficient to introduce a match stick. The capacity of lumen of appendix is 0.1–0.2 mL. The mucus secretion beyond the obstruction site in lumen can raise the intraluminal pressure of appendix

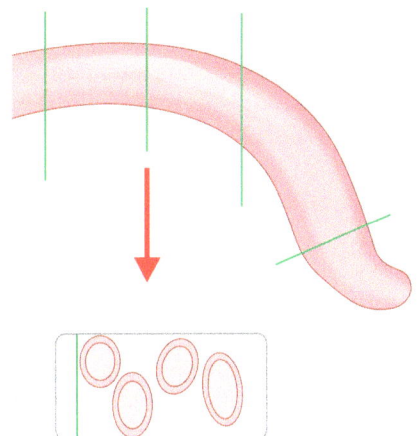

FIG. 12: Appendicular orifice and ileocecal valve.

FIG. 13: Lumen of appendix, at different sites.

considerably even by 0.5 mL mucus. The capability of appendicular mucosa to secrete mucus even in presence of raised in intraluminal pressure causes acute appendicitis, which is an important factor **(Fig. 13)**.

WHY APPENDIX IS PRONE TO INFECTION

It is due to following facts:
- It is a long narrow blind ended tube which encourages stasis of contents which leads to proliferation of bacteria.

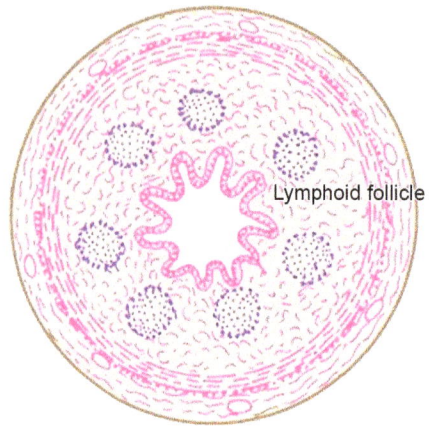

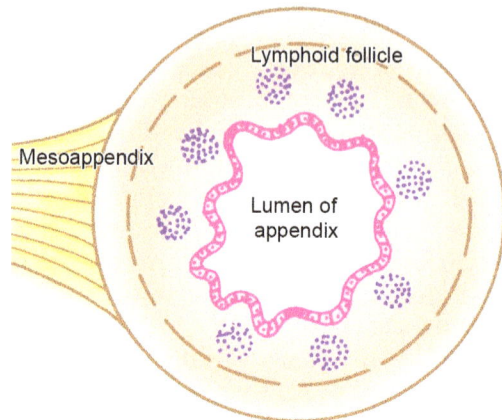

FIG. 14: Lymphoid follicles in the wall of appendix.

FIG. 15: Mesoappendix.

- Lymphoid follicles are present in the wall of appendix which catch bacteria **(Fig. 14)**.
- Lumen of appendix has a tendency to be blocked by hard stool (enterolith) which results in stasis.

MESOAPPENDIX OR MESENTERY OF APPENDIX

Appendix has a well-developed mesentery called 'mesoappendix'. It is continuous with the mesentery of the terminal ileum. It is a triangular fold of peritoneum. The appendix is suspended in peritoneal cavity by mesoappendix. It fuses with posterior layer of mesentery of ileum behind the terminal part of the ileum **(Figs. 15 and 16)**.

The tip of the appendix is not covered by mesoappendix, which is one of the reasons of early perforation of tip of appendix due to lack of protective covering. The thrombosis of appendicular artery develops due to inflammation of appendix as the artery is directly over it. The mesoappendix contains appendicular vessels and nerves. The mesoappendix in new born is transparent without any fat deposit but as we grow, gradually it becomes laden with fat. We identify the vessels in mesoappendix by seeing it against light. Fat-laden mesoappendix does not show vessels clearly.

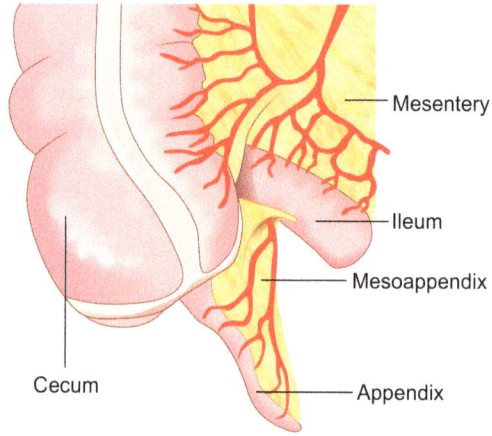

FIG. 16: Mesoappendix arising from mesentery.

The mesoappendix in normal cases goes all the way to the tip, or may even extend slightly beyond it, forming a knob-like projection; it, however, frequently appears to stop at some distance from the tip, extending, in some cases, according to Treves, and others, only to the middle of the appendix, or to the junction of middle and distal thirds.[10]

Appendicular Artery

The appendicular artery is a branch of lower division of ileocolic artery. It passes behind terminal ileum to enter mesoappendix, a short distance from the base of appendix from medial side and then it runs in the

CHAPTER 3 Surgical Anatomy

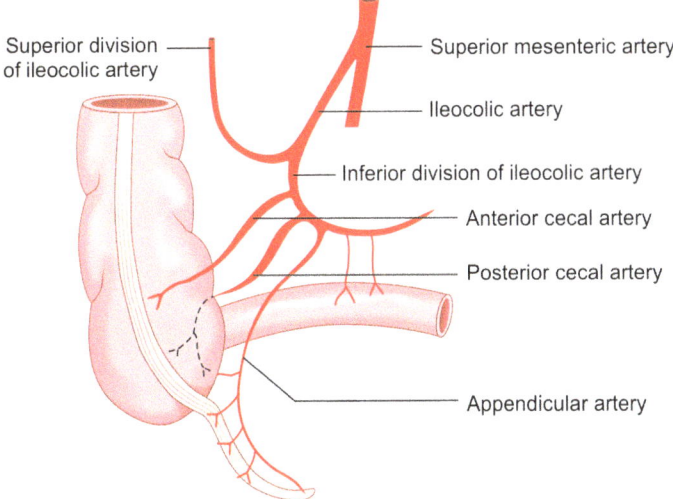

FIG. 17: Appendicular artery.

free border of mesoappendix, but at the tip of appendix it lies directly over the wall of appendix **(Fig. 17)**. Appendicular artery gives 3–4 branches in its course to appendix in mesoappendix. The appendicular artery is an end artery that is why the acute appendicitis results in gangrene and perforation once this artery is thrombosed and blocked causing necrosis of appendix, which is also known as gangrenous appendicitis. A recurrent branch is given by appendicular artery near the base of appendix which anastomoses with a branch of the posterior cecal artery. While putting purse string suture, this artery can be damaged and may cause big hematoma. The branches of appendicular artery form two main systems—the superficial in serous coat, and the deep in the submucosa. From this submucous system branches run towards mucosa.

Accessory Appendicular Artery (Artery of Seshachalam)

It is a branch of posterior cecal artery. It is quite commonly found. It supplies base of appendix. It sometimes bleeds a lot, if not properly ligated during appendicectomy. Tip and antimesenteric border of the appendix have least blood supply and therefore

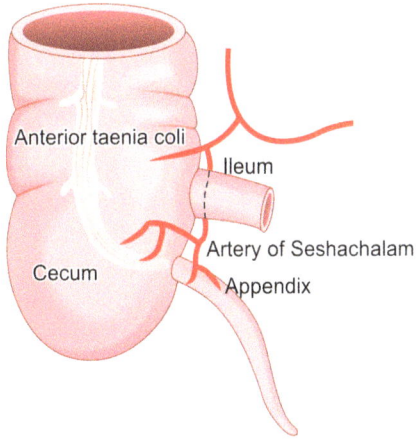

FIG. 18: Accessory appendicular artery (artery of Seshachalam).

these sites are prone to get gangrene and perforation **(Fig. 18)**. T Seshachalam, Indian Surgeon described this artery in 1930s.

VARIATIONS IN ARTERIAL SUPPLY OF APPENDIX

- Appendicular artery arising from ileocolic artery before it gives ilial and cecal branches (I and III).
- Duplicate appendicular arteries (II and IV).

CHAPTER 3 Surgical Anatomy

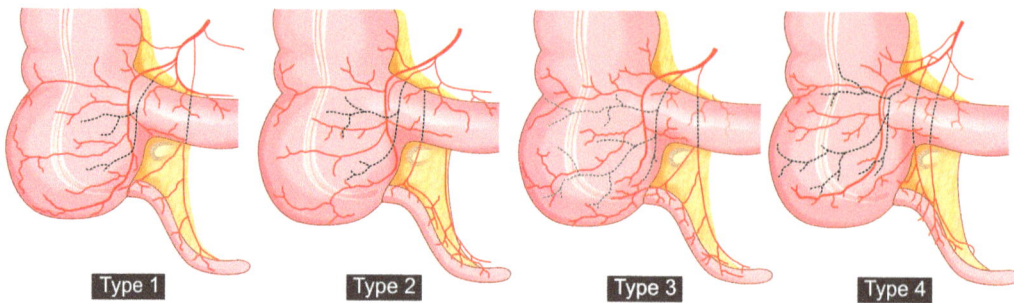

FIG. 19: Common variations in arterial supply of appendix. Type 1 one artery, supplying only the appendix, Type 2 two arteries, supplying only the appendix, Type 3 one or more arteries. Origin: Ileocolic, posterior ileocecal, mesenteric loop, etc. Proximal branch supplies a portion of the cecum. Type 4 two arteries, forming a loop in the mesoappendix from which the individual branches arise.
Source: Kelly HA. Appendicitis and Others Diseases of the Vermiform Appendix. Philadelphia: JB Lippincott Company; 1905.

Variations in appendicular artery are not rare and much common against our thoughts (**Fig. 19**).

VENOUS DRAINAGE OF APPENDIX

The veins draining the blood from appendix follow the arteries of appendix. The tributaries from appendix drain into ileocolic vein which drains into superior mesenteric vein which opens in portal vein. This is the part of portal circulation. The blood reaches liver via portal vein due to this reason suppurative appendicitis or appendicular abscess can lead to multiple pyemic abscess in liver (**Figs. 20 and 21**). Veins of the appendix are generally central to the arteries.

When we do appendicectomy, we crush the base of appendix with an artery forceps which blocks the lumen of veins also this avoids sending infected emboli to portal vein and liver.

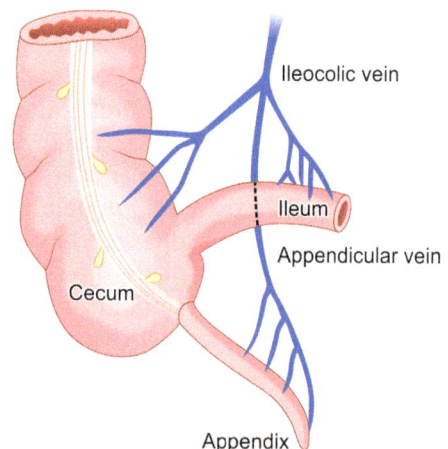

FIG. 20: Venous drainage of appendix.

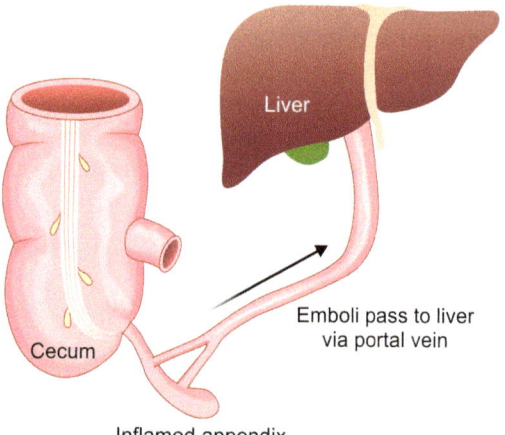

FIG. 21: Emboli from appendix reach liver via portal vein.

LYMPHATIC DRAINAGE OF APPENDIX

Lymph is drained from appendix to the regional lymph nodes by 4–6 lymphatic channels. These channels carry lymph:
- Directly to ileocolic lymph nodes.

- Some lymph passes first to appendicular lymph nodes in mesoappendix and then to ileocecal lymph nodes near the base of the appendix and then to ileocolic lymph nodes. Lymph from anterior surface of appendix and cecum reaches via anterior cecal vessels to anterior ileocolic lymph nodes and lymph from posterior surface of cecum and appendix reaches via posterior cecal vessels to posterior ileocolic lymph nodes. Ultimately the lymph reaches from ileocolic lymph nodes to superior mesenteric lymph nodes **(Figs. 22A and B)**. The lymphatics of appendix run into superficial, middle, and deep groups. Superficial group lie in serosa, middle group in between muscle coats and submucosa and deep group in mucosa.

The lowest lymph gland is situated over posterior cecal pouch is called Clado's gland or appendical gland. It receives lymph from the cecum and not from appendix. In a very few instances it received a small tributary from the caeco-appendical angle **(Figs. 22C and D)**.[11]

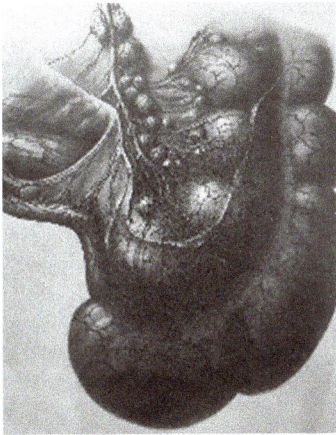

FIG. 22A: Lymphatic drainage of appendix. Posterior view of the ileocecal region, showing lymphatics of appendix and main lymph glands of ileocecal region.
Source: Kelly HA. Appendicitis and Others Diseases of the Vermiform Appendix. Philadelphia: JB Lippincott Company; 1905.

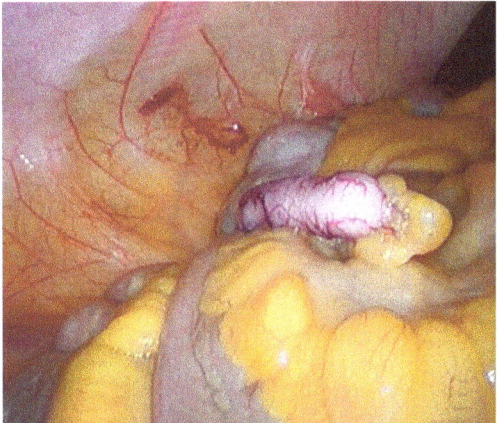

FIG. 22C: Lymph drainage of appendix.

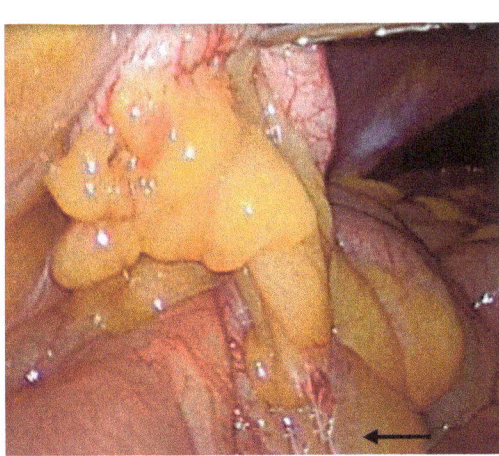

FIG. 22B: Enlarged appendicular lymph node.

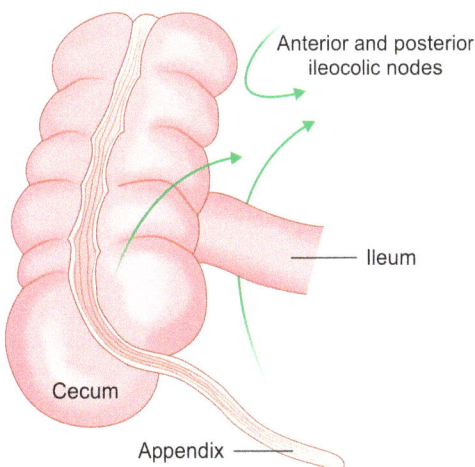

FIG. 22D: Lymphatic drainage of appendix diagrammatic presentation.

NERVE SUPPLY OF APPENDIX

- Sympathetic nerves come from thoracic nine (T9) and thoracic ten (T10) segments of spinal cord through coeliac plexus.
- Parasympathetic nerves come from vagus nerve.

The pain in initial stage of acute appendicitis is felt at umbilicus, it is 'referred pain' as the same segment of spinal cord (T10), supplies the umbilicus also. It is visceral pain.

Later on the pain shifts to RIF due to irritation and inflammation of local peritoneum. This pain is due to stimulation of nerve endings of local peritoneum and is called 'somatic pain'.

FOLDS AND RECESSES IN RELATION TO THE APPENDIX (FIG. 23)

- Superior ileocecal fold
- Superior ileocecal recess
- Inferior ileocecal fold
- Inferior ileocecal recess

Superior Ileocecal Fold and Recess

It is a commonly seen pair of fold and recess. Superior ileocecal recess is formed by superior ileocecal fold which is a vascular fold present between terminal ileum and ascending colon. The opening of recess directs down and medially.

Inferior Ileocecal Fold and Recess

This fold is a blood less fold and is also called 'bloodless fold of Treves'. It is between terminal ileum and base of appendix. The opening of this recess is downward **(Fig. 24)**.

JACKSON'S MEMBRANE (FIG. 25)

It is a peritoneal fold, attached from posterior abdominal wall to the anterior surface of cecum on lateral side. Sometimes it is required to cut to find out retrocecal appendix. It is vascular and has blood vessels which run parallel.

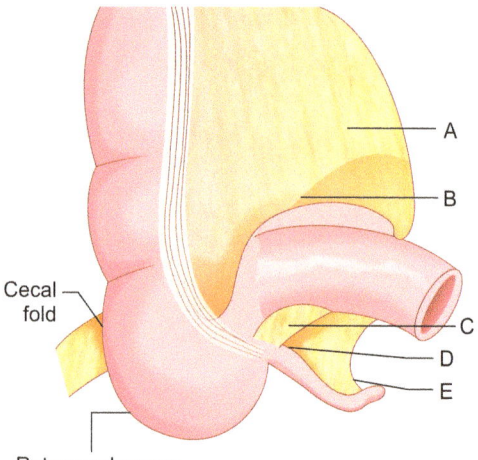

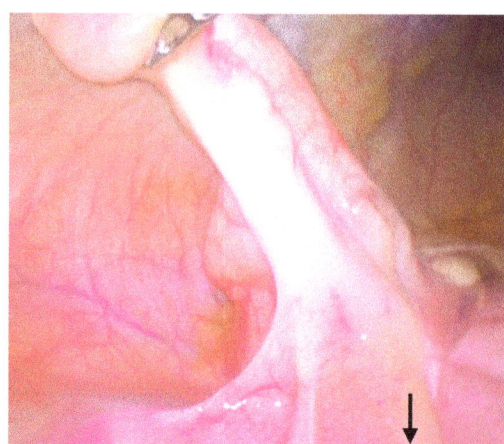

FIG. 24: Inferior ileocecal fold and recess.

FIG. 23: Folds and recesses in relation to the appendix. (A: vascular fold of cecum; B: superior ileocecal recess; C: inferior Ileocecal fold; D: inferior ileocecal recess; E: Mesoappendix)

CHAPTER 3 Surgical Anatomy

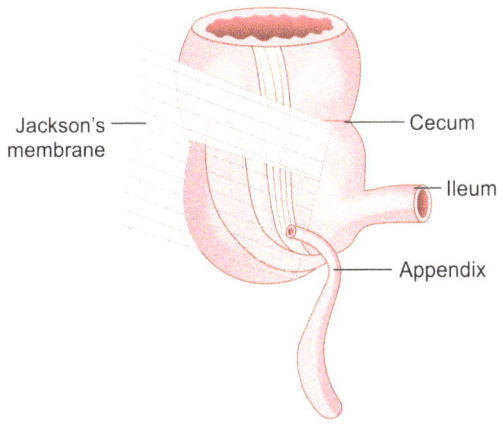

FIG. 25: Jackson's membrane.

In the majority of cases the first glandular station of the appendiceal lymphatics is in the mesentery of the ileocolic angle, from 1 to 3 cm above the ileum. The appendiceal glands, rarely more than two in number, are generally situated at the lower median side of the ileocolic chain of glands. In about three-fourths of the cases there are no glands in the mesoappendix, all the appendiceal lymphatics emptying directly into the mesenteric glands.[12]

The most capacious and the most constant of the fossae is the internal retrocolic, also called inferior ileocecal, which can only be demonstrated by lifting up the cecum, appendix, and ileum. It is then seen as a funnel-shaped pocket extending in an upward direction under the ileum and colon. From the depth of this fossa arises the posterior leaf of mesoappendix, and the entire appendix is oftentimes found curled up in this space, while its tip may point in various directions.[11]

Key Points

- Retrocecal is the commonest position of appendix.
- Appendicular artery is an end artery so necrosis and gangrene of appendix is common.

REFERENCES

1. Zetina-Mejía CA, Alvarez-Cosío JE, Quillo-Olvera J. Congenital absence of the cecal appendix. Case report. Cir Cer. 2009;77(5):407-10.
2. Williams SN, Bulstrode CJK, O'Connell PR. The Vermiform Appendix. In: Williams NS, Bulstrode CJK, O'Connell PR (Eds). Bailey and Love's, Short Practice of Surgery. 26th edition. New York: CRC Press; 2013. p. 1199.
3. Lally KP, Cox JR, Andrassy RJ. Appendicitis. In: Townsend CM (Ed). Sabiston Textbook of Surgery, Volume 2. 17th edition. Philadelphia: Saunders; 2004. p. 1381.
4. Ghorbani A, Forocezesh M, Kazemifar AM. Variation in anatomical position of vermiform appendix among Iranian population: an old issue which has not lost its importance. Anat Res Int. 2014:313575.
5. Denjalić A, Delić J, Delić-Custendil S, Muminagić S. Variations in position and place of formation of appendix vermiformis found in the course of open appendicectomy. Med Arh. 2009;63(3):100-1.
6. Rappaport WD, Warneke JA. Subhepatic appendicitis. Am Fam Physician. 1989;39(6):146-8.
7. Singh S, Jha AK, Sharma N, Mishra TS. A case of right upper abdominal pain misdiagnosed on computerized tomography. Malays J Med Sci. 2014;21(4):66-8.
8. Guinness World Records. (2006). Longest appendix removed. [online] Available from https://www.guinnessworldrecords.com/world-records/largest-appendix-removed. [Last accessed December, 2023].
9. Kelly HA. Appendicitis and Others Diseases of the Vermiform Appendix. Philadelphia: JB Lippincott Company; 1905. p. 27.
10. Kelly HA. Appendicitis and Others Diseases of the Vermiform Appendix. Philadelphia: JB Lippincott Company; 1905. p. 34.
11. Kelly HA. Appendicitis and Others Diseases of the Vermiform Appendix. Philadelphia: JB Lippincott Company; 1905. p. 21.
12. Kelly HA. Appendicitis and Others Diseases of the Vermiform Appendix. Philadelphia: JB Lippincott Company; 1905. p. 33.

CHAPTER 4

Histology of Appendix

*'What one knows, he sees, what one looks for,
he is more likely to see. Chance favors only the prepared mind.'*
—**Louis Pasteur**

INTRODUCTION

Histology, also known as microscopic anatomy or microanatomy[1], is the branch of biology that studies the microscopic anatomy of biological tissues[2-4] whereas in medicine, histopathology is the branch of histology that includes the microscopic identification and study of diseased tissue.[5]

Accurate diagnosis of a sickness sometimes requires histopathological examination of biopsied or resected tissue. Histopathology of appendix sample after appendicectomy details the correct diagnosis such as chronic appendicitis, subacute appendicitis, acute appendicitis, gangrene of appendix, perforation of appendix and tumor of appendix (benign or malignant). Negative appendicectomy is also confirmed by histopathological examination of appendix sample.

The appendix has the following layers which are similar to the intestine. These are from outside to inside (**Figs. 1 and 2**):

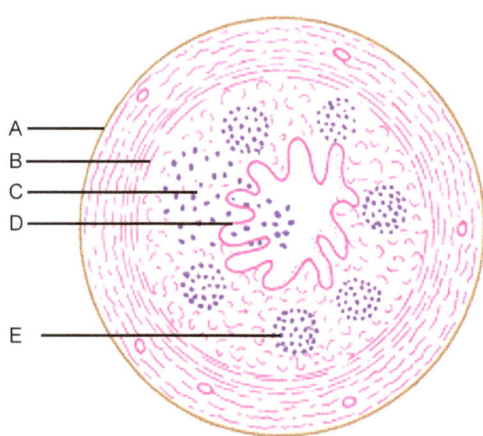

FIG. 1: Cut section of appendix; A–Serosa; B–Muscle coat; C–Submucosa; D–Mucosa; and E–Lymph follicle.

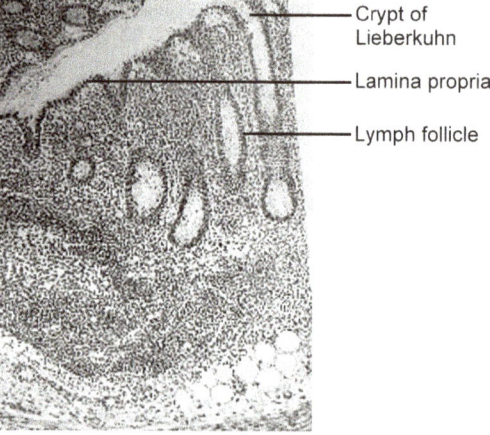

FIG. 2: Histology of appendix.
Source: Kelly HA. Appendicitis and Others Diseases of the Vermiform Appendix. JB Lippincott Company; 1905. p. 28.

- Serosa
- Muscle coat:
  - Outer longitudinal muscular coat
  - Inner circular coat
- Submucosa
- Mucosa

SEROSA (FIG. 3)

It is a complete investment of appendix, except a narrow strip along with the mesenteric attachment. There is a subserous layer of connective tissue. The serous layer surrounds the outer surface of appendix. The *mesoappendix* is the continuation of mesentery of the ileum and it wraps the appendix and mixes with the serosa of appendix.

MUSCLE COAT

It has outer longitudinal and inner circular muscle fibers as in small intestine but the muscle fibers in appendix are weakly developed in comparison to the intestine. They are deficient at some areas where serosa and submucosa are in contact. These gaps in muscle layers are called 'hiatus muscularis' through these gaps the infection from mucosa reaches fast to serosa and peritoneum. These gaps sometimes act as weak spots and perforation occurs here due to raised intraluminal pressure. Acquired diverticulum of appendix occurs through these gaps. The longitudinal muscle layer is thicker near base of appendix to form rudimentary taenia which is continuous with those of cecum and colon. The circular muscle layer is separated from longitudinal muscle layer by connective tissue. The muscularis mucosa is very thin in appendix.

SUBMUCOSA

It has 20–40 lymphoid follicles in adult. These lymphatic tissues decrease in size as the age advances. Follicular and parafollicular zones in submucosa contain B and T lymphocytes. The lymphoid masses are a local defense against infection. Lymphoid tissues in appendix are not present at birth, but develop at 2 weeks after birth. The number of lymphoid follicles is maximum during 12-20 years of age, 200, then number of lymphoid follicles reduces with age and almost they disappear by the age of 60 years. This is one of the reasons why acute appendicitis is rare after 60 years of age. Appendicectomy does not cause any change in person's immune response or cause any cancer. The appendix is also called as 'abdominal tonsil' due to its rich lymphatic tissue presence.

MUCOSA

The mucosa of appendix resembles that of colon. It has several longitudinal folds. The number of crypts of Lieberkuhn is less as compared to colon. Crypts of Lieberkuhn contain Kulchitsky cells or Argentaffin cells. The openings of crypts of Lieberkuhn are arranged around certain centers marked by a depression on the surface of the apices of lymph follicles. Nikolai Kulchitsky, first time described argentaffin cells which are responsible for tumor. As with rest of the colon, there are mucus secreting goblet cells throughout the mucosa.[6]

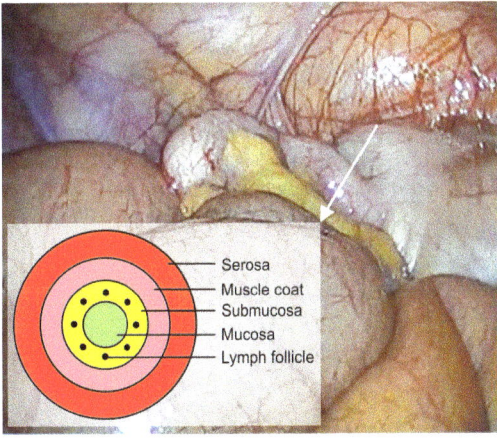

FIG. 3: Mildly inflamed appendix, cut section showing different layers.

CHAPTER 4 Histology of Appendix

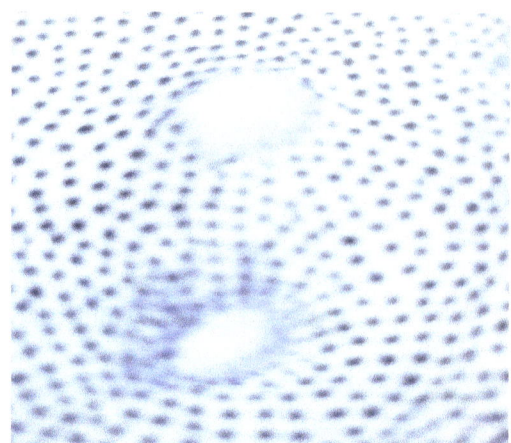

FIG. 4: The surface of mucosa showing opening of crypts of Lieberkuhn around apices of lymph follicles.

Special cells, called Paneth cells, after Joseph Paneth, physiologist and pathologist from Vienna, are found at the base of crypts of Lieberkuhn produce antimicrobial substances, and thus help in immunological defence **(Fig. 4)**.

Key Point
Appendix is a peculiar structure as its walls have plenty of lymphoid follicles and muscularis mucosa is very weak.

The thickness of the longitudinal muscular coat of the appendix varies in different individuals and also in the same specimen from 0.2 to 0.3 mm. The circular muscular coat measures from 0.2 to 0.5 mm in width. The thickness of the submucosa varies greatly in different individuals (0.2 to 0.8 mm or more). It is this layer which gains most in thickness during the process of obliteration. The submucosa consists of loose, wavy strands of fibrous, and elastic tissue which forms a framework for the blood, lymph vessels and nerves. In the interspaces are fat globules. The mucosa is bound to the submucosa by the vestiges of muscularis mucosa. The mucosa presents an irregularly folded appearance, the folds running parallel with the longitudinal axis of the appendix.[7]

REFERENCES

1. Microanatomy definition and meaning. Collins English Dictionary.
2. Histology/physiology. Encyclopedia Britannica.
3. Maximow, Alexander A; Bloom, William (1957). A Textbook of Histology, 7th edition. Philadelphia: WB Saunders Company.
4. Leeson Thomas S; Leeson C Roland (1981). Histology, 4th edition. WB Saunders Company. p. 600.
5. Stedman's medical disctionary, 27th edition. Lippincortt Williams & Wilkins. 2006.
6. Kelly HA. Appendicitis and Others Diseases of the Vermiform Appendix. JB Lippincott Company; 1905. p. 28.
7. Townsend CM, Beauchamp RD, Evers BM, Mattox KL. Sabiston Textbook of Surgery. Volume 3, 17th edition. Elsevier; 2004. p. 1381.

CHAPTER 5

Functions of Appendix

'Appendix is known more due to its misdeeds than its deeds.'
—**Vinod Kumar Nigam**

INTRODUCTION

Vermiform appendix is a small tubular structure attached with cecum. Earlier appendix was considered as a vestigial organ, serving no function, but now the view has changed. Appendix is found to be storing and developing body friendly flora of the intestine that can redevelop after its loss in the sicknesses of digestive tract. Appendix also plays a role in immune function as it contains lymphoid tissue. The appendix has been shown to have an important interaction with the intestinal flora.[1-3]

Though the appendix was considered as a vestigial organ but it is found that it is well developed in some animals, which doubts it being a vestigial organ. In view of its rich vascularity and histological differentiation, the appendix is probably a specialized rather than a degenerate or vestigial organ.

> The vermiform appendix is found in certain herbivorous animals and not in carnivorous animals, is not by chance, but it shows that the appendix has to do something functionally with plant origin food or vegetable matters. Probably appendix plays a role in digestion of vegetable food and the ability of digestion of vegetable food is poor in carnivorous animals.

It is not proved that the appendix has immunity-related role in body even though it has lymphoid tissue, but now most of researchers have started to consider appendix as an immunological organ that plays a part in body by secretion of immunoglobulin A (IgA) but appendicectomy does not lead to higher incidence of sepsis or other manifestations of immune compromise.[4] So it is not considered as a vestigial organ and it does not take active part in immunity of body but:

- Lymphoid follicles help in maturation of B-Lymphocytes.
- Appendix is a part of GALT (Gut-Associated Lymphoid Tissue) and forms globulin which is required for immune mechanism of body.

It is proved now that appendicectomy does not increase the incidence of carcinoma of colon which was doubtful in studies in 1960. The removal of appendix does not cause defect in immunoglobulin system functioning. So we can take following functions of appendix in consideration.

TO MAINTAIN GUT FLORA

William Parker, Randy Bollinger, and colleagues at Duke University proposed in 2007 that the appendix serves as a haven

CHAPTER 5 Functions of Appendix

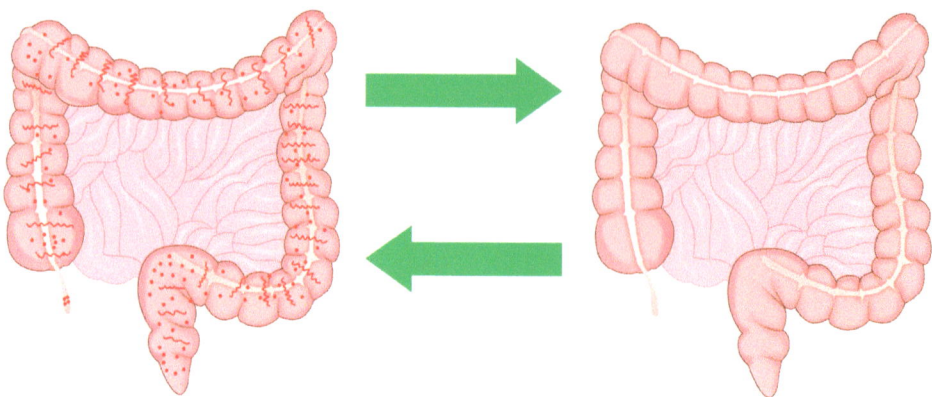

FIG. 1: Appendix acts as reservoir of bacteria. It repopulates the gut flora in the digestive system following a bout of dysentery or diarrhea.

for useful bacteria when illness flushes the bacteria from the rest of intestines.[5] This reservoir of bacteria could then serve to repopulate the gut flora in the digestive system following a bout of dysentery or cholera or to boost it following a milder gastrointestinal illness **(Fig. 1)**.[6,7]

> Vermiform appendix is found in man, in apes, in wombat, and in rodents. Appendix helps in self cleaning and pushing its secretions to the cecum **(Fig. 2)** and denying the entry of fecal material into its lumen. Barring this fact the microscopic anatomy of appendix shows the characteristic feature, rich in lymphoid tissue. This feature makes appendix to resemble tonsils. Appendix is therefore called as 'abdominal tonsil'.

IMMUNE FUNCTION

Appendix is an important part of mucosal immune functions through B and T cells to fight off pathogens.[8] Innate lymphoid cells of gut help the appendix to maintain digestive health.[9]

VESTIGIALITY

Earlier it was proposed that human appendix was a vestigial organ, as during evolution, cecum was thought to have shrunk in size and it's remnant was the appendix. After millions of years, the once necessary cecum

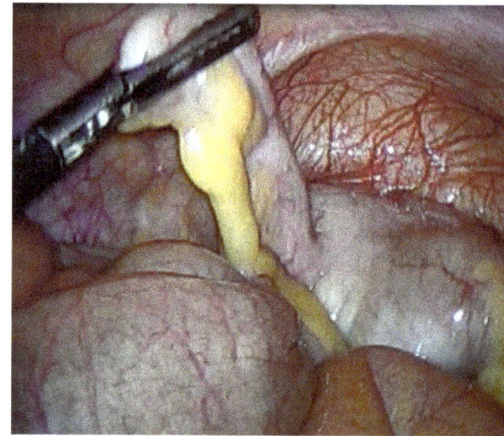

FIG. 2: Appendix empties its secretions directly into cecum without obstruction.

degraded to be the appendix of modern humans. Humans were having diet rich in foliates (cellulose-rich plants) but now take easily-digestible foods so a long cecum is not required to host bacteria digesting cellulose **(Fig. 2)**.

> The surface of the vermiform appendix is full of glands secreting a fluid which mingles with the faeces in the cecum, and by diluting these prevents their remaining stationary and doing harm. Glands of the same character are present in the cecum, but those of the appendix possess greater strength and usefulness. The fact that the appendix contracts at the same time as the cecum, prevents any foreign body from entering its lumen.[10]

Though there is no clear role of appendix in the causation of a human disease but studies have shown a correlation between appendicectomy and development of inflammatory bowel disease especially ulcerative colitis. Appendix delays the onset of ulcerative colitis. Association of the inflammatory bowel disease is not so clear as in ulcerative colitis.[11]

> **Key Point**
> Removal of appendix does not cause any immunological defect.

REFERENCES

1. Im Gy, Modayil RJ, Lin CT, et al. The appendix may protect against Clostridium difficile recurrence. Clin Gastroenterol Hepatol. 2011;9:1072-7.
2. Laurin M, Everett ML, Parker W. The cecal appendix: one more immune component with a function disturbed by post-industrial culture. Anat Rec (Hoboken). 2011;294:567-79.
3. Randal Bollinger R, Barbas AS, Bush EL, Lin SS, Parker W. Biofilms in the large bowel suggest an apparent function of the human vermiform appendix. J Theor Biol. 2007;249:826-31.
4. Jaffe BM, Berger DH. Schwartz's Principles of Surgery. 8th edition. McGraw Hill; 2005. P. 1199.
5. Everth ML, Patestrant D, Milller SE, Bollinger RR, Parker W. Immune exclusion and immune inclusion: a new model of lost bacterial interactions in the gut. Clin App Immunol Rev. 2004;5(5): 321-32.
6. Randal Bollinger R, Barbas AS, Bush EL, Lin SS, Parker W. Biofilms in the large bowel suggest an apparent function of the human vermiform appendix. J Theor Biol. 2007;249(4):826-31.
7. Zahid A. The vermiform appendix: not a useless organ. J Coll Physicians Surg Pak. 2004;14(4):256-8.
8. Rankin LC, Girard-Madoux MJ, Seillet C, Mielke LA, Kerdiles Y, Fenis A, et al. Complementary and redundancy of IL-22-producing innate lymphoid cells. Nat Immunol. 2016;17(2):179-86.
9. Darwin CR. The Descent of Man, and Selection in Relation to Sex. 1st edition. London: John Murray; 1871.
10. Lieberkuhn JN. De Valvula coli et usu processus vermicularis. Wishoff; 1739.
11. Brownicardi FC, Anderson DK, Billar TR, Dunn DL, Hunter JG, Mathew J, et al. Schwartz's Principle of Surgery. 9th edition. The McGraw Hill; 2010. pp. 2043-82.

CHAPTER 6

Diseases of Appendix

*'Appendicitis with complications can be fatal,
even when treated by the most experienced surgeon.'*
— **Vinod Kumar Nigam**

INTRODUCTION

The vermiform appendix is known because of its inflammation, appendicitis. Acute appendicitis is the most common and significant disease of appendix. Appendix can be involved in various pathologies. The appendix can have congenital abnormalities, inflammatory pathology and even cancer. Acute appendicitis is also very important that if it is not diagnosed and treated early can lead to serious complications which may prove sometimes life-threatening and even fatal. Pathologies related to vermiform appendix can be divided into three groups:
1. Congenital anomalies.
2. Inflammation (appendicitis).
3. Tumors of appendix (carcinoid and cancer).

Schnitzler was of the opinion that the so called chronic appendicitis did not exist. Deaver, on the other hand, believed chronic appendicitis to be a clinical entity and divided it into two distinct types—that which occur after acute appendicitis and that which has always taken the form of chronic inflammation without acute exacerbation. He felt that there could be a differential diagnosis in these two types of chronic appendicitis. He stated his belief that in cases of chronic peptic ulcer, chronic cholecystitis, ureteric colic, Dietl's crisis and chronic pelvic inflammatory disease that the appendix is commonly unjustifiably removed.

CONGENITAL ANOMALIES OF APPENDIX

*'Every child comes with a message that
God is not yet discouraged of man.'*
—**Rabindranath Tagore**

According to WHO, congenital disorders can be defined as structural or functional anomalies that occur during intrauterine life.

Congenital anomalies of appendix are quite rare—absence of appendix, duplication of appendix, and its diverticulum have been mentioned in literatures.[1-4]

AGENESIS OF APPENDIX (FIG. 1)

Absence of Appendix

It is a very rare occurrence, one in 100,000 cases. Sometimes it is not congenital but the appendix is auto digested after an attack of acute of appendicitis or appendicular abscess

CHAPTER 6 Diseases of Appendix

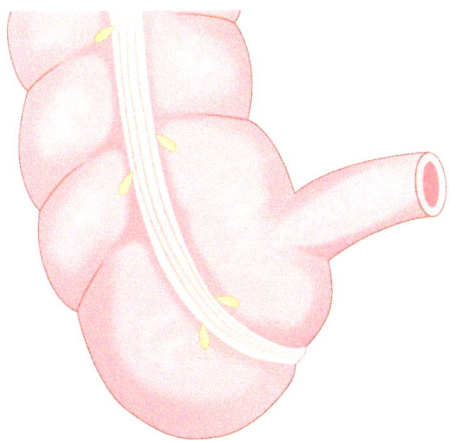

FIG. 1: Agenesis of appendix.

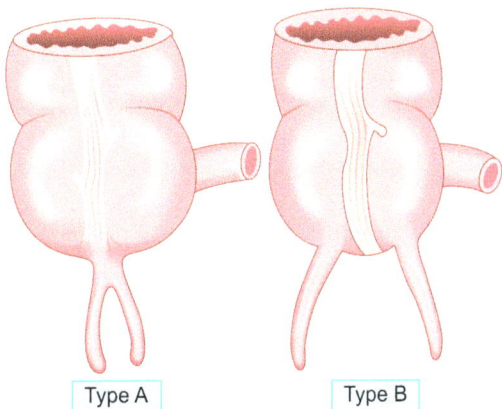

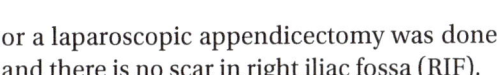

FIG. 2: Duplication of appendix.

or a laparoscopic appendicectomy was done and there is no scar in right iliac fossa (RIF).

DUPLICATION OF APPENDIX (FIG. 2)

It is also an extremely rare occurrence. A total of 10 cases are reported in literature so far. One case reported was having one normal appendix and the other one was inflamed. Maizels G has reported that failure to identify the presence of appendiceal duplicates has resulted in appendectomy being performed twice.[1,2]

Wallbridge Classification of Duplication of Appendix

- *Type A*: Partial duplication in a single cecum.
- *Type B*: Two separate appendices in a single cecum
- *Type C*: Double cecum with each one having one appendix.

Appendix in Left Iliac Fossa (Fig. 3)

It is found in situs inversus viscerum. It occurs one in 35,000 cases. It also occurs due to malrotation of gut.

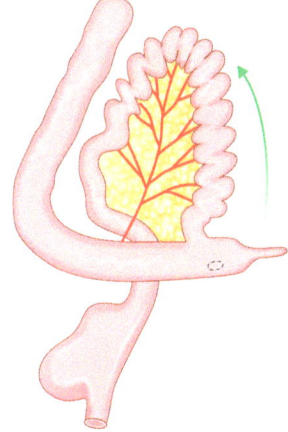

FIG. 3: Appendix in left iliac fossa due to malrotation of gut.

Subhepatic Appendix (Fig. 4)

It is the commonest type of all congenital anomalies of appendix. It is due to the arrest of downward migration of cecum. In this position it may be close to gallbladder so in such situation the acute appendicitis mimics acute cholecystitis.

Diverticulum of Appendix (Fig. 5)

Diverticula of appendix are rare. They are either congenital or acquired. The wall of congenital appendicular diverticulum

CHAPTER 6 Diseases of Appendix

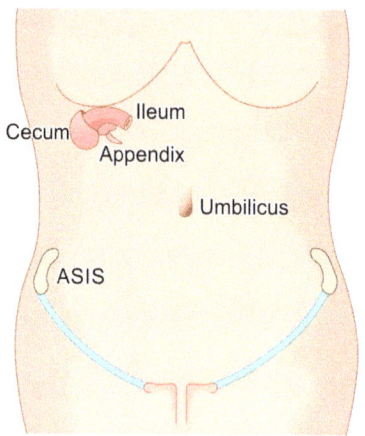

FIG. 4: Subhepatic appendix.

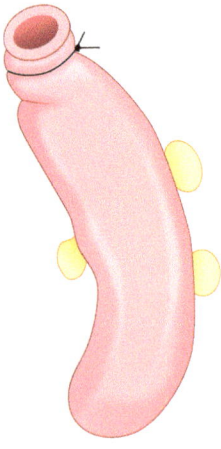

FIG. 5: Diverticula of appendix.

contains all layers. Congenital diverticulum is a rare entity, acquired diverticula occur more frequently. The mucosa of appendix balloons out from the weak spots in walls, 'Hiatus muscularis.' If the appendix with diverticulum develops appendicitis then perforation of appendix occurs early due to weak wall.

Key Point
Congenital anomalies of appendix are rarely seen.

APPENDICITIS

'Appendicitis is one of the most common etiological reasons of acute abdomen.'
—**Vinod Kumar Nigam**

Professor Howard mentions in his book, *'Appendicitis and Other Diseases of The Vermiform Appendix'* that SW Gay characterizes 'Appendicitis as the most treacherous of known diseases, insidious in its manifestations, uncertain in its career, and liable to sudden changes which at any moment may put the patient in a condition of extreme peril'.

The inflammation of vermiform appendix is called 'appendicitis'.

TYPES OF APPENDICITIS

Appendicitis can present in following forms:
- Acute appendicitis
- Subacute appendicitis
- Recurrent appendicitis
- Chronic appendicitis
- Grumbling appendix
- Pseudoappendicitis
- Residual appendicitis
- Appendicitis granulosa
- Appendicitis larvata

Acute Appendicitis

The acute appendicitis is the most common and dangerous type of appendicitis, others are milder version of acute appendicitis **(Figs. 6A and B)**.

Subacute Appendicitis

The subacute appendicitis is actually a milder form of acute appendicitis. If the acute appendicitis subsides before reaching to full blown appendicitis it is called subacute appendicitis. The symptoms subside and pain disappears. It may recur again. It is treated

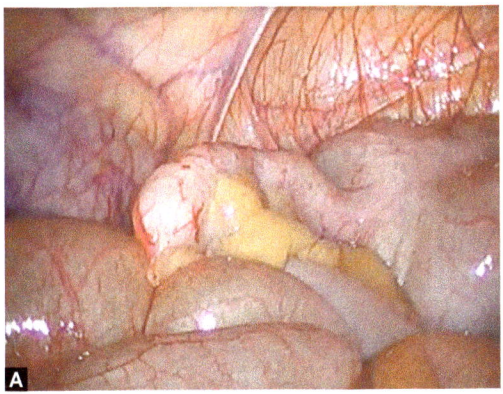 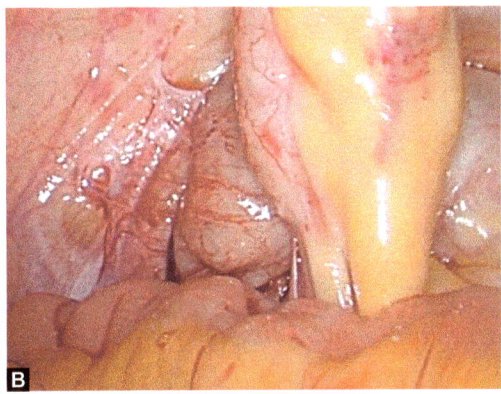

FIGS. 6A AND B: Acute and chronic appendicitis **(Video 1)**.

with appendicectomy which relieves the pain and prevents future complications.

Recurrent Appendicitis

It is a milder variety of appendicitis which occurs recurrently, there is a symptomatic interval between attacks. It is a common variety of appendicitis. The appendix shows obliteration of its lumen by fibrosis due to recurrent inflammation. Appendicectomy is the treatment of choice. Recurrent appendicitis occurs with an incidence of 8–14% following resolution of the acute episode. Out of 142 cases in 92% the removed appendix showed abnormality and 95% of these patients were cured.[5]

Chronic Appendicitis

Some researchers say that there is no entity called chronic appendicitis, it is actually a recurrent appendicitis. However, recent clinical data document the existence of this uncommon disease.[6,7]

In this type of appendicitis there is persistent RIF pain. The appendicectomy relieves the pain and other symptoms. Pain lasts longer and is less intense than acute appendicitis. Pain, nausea, anorexia, malaise, and pain with motion are frequent features. White blood cell (WBC) count and computed tomography (CT) scan are normal. The color of the appendix is reddish with white island areas. The appendix is rigid and bent over itself and often spiral **(Figs. 7A and B)**. The mesoappendix is thickened, shortened, and indurated. The histopathology of removed appendix shows chronic inflammatory cells infiltration in the wall of appendix. It may show old healed scar of previous inflammation. Appendix may show adhesions, kinks, and nodularity. Appendicectomy is the treatment of choice for chronic appendicitis.

> Chronic appendicitis develops either after an acute appendicitis episode or erupts in chronic form. Chronic appendicitis may occur in recurrent form, relapsing form or in residual form. Recurrent form of chronic appendicitis has repeated attacks of subacute or mild-acute attacks followed by a disease free interval. Relapsing form is a continuous form where patient is never free from symptoms. Residual form of chronic appendicitis is due to residual effects of previous attacks of acute appendicitis such as adhesions and angulations.

Grumbling Appendix

Recurrent bouts of pain in RIF are sometime called 'grumbling appendix.' It is usually a milder recurrent appendicitis. It is common in children. They are admitted several times in the hospital with pain in RIF. The grumbling of appendix is relieved by appendicectomy. It is associated with recurrent pain in RIF, general malaise, tenderness over appendix, and anorexia.[8]

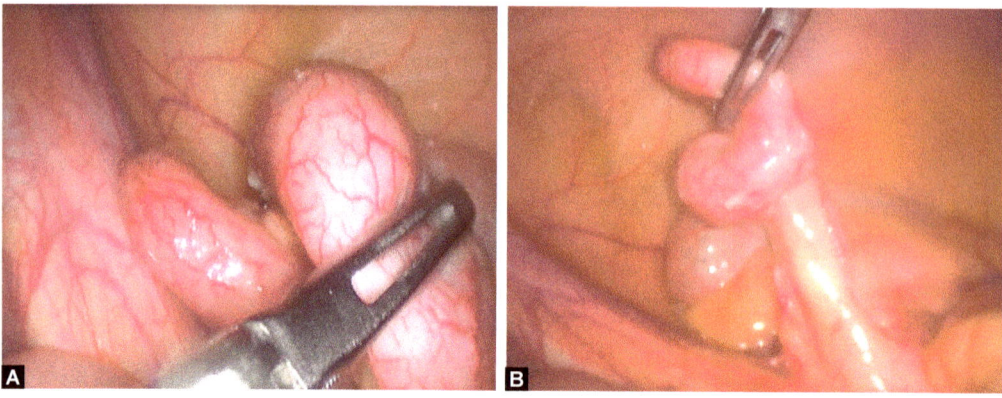

FIGS. 7A AND B: Chronic appendicitis, appendix is coiled **(Video 2)**.

Pseudoappendicitis

Pseudoappendicitis is due to acute ileitis. It is caused by following factors:
- Yersinia*
- Crohn's ileitis

Residual Appendicitis

Residual deformities of appendix develop after active inflammation subsides. After the attack of acute or chronic appendicitis it may be hypertrophy or atrophy, stricture, closer of lumen, cysts formation, dilation, kink, diverticula, adhesions, or fibrosis. This can cause recurrent pain in RIF.

Stump Appendicitis is also taken as residual appendicitis which occurs in the stump of appendix left after appendicectomy. It is a rare entity. It is difficult to differentiate clinically from acute appendicitis, this delays the diagnosis and treatment. This reminds us to avoid leaving a big stump during appendicectomy.

The ulcers inside the lumen of appendix in the wall develop due to acute inflammation of the appendix and they heal by connective tissue replacing the destroyed tissue. This fibrous tissue contracts like the cicatricial tissue anywhere and thus produces kinks, strictures, and angulations. If the appendicular luminal canal is partially occluded this cicatricial tissue causes complete obstruction by forming kinks, strictures, and angulations.

Appendicitis Granulosa

Riedel believes that acute appendicitis has always an insidious onset, one of the most important predisposing causes being a chronic primary disease, 'appendicitis granulosa.' Chronic inflammation of the appendix is essentially a hypertrophic process and produces a characteristic thickening and rigidity of its wall. In rare instances the inflammatory reaction seems to be confined to the mucous membrane, but, as rule, all the coats are more or less affected.[9,10]

Appendicitis Larvata

Clinical condition described by Lenzmann and by Ewald as appendicitis larvata....acute or chronic appendicitis exceedingly rarely results in a 'restitutio ad integrum' (restoration to original condition). In the mildest cases there is more or less connective—tissue

---

*Alexandre Emile Jean Yersin, 1863–1943, Bacteriologist, Paris, France, discovered the bacillus causing bubonic plague which was later named after him, 'Yersinia pestis.'

hyperplasia, and as a consequence a certain amount of rigidity and enfeebled muscular power persists.[11,12] This is also called as latent appendicitis.

Note: Nowadays after understanding more about appendicitis granulosa and appendicitis larvata we found that these are the other forms of, still ill – understood, chronic appendicitis.

Key Point

Acute appendicitis is most common and dangerous of all appendicitis.

ACUTE APPENDICITIS

'Appendicitis must be considered in the differential diagnosis of almost all cases of acute abdomen and must be excluded.'
—**Silen W**

Acute appendicitis may be divided into following groups clinically:
- Catarrhal
- Purulent
- Gangrenous
- Perforative

HISTORICAL BACKGROUND

'The best prophet of the future is the past.'
—**John Sherman**

The acute appendicitis is reported since 1500 AD, it used to be called as 'perityphlitis' which they used to mean as severe and fatal inflammation of the cecal region of large intestine. Jean François Fernel, a French physician and astronomer was first who reported a case of appendicitis in 1554 when he noted at autopsy the luminal obstruction, necrosis and perforation of appendix and cecum. He was first to describe this disease as 'perityphlitis'.[10,11]

Lorenz Heister (1683–1758) was a German anatomist, surgeon, and botanist who wrote, 'Chirurgie', a book on surgery that was translated into several languages. He coined the term 'tracheotomy' in 1718. He was the first physician to perform a post-mortem section of appendicitis, he wrote, 'When about to demonstrate the large bowel, I found the vermiform appendix of the cecum preternaturally black. As I was about to separate it, its membranes parted and discharge two to three spoonful of matter. It is probable that this person might have had some pain in the past.'
—**Maingot's Abdominal Operations**

Reginald Heber Fitz, Professor of Medicine, Harvard University, was credited for describing the acute appendicitis as a proper clinical entity for the first time. He presented a scientific research paper in the first meeting of Association of Physicians of America in 1886 entitled. 'Perforating inflammation of the vermiform appendix.' This paper helped doctors to diagnose more and more cases of acute appendicitis at early stage of acute appendicitis. He studied 25 patients and found that appendix was the primary site and source of inflammation in perityphlitis.[13,14]

French Surgeon Claudius Amyand performed the world's first successful appendicectomy at St. George's Hospital, London on an 11-year-old boy who swallowed a pin. It was a perforated appendix.

In 1889 Charles McBurney, Professor of Surgery, Columbia University College of Physicians and Surgeons, New York, described the clinical manifestation of acute appendicitis including the point of maximum tenderness in the RIF which later on was called as 'McBurney's point'.

Appendectomy for appendicitis is one of the advancements of surgery. Surgical treatment of appendicitis saves 261,134 lives per year in USA alone.[15]

> Harry Houdini was a Hungarian American magician and escape artist. He died of perforated appendix in 1926 after getting hammer like blows on his abdomen from J Gordon Whitehead in a show.

ACUTE CATARRHAL APPENDICITIS (FIGS. 8A AND B)

Catarrhal appendicitis is an inflammatory process affecting only the mucous lining of the appendix throughout the attack, and not involving the deeper layers. In all cases of acute appendicitis there is probably an early stage in which the reaction is limited to the mucous membrane, but in the majority of cases this is only momentary, and so speedily gives way to a general involvement of all the coats.[16]

Macroscopically, in acute endoappendicitis the appendix appears slightly thicker than normal, and owing to a more or less general edema it may be somewhat rigid. The superficial blood vessels, both those immediately beneath the peritoneum and those between the subperitoneal fibrous layer and the muscle, are prominent and tortuous, presenting a characteristic arborescent appearance. There is not, however, the diffuse redness of inflammatory tissue, on sectioning the appendix its canal is found to be patent, and, as a rule, is of uniform caliber **(Figs. 9A and B)**. The mucosa is swollen, edematous, diffusely injected, and granular in appearance.[16]

Histologically, the surface epithelium, which is generally intact, stains rather cloudily, and is infiltrated with leukocytes and

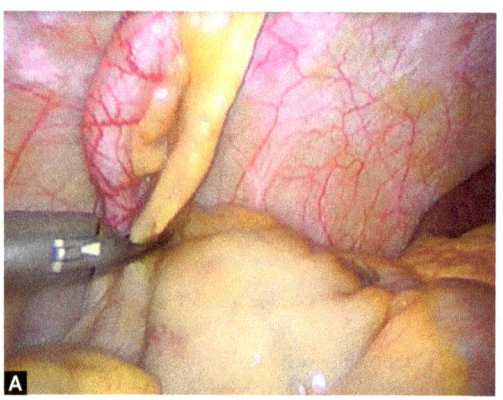 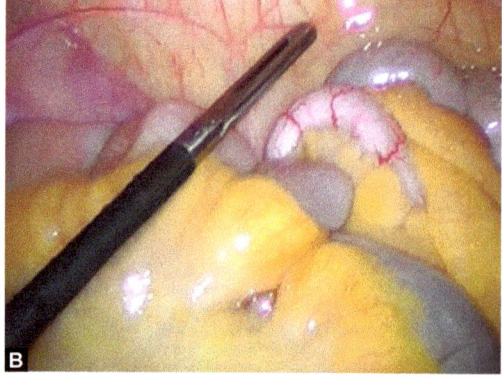

FIGS. 8A AND B: Acute and subacute appendicitis.

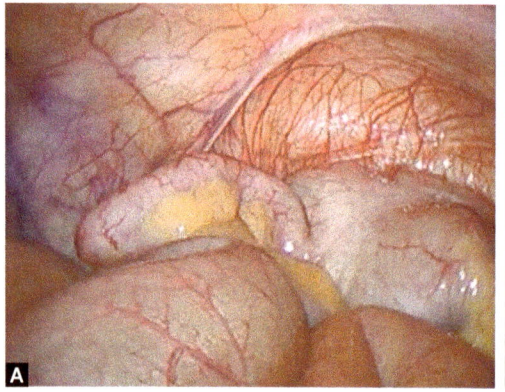 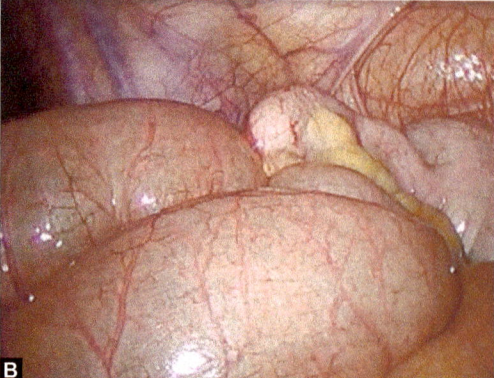

FIGS. 9A AND B: Acute catarrhal appendicitis.

occasional red blood cells. Slight exfoliation of the epithelium is frequently found, but the loss is soon repaired by cells derived from the surrounding epithelium, and especially from the neighboring glands. The stroma of the mucosa is hyperemic, edematous, and moderately infiltrated with leukocytes. The submucosa and the muscular coats of the appendix are perfectly normal, and its peritoneal covering, apart from the dilatation of its blood vessels, is unaltered.

> In most of the cases of acute catarrhal appendicitis the inflammatory process actually extends deeper to the mucosa very early and not that late. Appendix becomes thick, rigid, tense, increases in size, tip is clubbed, and color becomes bright or dark red.

In the gross specimen, the difference between an inflammation limited to the mucosa and the diffuse process is at once evident. In diffuse inflammation, the appendix shows a notable increase in all of its dimensions, and instead of the normal, pale, flaccid organ, of about the thickness of a goose quill, it may be twice the usual length, and is often as thick as the index finger, the tip being frequently slightly clubbed. The appendix is usually tense and rigid, and exceedingly hyperemic, the blood vessels standing out in high relief. Its color is a diffuse bright red or dark mahogany, mottled with subperitoneal extravasations of blood, and often presenting light yellowish or greenish-yellow areas due to localized foci of suppuration or necrosis.[17]

Simple catarrhal appendicitis may undergo complete repair, and in cases which presented clinical evidence of repeated attacks, the appendix, when removed in the interval, may appear quite normal.[18]

PURULENT APPENDICITIS

There is no sharp dividing line between purulent and nonpurulent appendicitis, and at any moment a nonpurulent process may become purulent. The nature of the inflammatory reaction is chiefly due to the virulence of the infection. A mild infection is commonly not suppurative, while a severe infection induces suppuration, unless the virulence of the infective material is so great that no migration of leukocytes occurs. In suppuration there is, first, necrosis of the tissue invaded, and second, the reaction of the tissue, producing cells which form the purulent exudates **(Figs. 10A and B)**. Suppuration is an evidence of the ability of the tissue to offer resistance to the invasion of the infective agent.[19]

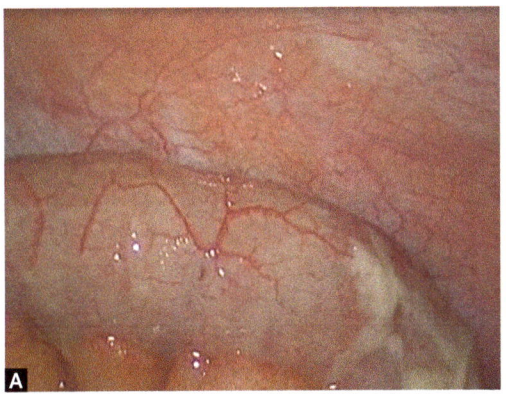
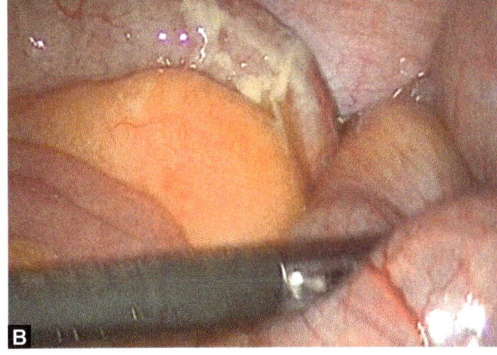

FIGS. 10A AND B: Purulent appendicitis **(Video 3)**.

One of the chief factors promoting suppuration is the existence of some earlier lesion which tends to obstruct the canal of the appendix. The acute swelling of the tissue at the outset of an attack results in complete closure of the stenosed area, and in consequence there is a damming back of the inflammatory exudates. The defective drainage, associated with the abnormal condition of the tissue, favor the development and exalts the virulence of the micro-organisms, and finally induces suppuration.[19]

GANGRENOUS APPENDICITIS

This condition is essentially characterized by the death and putrefaction of the tissues, and is due to the action of microbes upon tissue. The most important factors including gangrene are of those which act by obstructing the circulation, and so producing a local ischemia. Interruption to the blood current may occur in one of the small arteries which supplies only a limited portion of the appendix; or the main artery may be involved; or, in some instances, both the vein and artery, in which case the entire appendix becomes gangrenous. The obstruction to the circulation may be caused by thromboangiitis, twists, angulations, and compressions by adhesions or by hernial rings. Localized areas of gangrene may also be produced by pressure of concretions. The pressure of concretion, added to the acute edema which accompanies the early inflammatory changes compresses the tissue, and produces local ischemia with subsequent gangrene. Most frequently the tip of the appendix is affected, but it is not unusual to find several distinct areas of gangrene both in the proximal and the distal portions of the appendix. The role of bacteria in the production of tissue necrosis is an important one, and in cases where the gangrene of the appendix is partly due to mechanical influences, the heightened virulence of the contained bacteria, in the presence of the lessened vitality of the tissues, undoubtedly promotes the destructive process. The mesoappendix in acute inflammation becomes greatly thickened, due to the dilatation of the blood vessels, and the infiltration of the lax areolar tissue with the serous and cellular exudates. The tissue also becomes exceedingly friable, so that the ligature, although placed with the utmost care, often tears directly through it.[20]

The toxins of bacteria play role in causing gangrene of appendix even in absence of the obstruction of lumen and circulation by directly acting on interior of appendix due to harmful effect on the tissues. Bacteria which are putrefying are present in fecal material and they can cause gangrene in this way. If the inner lining of the appendix and other layers are already compromised then it is easier for the bacteria to cause gangrene in such a situation.

In appendix gangrene sometimes occurs only at proximal part and it may be due to the presence of a concretion. In this form of gangrene the appendix remains healthy except the proximal part connecting with the cecum. In such form of gangrene, the appendix may loose the attachment with cecum and fall off in the peritoneal cavity **(Figs. 11A and B)**.

PERFORATIVE APPENDICITIS

Perforation may take place in any variety of acute appendicitis, and in any stage of the attack. The rupture may be of pin-hole size or there may be a wide ragged aperture through which a large concretion can escape. The factors concerned in the production of a rupture are various; it may follow the eruption of an erosion to the peritoneal surface, the degeneration of the tissue due to purulent infiltration or it may be the result of thrombosis or embolism. If perforation occurs in appendix near its base then it may become completely detached from cecum and float free in the abscess cavity as can occur also in gangrene of appendix. It may get attached to any neighboring organs through adhesions. A tensely distended

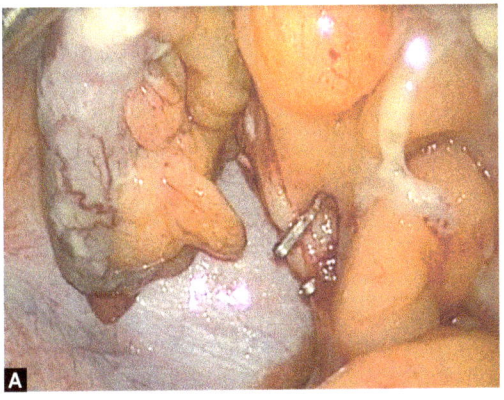
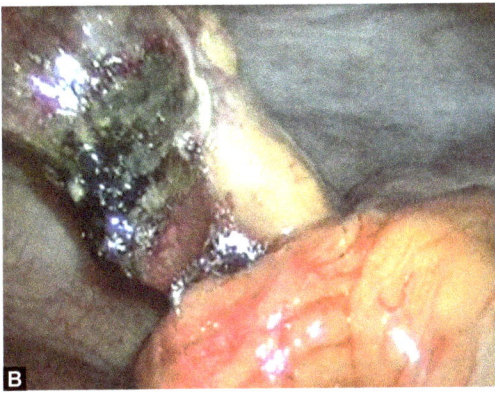

FIGS. 11A AND B: Gangrene of appendix tip A and proximal half B.

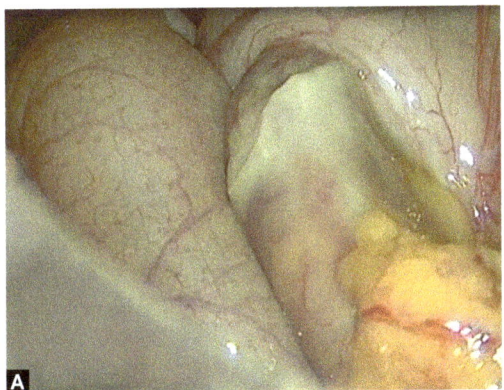
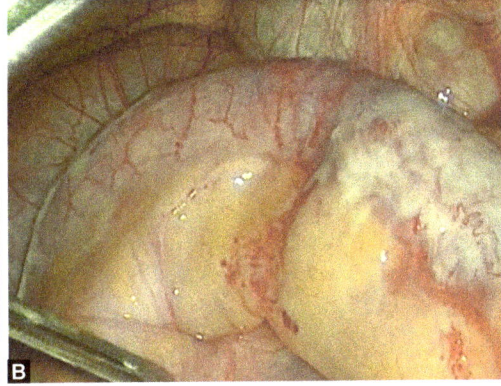

FIGS. 12A AND B: Perforative appendicitis.

empyema often terminates in rupture of the appendix walls, and it is particularly in such cases, where a large amount of highly virulent material empties into the abdominal cavity that the most fatal forms of the peritonitis result. One of the most important causes of rupture is the necrosis of the tissue, induced by the presence of concretions. The favorite location of the perforation is at or near the tip of the appendix, but it is not uncommon to find the perforation directly at the base, or at some intermediate point. A perforation at the base may involve the neighboring portion of the cecum and produce a wide opening through which the intestinal contents escape **(Figs. 12A and B)**.[21]

ETIOLOGY OF ACUTE APPENDICITIS

'To know that we know what we know, and that what we don't know we do not know, that is true knowledge.'
—Confucius

Common etiological factors of appendicitis:
- Diet
- Familial tendency
- Hereditary factor
- Nationality
- Viral infection
- Lumen of appendix

CHAPTER 6 Diseases of Appendix

- Socioeconomic status
- Obstruction of lumen of appendix
- Nonobstructive theory
- Purgatives
- Racial factor
- Epidemic of acute appendicitis
- Seasonal variation of acute appendicitis
- Trauma
- Menstruation

The appendicitis is one of the most common acute problems in medicine yet we do not know much about its etiology.

The real cause of acute appendicitis is still not known. We now understand the process of acute appendicitis well. The following contributing factors are important.

DIET

'Nothing will benefit human health and increase the chances for survival of life on earth as much as the evolution to a vegetarian diet.'
—**Albert Einstein**

Burkitt[22] found higher incidence of appendicitis in west and he attributed this to the low fiber and high sugar diet **(Figs. 13A and B)**.

It is found that the incidence of appendicitis is more in low fiber, meat rich, westernized diet consuming population than high fiber, vegetarian (cellulose) Indian diet consuming population. There is an increasing incidence of appendicitis when the diet changes to low-fiber western-type diet. But the role of diet in etiology of acute appendicitis has not been clarified and the role of dietary fiber is less convincing than was originally thought.[23] The reasons for and against it are:

- The low-fiber diet consuming persons have small stools, which take more time to pass through the intestine, this changes the bacterial flora of gut.
- The high-fiber diet increases the bulks of stool which takes less time to pass through intestine and bacterial flora change does not happen.
  Some people feel that role of high-fiber diet in prevention of acute appendicitis is highly exaggerated.
- The low-fiber diet reduces the mobility of the intestine, which predisposes for obstruction of appendix with a fecalith.
- The incidence of appendicitis is going down in the countries in west where intake of dietary fiber is gradually increasing.
- The appendicitis occurs in new born and pure vegetarians also which raises the doubt about the role of fiber rich vegetarian diet in keeping the incidence of appendicitis low.

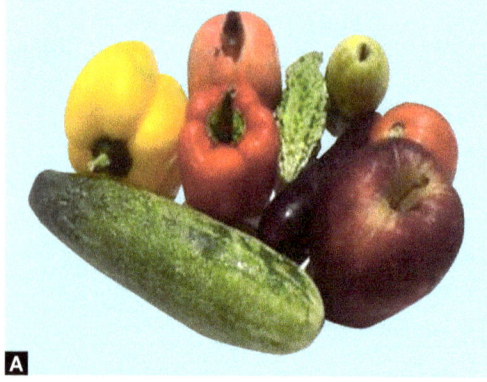 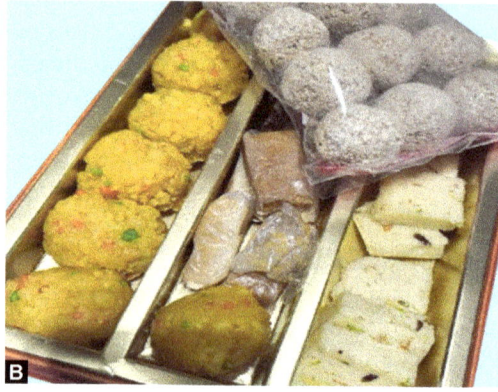

FIGS. 13A AND B: (A) Fruits decrease the chances of appendicitis; (B) Sugary and fatty foods increase the chances of appendicitis.

- There is an increase in incidence of acute appendicitis if high-fiber diet people change to low-fiber diet.
- There is also epidemiological evidence indicating that the consumption of green vegetables and tomatoes may be protective against appendicitis whereas potato consumption appears to be related to the disease. In elderly patients there is some evidence that chronic intake of nonsteroidal anti-inflammatory drug (NSAID) may increase the risk.[24]

FAMILIAL TENDENCY

Sometimes several members of the same family suffer from appendicitis, which may be a familial tendency (30%), or they are consuming same diet. It is seen in a long retrocecal appendix (which many members of the same family may have) where the blood supply of the distal part of the appendix tip is diminished which precipitates the appendicitis. Genetic factors theory can be explained by following factors:[23]
- Shared dietary habits
- Genetic resistance to bacterial flora
- Inheritance of fibrous band anomalies in the appendix.

> A McCosh (American Journal of the Medical Sciences, May, 1897) reports three cases in three successive generations, and Finney had five cases in one family, the father, two sons, and two daughters being affected. In one case of John Hopkins Hospital cases a girl, 12 years of age, was operated on for acute appendicitis while her father was still in the ward convalescing after an operation, also performed during an attack.

HEREDITARY FACTOR

Sometimes a particular anatomical position of the appendix is found in many members of the same family, which is inherited. The familial anomaly may be the cause of acute appendicitis. A family predisposition is explicable upon the ground of anatomic peculiarities and constitutional predisposition. It is well known that in some families there is a marked tendency toward affections of the lymphoid tissues. As a rule, the affection appears in the various members of the family at the different periods but there are a considerable number of observations referring to its developments in two or more at the same time.[25]

> Leannander (Beit. z. klin. Med. u. Chir., 1895) characterizes appendicitis as a family disease, and most physicians of wide experience are impressed with the remarkable frequency of its occurrence in members of the same family. Brothers and sisters are affected more often than parent and child, although the latter association is not uncommon.[25]

NATIONALITY

Though this factor seems to be of not much importance but some researchers have found that appendicitis is much less common in colored people (Africans) than white people. Some found it rare to see appendicitis in Africans. Various nations have different incidents of acute appendicitis. Incidence is taken as number of cases per 100,000 people.

> The statistics of The Johns Hopkins Hospital show that, while the number of admissions of colored to white averages about 1 to 4, the number of cases operated upon for appendicitis is 1 to 12 according to Howard A Kelly.

VIRAL INFECTION

Relationship of viral infection and acute appendicitis is based on the following factors:
- Appendicitis seems to have seasonal variations as viral infection has.
- Raised viral antibodies have also been found during appendicitis.
- Lymphoid hyperplasia in submucosa of appendix is commonly seen on

histopathology in appendicitis. Viral infection may enlarge the lymphoid tissue causing blockage of the lumen of appendix leading to appendicitis.

Viral infection causes mucosal inflammation which gets secondarily infected leading to acute appendicitis. Most commonly appendicitis is found in association with influenza, leading to catarrhal appendicitis.

> Leudet (Leudet. Arch.gen.de med., 1859; 104:137-316) describes a case of perforative appendicitis accompanying varioloid. The association of appendicitis with scarlet fever has been frequently observed. An interesting example was communicated to me as follows: A boy, 8-year-old, was taken ill with a severe attack of scarlet fever accompanied by abscess of neck gland and 3 weeks later was operated for acute appendicitis.

LUMEN OF APPENDIX

The lumen of appendix is quit narrow and so it is prone to get obstructed. Approximately 60% of inflamed appendix removed during appendicectomy for acute appendicitis show blockage of lumen. The blockage is most commonly found due to a fecalith but rarely neoplasm of cecum (<1% is also responsible).

SOCIOECONOMIC STATUS

- Appendicitis is more common in rich and upper middle class people. The reason for this is known as probably they tend to take more protein as the main dish and try to ignore vegetables there by take a low-fiber diet or high-caloric diet.
- The role of personal hygiene and domestic overcrowding is considered as the one of the reasons of infection.

OBSTRUCTION OF THE LUMEN OF THE APPENDIX

Obstruction of the lumen of the appendix is the most common factor in causing acute appendicitis. Wangensteen studied the anatomy of appendix and postulated that mucosal folds and sphincter-like orientation of muscle fibers at appendiceal orifice make the appendix susceptible for obstruction. The cause of obstruction of lumen may be in the lumen, in the wall or outside the wall of appendix. Lymphoid hyperplasia and fecalith are the most common factors in appendicular lumen obstruction, 60% obstruction in teens is due to submucous lymphoid hyperplasia and 35% in older adults and children.

Causes of Obstruction

- *In lumen*:
    - Fecalith
    - Worm
    - Foreign body, i.e., seeds of fruits
- *In the wall*:
    - Hyperplasia of lymphoid follicles
    - Fibrosis and stricture due to previous appendicitis—if a normal appendix gets adherent to a neighboring organ or a previous operation scar, it becomes prone to inflammation.
    - Neoplasm
    - Crohn's disease
    - Distal colonic obstruction
- *Outside the wall*:
    - Adhesions
    - Kinks
    - Bands

Fecalith

It is a mass of inspissated fecal material and it is made up of:
- Fecal material
- Calcium phosphate
- Bacteria
- Epithelial debris
- *Foreign body*: Foreign body causing appendicitis is rare, but Fitz, in 1886 found foreign bodies in 12% cases of perforative appendicitis. Gallstones are also found as enterolith inside the appendix. The clinical evidence in some of these cases so strongly supports the gallstone theory as to leave no doubt in the mind of observer.

CHAPTER 6 Diseases of Appendix

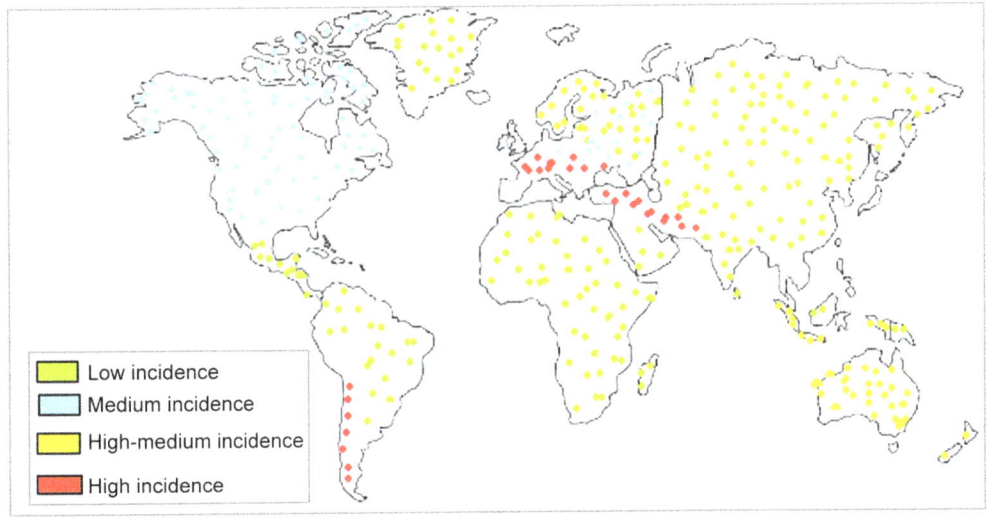

FIG. 14: Global distribution of appendicitis.

Global distribution of appendicitis varies according to various factors such as geographic site, eating habits and environmental factors **(Fig. 14)**.

Fecaliths are the most common causes of appendicitis. They are found in 40% cases of acute appendicitis, 65% cases of purulent appendicitis with rupture and nearly 90% of cases of gangrenous appendicitis with rupture.[26] It is also found that histologically normal appendix having fecalith and appendicitis may show no fecalith obstruction.[27,28] A fecalith in combination of localized RLQ pain is highly diagnostic of appendicitis.[29] The fecalith is also called enterolith **(Figs. 15A and B)**.

Worms

Usual parasites found in appendix are following:
- Pin worm (oxyuris vermicularis)
- Ascaris lumbricoides
- Enterobius vermicularis
- Strongyloides stercoralis
- *Echinococcus* granulosus
- Entamoeba histolytica

The most common intestinal parasite causing obstruction of appendix lumen is pinworm (Oxyuris vermicularis). Careful examination of stools for worms and ova is important.

Presence of parasite in the lumen of appendix sometimes produces difficulty in ligation or stapling of base of appendix. All such cases must be given deworming treatment post appendicectomy and cases of amebiasis with antiamebic therapy.

NONOBSTRUCTIVE THEORY

This is due to bacterial infection in the wall of the appendix without obstruction of its lumen **(Figs. 16A and B)**. It is due to following factors:
- Hematogenous spread of generalized infection.
- Vascular occlusion
- Diet with low roughage
- *Disorders of digestion*: Many persons suffering with appendicitis give history of indigestion or constipation or diarrhea.

Purgatives

Acute appendicitis sometimes is precipitated by administration of purgatives, and it can cause perforation of the appendix in a patient suffering with acute appendicitis. That is why purgative is contraindicated in RIF

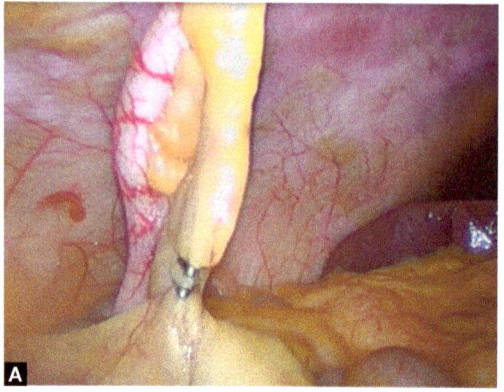 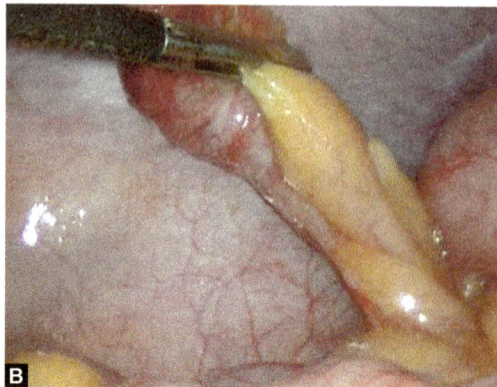

FIGS. 15A AND B: Obstructive appendicitis.

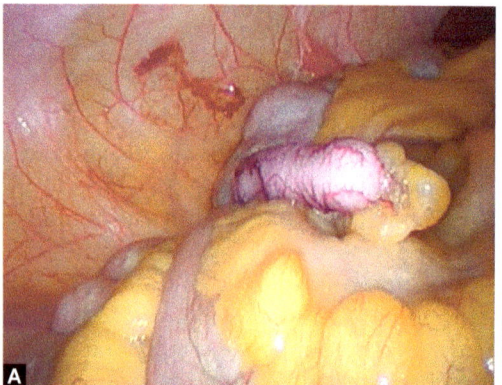 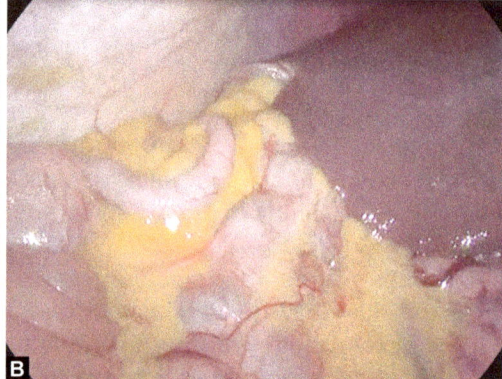

FIGS. 16A AND B: Nonobstructive appendicitis.

pain as generally it is said 'Purgation means perforation.'

Racial Factor

It is seen that appendicitis is most common in white Westerners than dark-colored Asians and Africans.

Epidemic of Acute Appendicitis

Epidemic of acute appendicitis is also reported. It usually occurs in institutionalized children.

Seasonal Variation of Acute Appendicitis

In Europe, it has been observed that between May and August, more cases of acute appendicitis are reported in hospitals. In some western countries a link between viral infection and appendicitis is found which also explains the seasonal variation.

Trauma

Many researchers believe that blunt trauma can cause appendicitis. Straining at weight lifting may also can be a causative factor.

An interesting case was reported by Baltimore Daily Sun, July 29, 1902: A boy, 12 years old, died at St. Joseph's Hospital, after an operation for appendicitis, immediately following a blow upon the abdomen given by a companion during a quarrel. The assailant was arrested on the charge of assault, and then released, but on the death of the patient he was re-arrested to await the verdict of the coroner's jury. The city physician, NG Keirle, testified that 'the autopsy showed inflammation of the appendix which had given rise to appendicitis. The appendicitis could have been occasioned by a blow.'

Menstruation

The intimate relation existing between the menstrual periods and appendicitis has been frequently noted, not only when the appendix is situated in the pelvis, but also when it is retrocecal. The probable explanation lies in the fact that the congestion of the whole splanchnic area which accompanies the lowered blood-pressure of the peripheral circulation during menstruation creates a favorable soil for the activities of the micro-organisms contained in the appendix. I have observed this association in several instances, in some of which the recurrent appendiceal attacks invariably occurred at the menstrual period.

> **Key Point**
>
> Commonest cause of acute appendicitis is obstruction of its lumen by fecalith or enterolith.

PATHOLOGY OF ACUTE APPENDICITIS

'To be conscious that you are ignorant is a great step to knowledge.'
—**Benjamin Disraeli**

Acute appendicitis starts as inflammation and then converts to infection of appendix. The infection in appendix develops from the bacteria contained in the contents of appendix. No single organism is found responsible for acute appendicitis. Usually it is a mixed infection with aerobic and anaerobic bacteria. The obstruction of the lumen accelerates the process of infection as the contents become stagnant and bacteria multiply fast.

The bacteria gain access to the wall of the appendix through a breach in the continuity of mucosa of appendix.

> The cecum is the point which offers the very best conditions in entire intestinal tract for the development of bacteria. Here the reaction is favorable to the growth of bacteria and sufficient undigested food is present to supply the nutriment necessary to their increase by direct continuity the bacteria spread from the cecum to the lumen of appendix, hence, we have the most favorable conditions for the rapid development of bacteria through to the walls of appendix and the initiation of an inflammatory process. (Howard A Kelly, Appendicitis and Other Diseases of the Vermiform Appendix).

The infection and inflammation spread in the wall of the appendix from inside to outside (from mucus membrane to the serosa) that is why some time at early stage of appendicitis appendix looks normal from outside but on exploration it is found inflamed from inside, it is called 'macroscopic normal appendix' but microscopically it is diseased.

BACTERIOLOGY

The infection in appendix is a mixed infection by anaerobic and aerobic organisms. In 85% cases the organism responsible is *Escherichia coli* (*E. coli*).

- The appendiceal flora remains constant throughout the life except *Porphyromonas gingivalis* which is seen only in adults.[30] Porphyromonas is a gram-negative, rod shaped, anaerobic, pathogenic bacterium. It is found in periodontal disease, gastrointestinal tract, and respiratory tract.
- Peritoneal fluid cultures show bacteria in <50% of cases in nonperforated appendicitis and in >85% cases of perforated or gangrenous appendicitis.[31,32]
- It is usually caused by organisms normally residing in appendix.
- *Enterococcus* is also responsible for appendicitis infection in large number of cases.
- In 1938, Altemeier demonstrated polymicrobial nature of the perforated

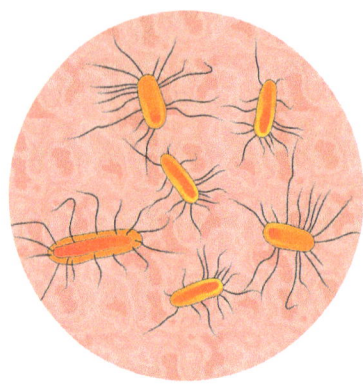

FIG. 17: *Escherichia coli.*

appendicitis.³³ Now due to this, the routine peritoneal culture in perforated appendicitis is questioned.³⁴

The bacteria commonly contained in appendix in acute appendicitis are given below. The commonest bacteria is *E. coli* **(Fig. 17)**.

COMMON ORGANISMS SEEN IN PATIENTS WITH ACUTE APPENDICITIS

Aerobic and facultative	Anaerobic
Gram-negative bacilli	Gram-negative bacilli
Escherichia coli	*Bacteroides fragilis*
Pseudomonas aeruginosa	*Bacteroides* species
Klebsiella species	*Fusobacterium* species
Gram-positive cocci	Gram-positive cocci
Streptococcus species	*Peptostreptococcus* species
Streptococcus species	Gram-positive bacilli
Enterococcus species	*Clostridium* species

Foul smelling odor in perforated appendix is not due to *E. coli* or anaerobic bacilli as it is commonly and wrongly believed, but is due to anaerobic streptococci.

In the majority of cases several species of organisms were isolated side by side, no matter whether the lumen of the appendix only was examined, or a localized peritonitis around the appendix, or a general inflammation of the peritoneum was present.

Routine culture of intraperitoneal samples in patients with either perforated or non-perforated appendicitis is questionable, the peritoneal fluid culture should be reserved for immunosuppressed patients and those who developed abscess after appendicitis.

TYPES OF ACUTE APPENDICITIS

Acute appendicitis is of two types:
1. Obstructive acute appendicitis
2. Nonobstructive acute appendicitis

Obstructive Acute Appendicitis

In most of the cases of acute appendicitis, the obstruction of its lumen is the main and essential reason. Obstruction is found in 50–80% cases of acute appendicitis. Gangrene and perforation of appendix usually does not occur if the appendix is not obstructed.

When obstruction happens due to lymphoid hyperplasia or other obstructing agents the intraluminal pressure in appendix increases due to continuous mucus secretion and inflammatory exudates formation and a closed-loop obstruction is produced. Secretion of even 0.5 mL fluid distal to obstruction raises intra-luminal pressure to quite high level. Rapid distension of appendix ensues because of its small luminal capacity, and intraluminal pressure can reach 50–65 mm Hg.³⁵⁻³⁸

The distension of appendix stimulates nerves endings of visceral afferent nerve fibers, producing dull, vague, diffuse pain in mid-abdomen, or lower epigastrium,²⁶ it also causes reflex nausea and vomiting. The raised intraluminal pressure does not decrease or stop further mucus secretion. The raised intraluminal pressure obstructs the lymphatic drainage from wall of the appendix, which leads to the edema of the wall. The high intraluminal pressure and edema cause superficial ulcerations in the wall which become port of entry for the bacteria to the wall of appendix from the luminal contents.

The further increase in intraluminal pressure causes venous obstruction which further increases the edema of the wall. Now the increased intraluminal pressure, venous obstruction, and increasing edema of the wall cause compromise of arterial blood flow which leads ischemia of the wall. Further bacterial invasion causes full blown acute appendicitis.

> The appendicitis can get resolved by person's immunity and antibiotics or can lead to gangrene and perforation. The appendicular mass can resolve with conservative treatment or can become appendicular abscess.

The further development leads to acute gangrenous appendicitis and then the further increase in intraluminal pressure causes perforation of the wall of the appendix, leading to local or general peritonitis. The body tries to limit the damage and tries to prevent the spread of infection to other parts of peritoneal cavity. So loops of small intestine, greater omentum, and cecum come close and become adherent to wall-off the appendicular lesion to avoid peritoneal contamination. This leads to formation of appendicular mass or lump. The omentum is therefore called 'abdominal policeman', as it helps to contain the problem.

Rarely the obstructed appendix becomes mucus filled sac called 'mucocele of appendix' when infection subsides and sometime it become 'empyema of appendix', when the obstructed appendix become filled with frank pus.

The most dreaded complication of appendicitis is perforation of a gangrenous appendix leading to generalized peritonitis. Sir David Wilkie, Professor of Surgery, Edinburgh, Scotland (1882-1938) stated that close examination of gangrenous appendicitis directly after their removal shows conclusively that they usually belong to the obstructive group.[39] Usually the perforation occurs at the tip of the appendix due to poor vascularity or at the site of obstruction due to pressure necrosis or at antimesenteric border.

Fate of appendicitis can lead to resolution, operation, perforation, peritonitis, fecal fistula, appendicular mass, abscess **(Flowchart 1)**.

This appendicular condition leads to enlargement of cecum due to cecal localized ileus, caused by the inflammatory process. The cecal content is stored and is not conducted to the right colon. The presence of fecal loading inside a large cecum is identified in the plain abdominal radiography as a specific sign of acute appendicitis **(Figs. 18A and B)**.[40-42]

Nonobstructive Appendicitis (Catarrhal Appendicitis)

The infection occurs in the wall of appendix from the mucosa and the process of inflammation is slow **(Figs. 19A and B)**.

Nonobstructive appendicitis is usually a catarrhal type of appendicitis.

Generalized peritonitis is not a common finding with nonobstructive appendicitis but it can occur. It occurs due to:
- Transmigration of bacteria to the peritoneal cavity through the wall of the appendix
- Rarely due to perforation of the appendix.

Macroscopic Changes

In normal looking appendix only mucosa is inflamed so every normal looking appendix must be opened to see mucosa.
- Early stage of acute inflammation—appendix is swollen with hyperemic serosa.
- Late stage of acute inflammation—surface is coated with fibrinopurulent exudates with prominent vessels. In later stages edema, necrosis, and gangrene develop.

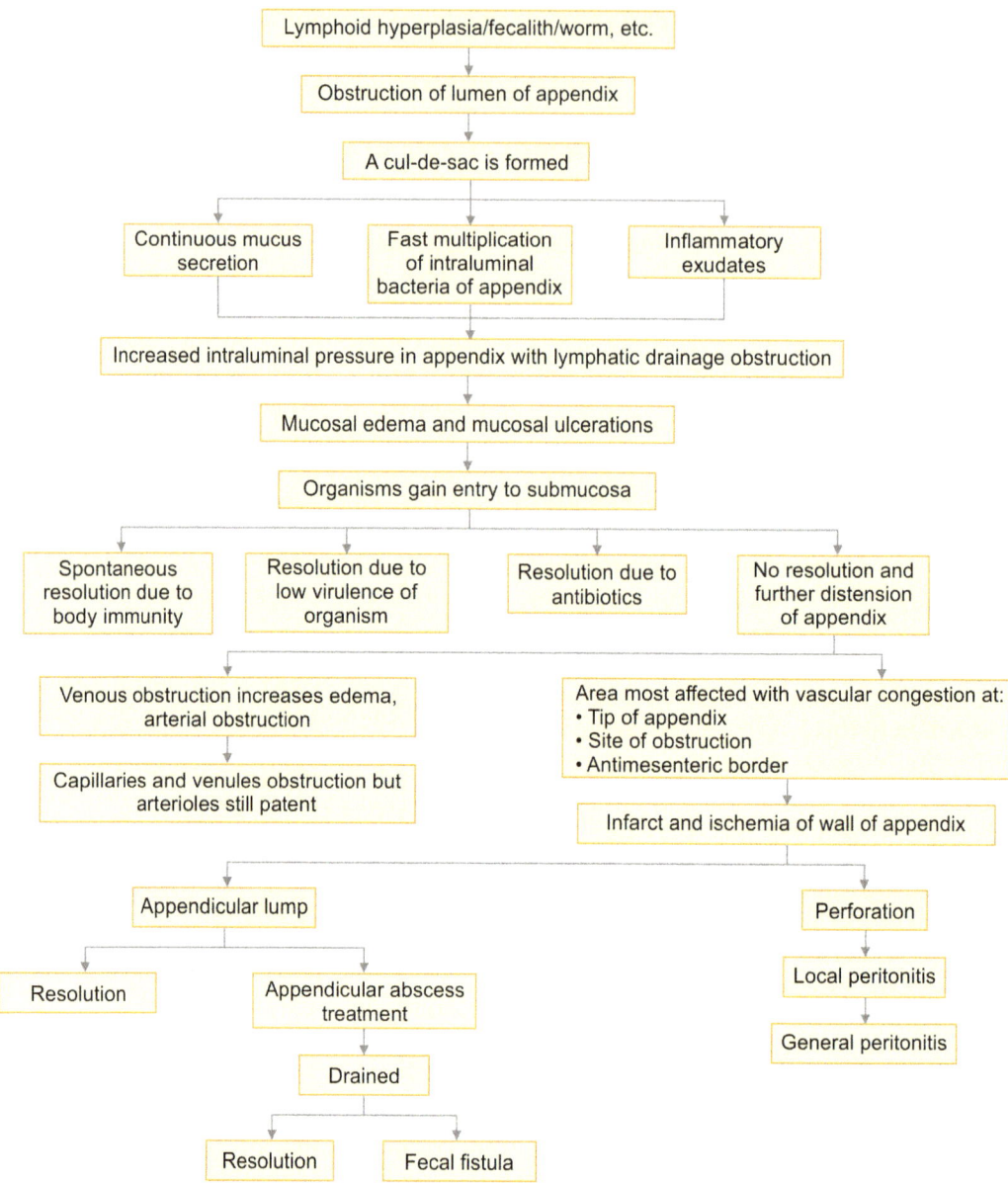

FLOWCHART 1: Sequence of events in acute obstructive appendicitis.

Microscopic Changes

- Neutrophilic infiltration of muscularis mucosa is characteristic of acute appendicitis.
- Congestion, edema, microabscesses, immobilized blood vessels, necrosis, and gangrene may be seen.
- Cause of obstruction is also confirmed.

Many patients, who are forced for operation with acute appendicitis, give a history of previous similar, but less severe, attacks of right lower quadrant pain. Pathologic examination of the appendices removed from these patients often reveals thickening and scarring, suggesting old, healed, and acute inflammation.[43-45]

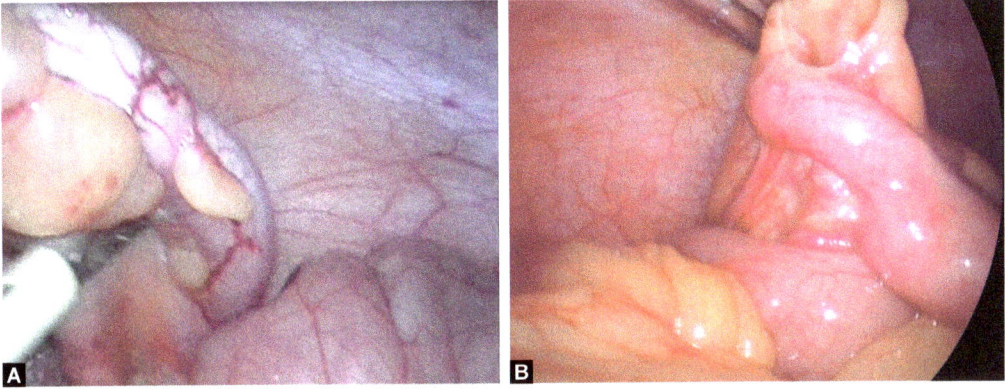

FIGS. 18A AND B: Obstructive appendicitis.

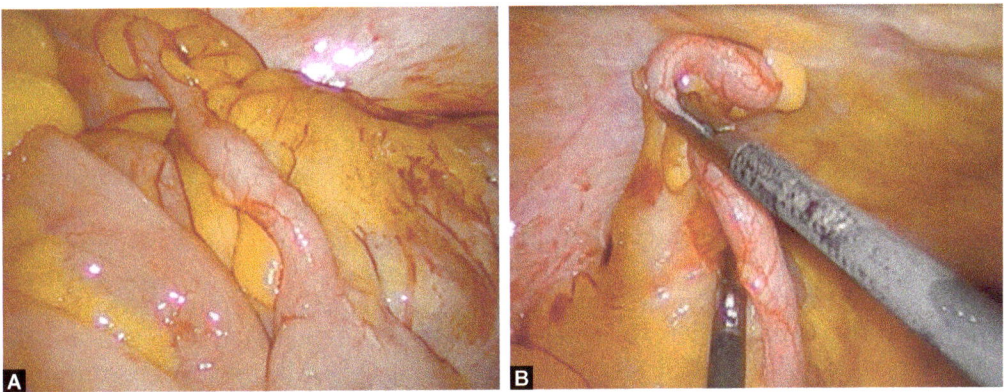

FIGS. 19A AND B: Nonobstructive appendicitis.

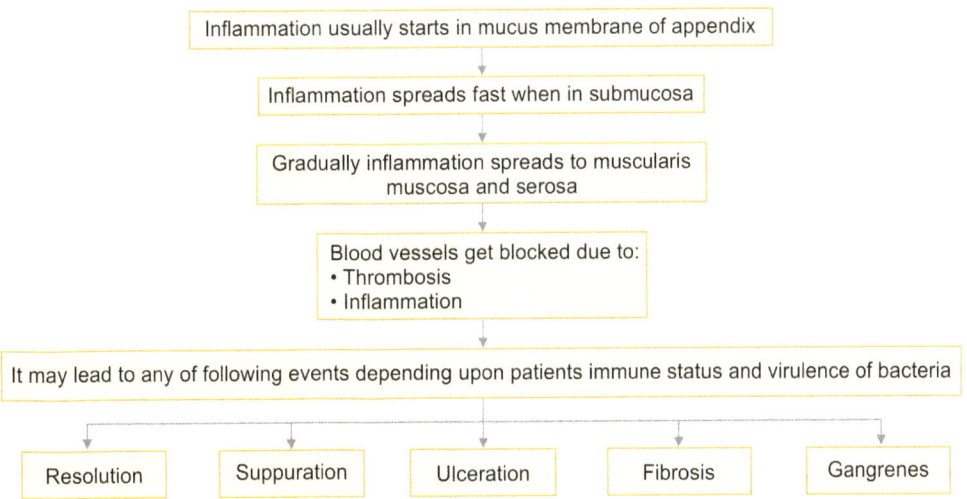

FLOWCHART 2: Sequence of events in nonobstructive appendicitis (it is much slower process than obstructive appendicitis).

Appendicitis can eventually may resolve or develop complications **(Flowchart 2)**.

CHAPTER 6 Diseases of Appendix

> **Key Point**
>
> Gangrene and perforation of appendix are common in obstructive appendicitis and uncommon in nonobstructive appendicitis.

CLINICAL FEATURES OF ACUTE APPENDICITIS

'It is a matter of common experience to find a mild attack which is subsiding, develop symptoms of the gravest significance; while in other instances, the most ominous symptoms are sometimes followed by a speedy recovery.'
—SW Gay

INCIDENCE

The lifetime incidence of acute appendicitis is 6.7–20%, with lifetime risk of appendectomy of 12% for men and 23% for women.[46,47]

Acute appendicitis represents about 17% of all cases of acute abdominal pain presented to hospital.[48]

Acute appendicitis is the most common emergency in surgery where a general surgeon is called. It is the commonest cause of acute abdomen in young adult.

It is more common in western countries than India probably due to diet, which is more vegetarian and with high roughage contents.

By adulthood one in six people will have undergone removal of this appendix. Nowadays the disease is increasing in the developing areas of the world, but decreasing in western countries, probably due to changing food habits.[49]

The incidence of acute appendicitis in population is most frequently seen from 2nd to 4th decade with a mean age of 31.3 years and a median age of 22 years.[50,51]

- Appendicectomy is one of the most common operations performed in general surgery
- Lifetime rate of appendicectomy is 7% for population, it is 12% for men and 25% for women.
- The rate of appendicectomy for appendicitis is 10 per 10,000 patents per year[52] and is constant.
- Rate of misdiagnosis of appendicitis is 15.3%, higher in women (22.2%) than men (9.3%)[51]
- Negative appendicectomy rate for female, if fertile age is 23.1% and is highest in females above 80 years.[53]

Classical Acute Appendicitis

'Whatever the clinical presentation, whatever the abdominal findings, always keep acute appendicitis at the back of your mind in acute abdomen.'
—Moshe Schein

History and physical examination are most important tools in the diagnosis of the acute appendicitis. Ask the patient about exact time of pain occurrence in clear terms such as 6 am or 7 am and not as morning or yesterday as every hour is important. Ask about exact time of pain, character of pain (colicky or dull), site of pain, migration of pain, and radiation of pain, anything increasing the pain as movement or coughing; while coming to hospital the movement of vehicle was causing pain to increase or not. Ask about vomiting, how many times, type (projectile) **(Fig. 20)**.

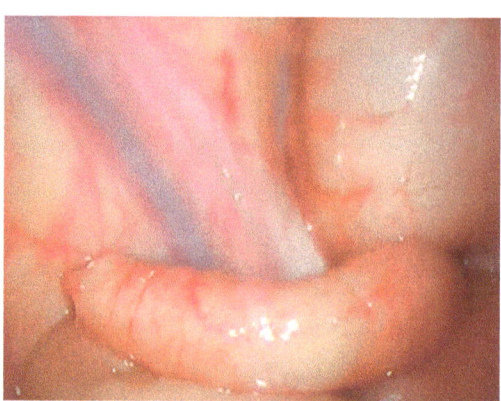

FIG. 20: Acutely inflamed appendix.

CHAPTER 6 Diseases of Appendix

> Acute appendicitis may have a sudden onset; or it may be insidious in character, being ushered in with symptoms of moderate severity which steadily grow worse; or it may possibly exhibit occasional remissions. In a number of cases a feeling of general malaise precedes the onset of the attack. The early symptoms may include pain, tenderness, rigidity, muscle spasm, nausea, vomiting, and constitutional disturbance; distention and tumor may also be present. The time at which these symptoms appear, however, is variable, and some of them may never occur at all. The most constant, most characteristic, and most important symptoms of all are pain and rigidity.
>
> —**Howard A Kelly**

Whether pain preceded vomiting or not, ask about fever, was it high and associated with rigors, was there diarrhea or constipation or absolute constipation? Ask previous history of such pain. Ask about menstrual periods and the date of the last menstrual period. Ask about drugs, the purgative, taken to relieve constipation **(Figs. 21A and B)**.

Age

The maximum incidence occurs in second and third decades, mean age is 31.3 years. Acute appendicitis is rare in infancy; it is uncommon before the age of 2 years but no age is exempted from it. The incidence of acute appendicitis gradually decreases after the middle age. The peak incidence occurs between 20 and 30 years and median age is 22 years. This is also the age of peak increase in size and number of lymphoid follicles. This indicates the relation between incidence of acute appendicitis and amount and number of lymphoid follicles. The incidence of acute appendicitis becomes very low after 60 years of age almost a rarity, 70% of appendicitis occurs <30 years of age.

Mortality rate of acute appendicitis is 0.8%, such patients are either very young or very old.

> Acute appendicitis may develop suddenly or it may develop gradually. Symptoms of acute appendicitis may be mild, moderate, or severe and it may grow worst from milder or not often, but may resolve. One of my patients had sudden pain, 'like a shot of a gun', he fell down on the ground and fainted. Operation revealed an obstructive acute appendicitis. (Appendicitis and Other Diseases of the Vermiform Appendix, p. 154)

The incidence of acute appendicitis in male and female is age related. Before the puberty it is equal among both sexes, in second and third decades the male and female ratio is 3:2. After the third decade the incidence among males declines and becomes equal gradually.

Acute appendicitis is more common in teenaged girls.

Highest incidence of appendicitis in males is at early years, whereas in female it is later years.

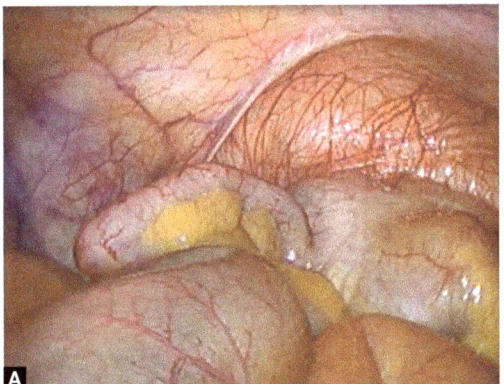
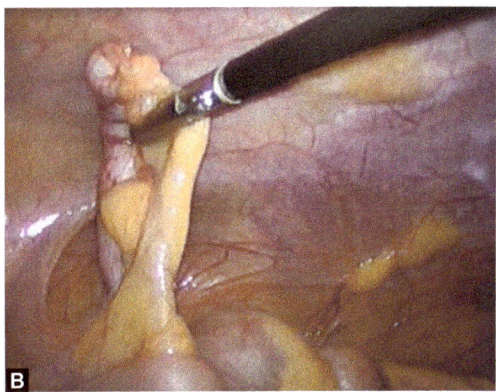

FIGS. 21A AND B: Acute appendicitis.

Association between menstruation and appendicitis is frequently noted. Some researchers indicate that the probable explanation lies in the fact that condition of the whole splanchnic area which accompanies the lowered blood pressure of the peripheral circulation during menstruation creates a favorable soil for the activities of the microorganisms contained in the appendix (Howard A Kelly).

> Some people still believe in a theory by Byron Robinson that appendicitis is more common in males….. the relation of the appendix to the psoas muscle may explain the greater frequency of appendicitis in males. The psoas in them is longer, broader, and more developed generally, thus offering a greater surface for contact with the appendix. This disparity is further increased by the shape of the pelvis which is long and narrow. (Byron Robinson. Annals of Surgery.1901;33:407)

SYMPTOMS

'The wider the experience of surgeon in dealing with the protean forms of this disease, the less confidence will he have in formulating any definite conclusions regarding the interpretation of its individual symptoms, and particularly concerning their prognostic value. But, although this fact should always be born in mind, it must be added that with few exceptions appendicitis ought always to be recognized.'
—**Howard A Kelly**

Important symptoms of acute appendicitis:
- Pain
- Nausea
- Vomiting
- Anorexia
- Fever
- Murphy's syndrome
- Constipation or diarrhea

Pain

Pain in acute appendicitis usually starts in the early morning. The patient sleeps well in the night and pain wakes him up in the early morning.

The pain in appendicitis is produced by distension of its lumen or spasm of its muscle due to stimulation of visceral nerve endings responsible for pain.

First the pain is felt at the umbilicus. It is referred pain as both the umbilicus and the appendix receive their nerve supply from thoracic ten (T10) segment of spinal cord. Appendix receives its sympathetic nerve supply from T10 via celiac plexus and the umbilicus by somatic nerves via vagus nerve. This is referred pain and is vague pain. The explanation of referred pain is that the nerve fibers from diseased organ and the area where the referred pain is felt (here umbilicus) ascend to cerebral cortex and cerebral cortex sometimes becomes incapable of differentiating between the causative site and referred site that is why some patients complain of umbilical pain. This umbilical pain is seen in appendicitis irrespective to any position of appendix. One can explain this visceral pain by midline radiation of delta nonmyelinated fibers that have very poor localization.

The pain increases gradually as the inflammation increases. The pain later migrates to the RIF. This shift of pain is due to involvement of the parietal peritoneum by inflammation over the appendix. As the inflammation increases pain spreads. The visceral layer of peritoneum is insensitive to pain but parietal peritoneum is sensitive to pain that is why in early stage of inflammation when parietal peritoneum is not involved the pain is not felt in RIF and is only felt at umbilicus. When parietal peritoneum is involved the pain is conveyed by alpha fibers at the RIF.

CHAPTER 6 Diseases of Appendix

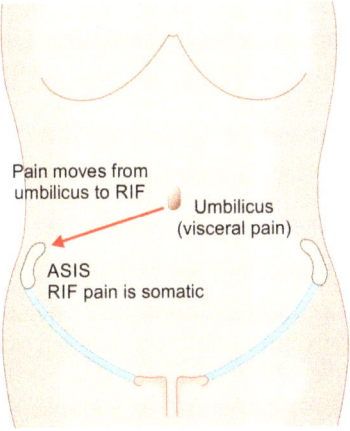

FIG. 22: Migration of pain in appendicitis.

Initial pain is visceral pain which is felt at umbilicus and later on pain is somatic pain which is in RIF. It is called 'shifting pain' of acute appendicitis. The history of shifting pain from umbilicus to RIF if present is very important symptom to diagnose acute appendicitis. The visceral pain in acute appendicitis is dull, diffuse and vague in umbilical, paraumbilical, and lower epigastrium region. 25% patients have no visceral pain and present with localized pain (Fig. 22).[54]

Sudden movement or coughing increases the pain, even walking increases pain. The diminution of pain is not always a good news. In acute appendicitis sudden disappearance of pain may be due to perforation of gangrenous appendix or obstructive appendicitis.

In pelvic appendicitis the pain is aggravated when right obturator internus muscle is stretched by flexion and medial rotation of right thigh. It is due to fact that inflamed appendix is touching the obturator internus muscle.

Pain severity and associated nausea and vomiting depend upon degree of distension of appendix.

In retrocecal appendicitis pain is aggravated or even caused when psoas major muscle of right side is stretched by extension of right hip joint. This is not often seen in obese patients.

The distension of lumen of appendix also stimulates the peristalsis in appendix which produces cramp-like pain as in acute gastroenteritis or in ureteric colic so the visceral pain may be cramp-like pain super imposed on dull pain.

Anorexia

It is a constant feature in every patient of acute appendicitis. It is more marked in infants and children than adults. It is difficult to find a case of acute appendicitis without anorexia. If anorexia is absent, the diagnosis of acute appendicitis is reconsidered.[55]

Hiccough is rare, but is present in generalized peritonitis due to irritation of peritoneal surface of diaphragm.

> Anorexia is a reliable and permanent feature of acute appendicitis, usually it is the first sign. If anorexia is not present then the diagnosis of acute appendicitis may be deferred.

Nausea

It is a common symptom in both types of obstructive and nonobstructive appendicitis. Nausea and vomiting occur in 70% patients of appendicitis.

Vomiting

It occurs due to reflex pylorospasm which is protective as body does not want food to reach site of inflammation, i.e., appendix. It is more marked in obstructive appendicitis than nonobstructive appendicitis. It follows the abdominal pain. It is more marked in children than adults. Vomiting is not persistent; it subsides when stomach becomes empty. If vomiting precedes the pain, the diagnosis of acute appendicitis should be questioned.[56]

Fever

It is due to bacterial infection and is of low grade (<100°F). Fever is the last symptom after pain and vomiting. So it is not present in initial sickness. In 20% patients there is no fever. Higher fever indicates that a complication has occurred or that another diagnosis should be considered.[34] High and persistent temperature relates to the severity of infection and local or metastatic collection of pus.

> The temperature varies in different cases and so it is not a very reliable feature of acute appendicitis, but in association with other features it may be important for observing the progress or recovery of appendicitis.

Murphy's Syndrome*

Pain first, followed by vomiting and then by fever is called 'Murphy's triad of acute appendicitis' or 'Murphy's syndrome' after John Benjamin Murphy. He used to say that 'If vomiting precedes the pain, probably you are not dealing with acute appendicitis'. It is not a must to find Murphy's triad in every case of acute appendicitis **(Fig. 23)**.

Constipation or Diarrhea

Constipation is a common feature in acute appendicitis except in pre- and post-ileal appendicitis where diarrhea occurs due to irritation of ileum. In pelvic appendicitis patient may have 'tenesmus' (ineffectual straining at defecation with passage of mucus and blood only). Due to irritation of rectum diarrhea occurs in 10% patients of acute appendicitis, causing doubt of acute gastroenteritis and delay in diagnosis of acute appendicitis and appendicectomy.

Hematuria

It is not a common finding and when occurs it is due to irritation of the right ureter, especially in retrocecal appendicitis. Patient may feel strangury (painful and frequent attempts at micturition passing only small quantity of urine) if the appendix is touching urinary bladder or ureter in pelvic appendicitis or retrocecal appendicitis.

> **Key Point**
> Murphy's triad of acute appendicitis pain, vomiting and pyrexia in that sequence is almost diagnostic. PAIN → PUKING → PYREXIA (PPP)

EXAMINATION

Examination of the patient of acute abdomen attracts the attention of the posture of the patient—the dorsal decubitus with right leg slightly flexed and avoiding any movement.
- *Inspection:* Abdomen appears normal or slightly distended. Respiratory movements of abdominal wall are slow and mild.
- *Palpation:* Knees and thighs to be flexed and relaxed. Gradually speaking clearly ask the patient questions about features of the disease while your right hand is passed over whole abdomen except RIF and slightly press here and there. This way gain the confidence of the patient and then with finger tips press at McBurney's point, patient may wince or cry with pain, feeling tenderness, rigidity, and muscle guarding.

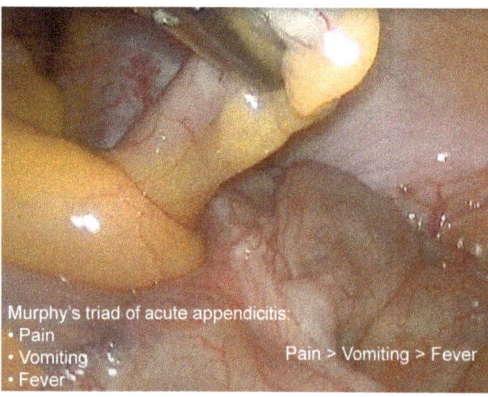

FIG. 23: Murphy's triad of acute appendicitis.

---

*John Benjamin Murphy (1857–1916), Professor of Surgery, Northwestern University, Chicago II, USA. He described this syndrome in 1903.

- *Percussion:* It shows normal tympany but dullness if appendicular mass or abscess is present.
- *Auscultation:* It shows reduction or absence of bowel sounds if ileus is present.

In olden days an instrument called 'piezometer' was used to measure the amount of pressure required to produce pain. It has become obsolete now.

SIGNS

'Exquisite tenderness is not easily feigned, and, if the patients' attention is diverted, can be accurately gauged.'
—MH Richardson

Important signs of acute appendicitis	
• Pyrexia • Tachycardia • Coated and dry tongue • Limited respiratory movements • Pointing test • Tenderness • Rebound tenderness (Blumberg's or release sign) • Muscle guarding	• Cough sign (Dunphy's* sign) • Rovsing sign • Hyperesthesia in Sherren's triangle • Cope's psoas test • Cope's obturator test • Bed shaking test of Bapat • Baldwin's test • Tenderness on digital rectal examination (DRE) • Bastede Sign • Markle sign or jar tenderness

Key Point

The appendicitis is diagnosed by surgeon's hands more than any investigations or ultrasound.

Pyrexia

Usually the patient looks unwell with low grade pyrexia. The temperature is not very high but in children temperature may be high. It is between 90° and 100°F. The temperature may be normal in uncomplicated and early appendicitis. When generalized peritonitis occurs temperature goes up to 102–103°F. It must be remembered that pyrexia is not an early sign in acute appendicitis. In acute appendicitis pyrexia comes after pain and vomiting so it is the last sign of the three, i.e., pain, vomiting, and fever (Murphy's syndrome).

A child at the Johns Hopkins Hospital, aged 4 years, was seized after a hearty dinner with violent abdominal cramp, lasting some hours. She passed a comfortable night, however, and in the morning felt well, but her temperature was 104°F and her pulse 160. At 10 am the abdominal pain returned and grew steadily worse: the abdomen seemed slightly swollen and tender, and the temperature was 105°F. A diagnosis of enterocolitis was made and an oil enema given. The next morning paroxysmal pain continued, referred by the child to the epigastric region. She lay with her knees drawn up. The abdomen was swollen and tender, especially in the right ileocecal and lumbar regions; the tongue was dry and coated, the temperature 104°F and the pulse 140, the leukocytes 32,000. Operation revealed a general septic peritonitis. The appendix showed an acute hemorrhagic inflammation with slight necrosis of the mucosa. Death occurred before the incision was closed.

(Appendicitis and Other Diseases of the Vermiform Appendix)

Tachycardia

It is a good diagnostic guide in acute appendicitis. Sometimes when the pain is not severe and the patient cannot locate the abdominal pain properly, pulse plays an important role in suspecting acute appendicitis. Pulse rate is usually slightly elevated between 80 and 90 beats/min. Temperature and pulse rate are usually not elevated in first 4–6 hours, the pulse increases in proportion to the temperature rise.

---

*Osborne Joby Dunphy (1898–1989), a British American physician observed this sign for the first time.

> A high tachycardia or very rapid pulse is not a good sign, it may be a grave sign. Tachycardia out of proportion to fever is also a grave sign.

Coated and Dry Tongue

Rough, brownish coated, and dry tongue—it indicates toxemia. Even in early acute appendicitis tongue may be thickly coated and dry as patient might have vomited several times and is dehydrated.

Limited Respiratory Movements

Movement of abdominal wall during respiration may be limited in RIF in acute appendicitis due to localized irritation of peritoneum from the inflammation. The vigorous respiratory movements will shake the inflamed parietal peritoneum and will cause pain so the movement of abdominal wall is limited. It is also a protective phenomenon.

Pointing Test

This test confirms RIF inflammatory pathology, patient is asked to indicate the site of pain by tip of a finger, he indicates toward RIF. If the pain is diffuse then patient will use his whole hand instead one finger to point toward site of pain **(Fig. 24)**.

Method of Test

- Ask the patient to lie down.
- Ask to indicate the site of maximum pain. If it is also the point of maximum tenderness this is the site of inflamed organ.

Tenderness

In acute appendicitis, the RIF is tender. The maximum tenderness is elicited at McBurney's point. The tenderness can be best elicited in left lateral position when coils of small intestine shift to the left exposing the appendix direct to palpation. The abdominal wall also becomes relaxed in this position **(Fig. 25)**. Tenderness persists even after cessation of pain till the inflammatory process is present.

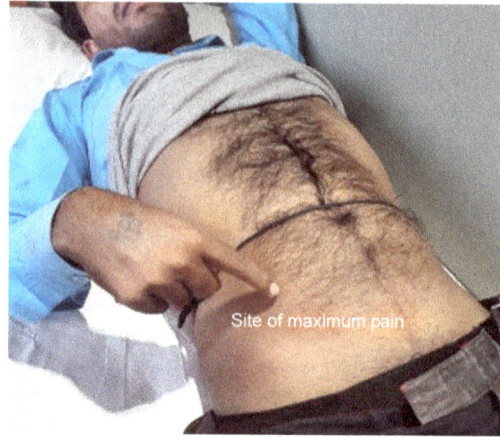

FIG. 24: Pointing test.

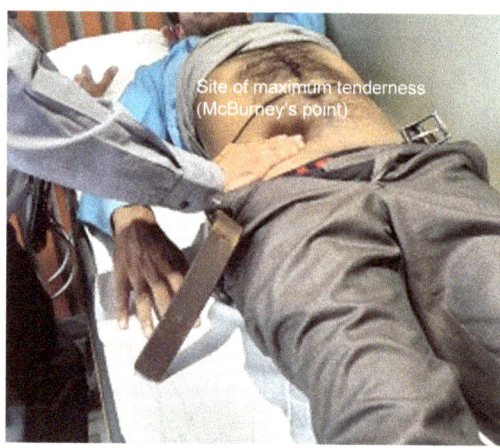

FIG. 25: Tenderness at McBurney's point.

> Tenderness on pressing RIF is one of the most important signs of acute appendicitis. It is very significant that if it is absent surgeon is doubtful of the diagnosis of acute appendicitis.

Rebound Tenderness (Blumberg's Sign*)

The RIF is palpated with flat of right hand. With each expiration hand on abdomen is gradually pressed down the abdomen. Then the hand is suddenly withdrawn completely, so the abdominal musculature springs back suddenly to its original position, patient will cry or will wince due to pain. This pain is due to sudden movement of inflamed parietal peritoneum **(Figs. 26A and B)**.

Muscle Guarding

Spasm or rigidity is the involuntary tightening of the abdominal musculature that occurs in response to underline inflammation. This stiffness can be felt when touched or pressed.

Guarding in contrast is a voluntary contraction of the abdominal wall musculature to avoid pain.

> Next to pain, rigidity is the most important and dependable sign of acute appendicitis. Richardson expressed about rigidity that 'Rigidity with distinctly localized pain strongly suggests appendicitis, with fever it almost proves it, and with tumor it fully establishes the diagnosis.'

In acute appendicitis, the site of muscle guarding varies according to the position of the appendix.

- In paracecal appendicitis guarding is in RIF.
- In retrocecal appendicitis it may be present over flank and even on back muscle and RIF may be totally free. In pelvic appendicitis there may not be any rigidity in anterior abdominal wall. In preileal and postileal appendicitis guarding may be near umbilicus.
- Muscle guarding is an indication of irritation of parietal peritoneum. It is a protective mechanism for inflamed organ not to get hurt. It is important to differentiate the involuntary muscle rigidity of acute appendicitis from voluntary muscle guarding. Involuntary muscle rigidity indicates local parietal peritonitis due to underlying inflamed appendix. Voluntary muscle guarding is brought by the patient himself due to fear of being hurt. In every case of acute appendicitis there is some degree of voluntary muscle guarding. It is more so in children. To elicit muscle guarding, patient's confidence must be gained by your polite manners and behavior. Ask

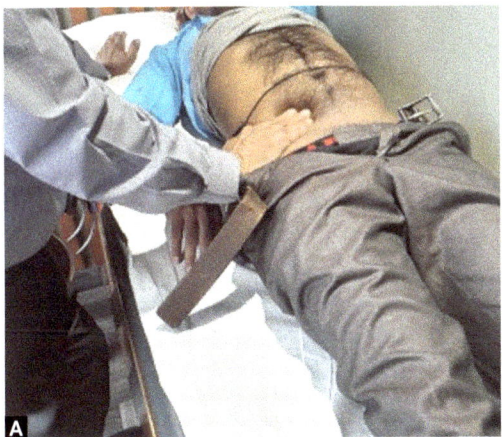 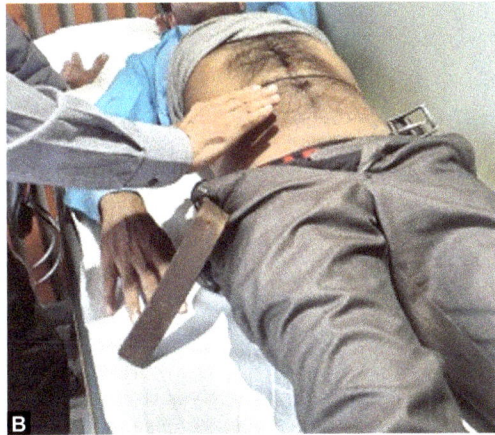

FIGS. 26A AND B: Testing rebound tenderness.

---

*Jacob Moritz Blumberg (1873–1955), Surgeon and Gynecologist in Berlin and later in London reported this sign for the first time.

the patient to open the mouth and do deep breathing. This will make voluntary muscle guarding to disappear. The muscle guarding usually corresponds to the area of tenderness. It is directly proportional to the severity of inflammation.

Patient will complain of pain or will wince with pain when asked to extend right thigh as inflamed retrocecal appendix remains in contact with psoas major muscle, which becomes contracted during flexion of hip joint. Tenderness, muscle guarding, rebound tenderness, and perforation usually develop after 24–36 hours of onset of symptoms.

Method of Eliciting Muscle Guarding

- Make patient comfortably lie on bed.
- Sit on right side of patient bed on a stool.
- Gently keep the flat of right hand on his abdomen on left upper quadrant (LUQ) abdomen, palpate it then move hand toward RIF you will feel firmness of muscles.

> The surgeon is constantly reminded that in practice, the classic presentation of acute appendicitis is not present in all patients…….
> Because appendicitis is so common, a high index of suspicion for appendicitis is warranted in all patients with abdominal pain.
> —Douglas S Smink and David (Maingot's Abdominal Operations)

Pain in Right Iliac Fossa on Coughing (Dunphy's Sign[*])

Ask the patient to cough and he will indicate to RIF for pain. It is due to the movement of inflamed parietal peritoneum. It differentiates acute appendicitis from right-side ureteric colic, where pressing the loin with hand gives relief but not in appendicitis. This sign is named after Osborne Joby Dunphy (1898–1989, a British-American physician).

Rovsing Sign[**]

The palpation of left iliac fossa (LIF) produces pain in RIF. It is due to the displacement of colonic gases and small bowel coils, causing movement of inflamed appendix. It is named after Niels Thorkild Rovsing, who observed and explained it initially **(Fig. 27)**.

Method of Eliciting Sign

- Ask the patient to lie down comfortably on bed.
- Sit on right side of bed on a stool.
- Put whole flat palm and finger of right hand on LIF and gradually press. Slowly increase the pressure he will wince with pain, ask him where is the pain, and he will point toward RIF.

Hyperesthesia in Sherren's Triangle

It is due to irritation of lower abdominal nerves. The 'Sherren's triangle' is formed by line joining ASIS, umbilicus, and pubic symphysis. It can be sometimes first-sign in early appendicitis.

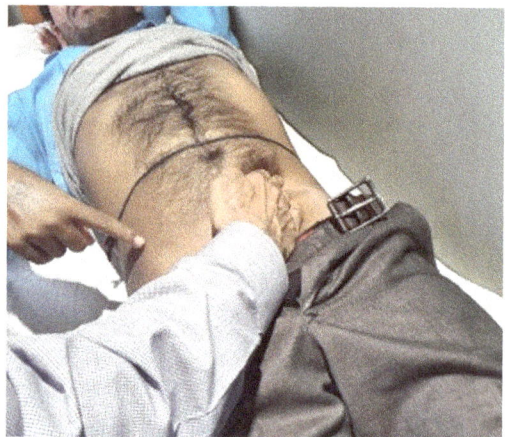

FIG. 27: Rovsing sign.

---

[*] Osborne Joby Dunphy (1898–1989), a British-American physician observed this sign for the first time.
[**] Niels Thorkild Rovsing (1862–1937), Professor of Surgery, Copenhagen, Denmark.

muscle and moves the inflamed appendix lying over it. It is named after Sir Vincent Zachary Cope, (1881–1975), Surgeon, St. Mary's Hospital, London, England.

Method of Eliciting Test

- Ask the patient to lie down on left side, right side up laterally.
- By left hand hold right ileum area.
- Ask to extend the thigh voluntary by patient or do it yourself with your right hand. It will cause pain.

Cope's[*] Obturator Test

It is seen in pelvic appendicitis, which causes irritation of the internal obturator muscle so flexion and medial rotation of thigh produces pain in hypogastrium due contraction of internal obturator muscle which moves the inflamed appendix.

Method of Doing Test

- Ask the patient to lie down supine.
- Hold the knee by left hand and foot by right hand. Flex the hip joint 90° and then move the foot away from patient's body, it will rotate the thigh medially and will make obturator internus muscle tense and patient will wince with pain.

Bed Shaking Test of Bapat[**]

Foot end of the bed is moved slightly and this will evoke pain in RIF by shaking the inflamed appendix suddenly.

Baldwin's Test

In retrocecal and pelvic appendicitis, there may not be any tenderness or muscle rigidity at the McBurney's point.

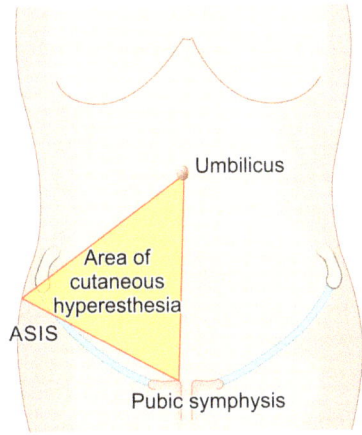

FIG. 28: Sherren's triangle.

> Cutaneous hyperesthesia is regarded as a symptom of great importance. Where cutaneous hyperesthesia, muscular rigidity and localized or general pain are present, peritonitis always be found. It is sometimes exceedingly vivid, making further palpation impossible. (BLOS. Beitz.z.klen.Chir. Volume 32:420) **(Fig. 28)**.

Method of Eliciting Sign

- This can be elicited by gently picking up a fold of skin and lifting it off the abdomen or by gently scratching the abdominal wall by finger nails.
- If this hyper-aesthesia disappears during illness it indicates bursting of gangrenous appendix.

Cope's Psoas Test

It is seen in retrocecal appendicitis. The retrocecal appendicitis causes irritation of psoas major muscle. The psoas major muscle causes flexion of hip so the attempts to extend hip causes pain as it stretches the psoas

---

[*]Sir Vincent Zachary Cope, (1881–1975), Surgeon, St. Mary's Hospital, London, England. He described 'Acute Abdomen in Rhyme' as:

Distension, rigidity, vomiting, pain,
Are actors abdominal which often deign
To act on behalf of the chest, spine or brain,
Or general ills of which typhoid's the main.

[**]RD Bapat, Professor Emeritus of the Seth GS Medical College and King Edward Memorial Hospital, Mumbai.

Method of Doing Test

- Patient lies supine.
- The left hand is placed and pressed at right flank of patient, now the patient is asked to raise right lower limb off the bed keeping right knee extended. He will feel pain in RIF. The tenderness and rigidity may not be present or may not be so prominent in RIF. History of diarrhea, fever, strangury, and tenesmus makes the clinical picture very confusing. Surgeon must give importance to the history, which with proper examination will make up to reach to diagnosis of pelvic appendicitis. History of periumbilical pain, Rovsing sign, Copes obturator test, and DRE will diagnose pelvic appendicitis. DRE is very helpful as tenderness on the right side of recto-uterine pouch in females and rectovesical pouch in males is present in pelvic appendicitis. A tender boggy lump or a cystic swelling in digital rectal examination is diagnostic of appendicitis with pelvic abscess.

Tenderness on Digital Rectal Examination

No examination is complete in acute abdomen without DRE. Tenderness in right rectal wall is present in pelvic appendicitis. It is found in 25% cases. It also excludes pelvic lesions in females. 'If you do not put your finger in rectum you will put your foot.'[24] Rectal examination is of little value in establishing the diagnosis of acute appendicitis but can be useful to determine the presence or absence of a mass.[57]

Bastede Sign

Pain and tenderness elicited on RIF by pushing air through rectal tube. This test is not done now due to risk of perforation.

Markle Sign or Jar Tenderness

It is a sign in acute appendicitis. Pain in the RLQ of abdomen is elicited by dropping from standing on toes to the heels with a jarring landing. It is found in the patients with localized peritonitis due to acute appendicitis. It is named after George Bushar Markle IV (1921–1999), who was an American surgeon. This article was published in American Journal of Surgery in 1973.

> **Key Point**
> The most important signs in diagnosing acute appendicitis are tenderness and rebound tenderness in RIF.

OTHER IMPORTANT POINTS IN CLINICAL FEATURES OF APPENDICITIS

Appendicular Dyspepsia

Appendicular dyspepsia is a common presentation of recurrent appendicitis. It is the gastric symptom which predominates in it. Dyspepsia resembles the symptoms of diseases of stomach, duodenum, and gallbladder. Usually the symptoms of milder appendicitis are anorexia, nausea, epigastric discomfort, flatulence, and dyspepsia. It does not improve with antacid or H2 receptor antagonist or PPI.

Cause of Appendicular Dyspepsia

The infected lymph from appendix is drained to subpyloric lymph nodes which irritates the pylorus and causes symptoms of dyspepsia. Treatment is appendicectomy.

Annotation of Notes

- Write your notes clearly and in brief.
- Describe important clinical findings associated with simple line diagrams.
- On re-examination of patient update your note and illustration.
- Always write your diagnosis and differential diagnosis, it is a good habit. If you receive any investigation reports on telephone or any advice on telephone always write on case sheet.

History Gives Clue in Acute Appendicitis

In most of the cases of acute appendicitis the pain starts as poorly localized abdominal pain, frequently it is central or periumbilical pain. This pain may mimic the pain of small bowel obstruction but the intensity is much less. Patient may give history of similar pain earlier, which was settled spontaneously without treatment. In this early stage pain or discomfort is associated with anorexia and nausea. He may not give history of vomiting. As the inflammation increases the periumbilical pain, which is a visceral pain shifts to the RIF due to involvement of parietal peritoneum. This is somatic pain. This history of visceral-somatic pain sequence is seen in >50% of confirmed cases of acute appendicitis. At this stage patient feels accentuation of pain by coughing and movement. While coming to hospital patient must have felt pain by sudden movements and jerks and jolts of car. Patient walks slowly and slightly bends forward to protect the inflamed organ. This typical history, if taken properly diagnoses the acute appendicitis.

Other patients have atypical pain, which may be either visceral or somatic and poorly localized. It is common in elderly patients and in pelvic appendicitis.

> In the early stages of acute appendicitis, it is found that surgical intervention could save many cases developing complications and proceeding to dangerous stage even leading to death, but it is difficult or impossible to determine the fate, resolution or dangerous complications such as perforation and gangrene.

In first few hours there is no tachycardia or fever but after 6–8 hours patient develops mild pyrexia, approximately 99°F and tachycardia, below 90 beats/minute pulse rate.

CLINICAL FEATURES ACCORDING TO THE TYPE OF APPENDICITIS

'Half of us are blind, few of us feel, and we are all deaf.'
—**Sir William Osler**

Not to forget
- Appendicitis is common in 20–30 years of age.
- Gangrene and perforation of appendix are common in obstructive appendicitis and rare in nonobstructive or catarrhal appendicitis.
- Pneumoperitoneum is uncommon in appendicular perforation, but common in duodenal perforation.
- Appendicitis in child <2 years is uncommon, but if happens then perforation, peritonitis, and poor prognosis are common.
- Appendicitis is found in LIF in a case of situs inversus and mimics acute diverticulitis.
- Mortality rate in appendicitis is <1%.
- If normal appendix is found on operation is called 'Lilly White Appendix', if appendix is found directly on introduction of laparoscope in abdomen it is called, 'hand shake appendix'.

OBSTRUCTIVE APPENDICITIS

- The onset of symptoms is abrupt and then symptoms progress fast.
- Pain is severe.
- Pain is of colicky nature.
- Vomiting is common.
- Temperature may be normal.
- Patient immediately goes to bed as cannot perform usual day-to-day duty due to tiredness and pain.
- Tenderness is more.
- It is more dangerous variety.
- The obstruction makes the appendix a closed loop, so the contents stagnate

and walls get infected fast and it rapidly progresses to perforation and gangrene.
- It may mimic acute intestinal obstruction **(Fig. 29A)**.

> A sudden onset of violent pain, high temperature, tachycardia, vomiting indicates a dangerous condition due to acute appendicitis.

NONOBSTRUCTIVE APPENDICITIS

It is also called as 'acute catarrhal appendicitis.'
- The onset and progress is slow and not so abrupt as in acute obstructive appendicitis.
- Pain is less and of dull type or constant burning pain rather than colic.
- Vomiting is not much and may be absent.
- Fever is usually present which may be normal in obstructive appendicitis.
- Patient carries out his usually day-to-day duties but with discomfort in abdomen, nausea, vomiting, and anorexia. He is not much sick **(Fig. 29B)**.

> It is understood that if the attack of acute appendicitis begins with slight or moderate signs and symptoms associated with mild constitutional features probably we are dealing with a catarrhal or nonobstructive appendicitis.

- Tenderness is not much.
- It is not so dangerous variety as the acute obstructive appendicitis.
- Usually does not lead to gangrene and perforation.
- Does not mimic acute intestinal obstruction.
- Inflammation spreads from mucosa to serosa slowly and appendix becomes congested.
- The inflammation ends in:
  - Resolution or
  - Fibrosis or
  - Suppuration or
  - Gangrene
- Nonobstructive appendicitis can be acute, subacute, chronic, or recurrent.

> **Key Point**
>
> Acute obstructive appendicitis is the commonest variety and dangerous too.

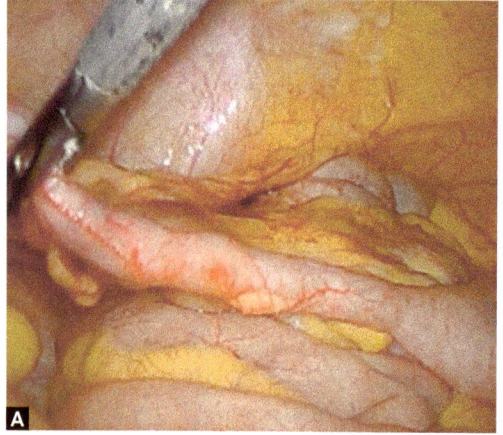 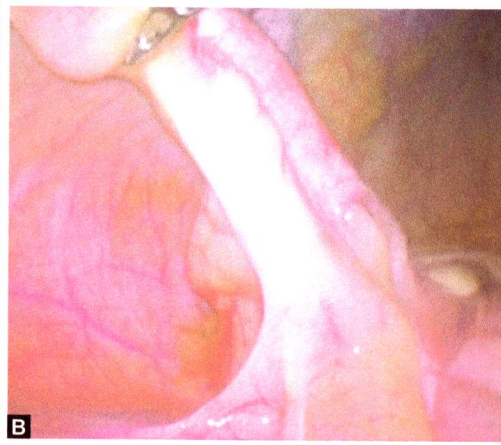

FIGS. 29A AND B: (A) Obstructive appendicitis; (B) Nonobstructive appendicitis **(Video 4)**.

CLINICAL FEATURES ACCORDING TO THE POSITION OF THE APPENDIX

'It is better to be approximately right, than be precisely wrong.'
—**Warren Buffet**

Characteristic features in different anatomical positions of appendix in acute appendicitis:
- Retrocecal appendicitis—silent
- Pelvic appendicitis—diarrhea
- Pre-ileal and post-ileal—diarrhea
- Sub-hepatic—pain above RIF as in cholecystitis and RIF is pain free

RETROCECAL APPENDICITIS

This may be silent without any tenderness and rigidity in the RIF, that is why called 'silent appendix.' It is due to distended cecum with gas lying anterior to the appendix so the pressure exerted cannot pass up to appendix. In such cases, deep tenderness may be present in loin and muscles of loin (i.e., quadratus lumborum) may be found in spasm. Here the inflamed appendix lies over psoas major muscle so it may be in spasm causing flexion of hip joint, the extension of hip joint causes pain. If the irritation of psoas major muscle is not much then instead extension, hyperextension of hip may cause pain as extension may not cause sufficient stretching of psoas muscle.

The fact that a retrocecal position of the appendix demands special consideration, and may mislead the operator who is on upon his guards,........If we could, with the fare degree of certainty, predict in a large percentage of cases that the appendix and the abscess were to be found in a retrocecal position, such knowledge would be off material and to the surgeon in guiding his exploration. (Appendicitis and Other Diseases of the Vermiform Appendix)

In retrocecal appendicitis if the appendix is totally and completely retroperitoneal then there is no rigidity and tenderness in anterior abdominal wall. There may be tenderness and rigidity in right flank and more posteriorly. To elicit such tenderness patient has to be rolled to left side **(Figs. 30A and B)**.

If the appendix is in direct contact with right ureter, patient may feel pain radiating from loin to groin and may have hematuria. This may confuse the surgeon with ureteric colic but initial history of pain around umbilicus, Rovsing sign, psoas test, and examination in left lateral position will

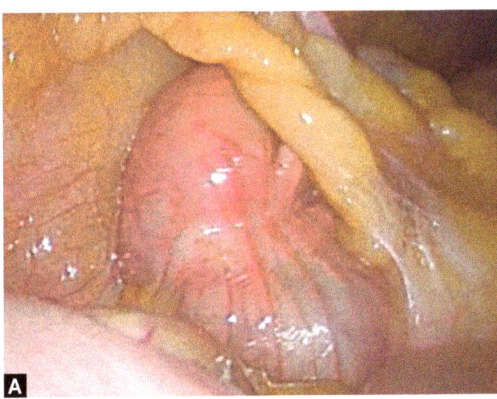
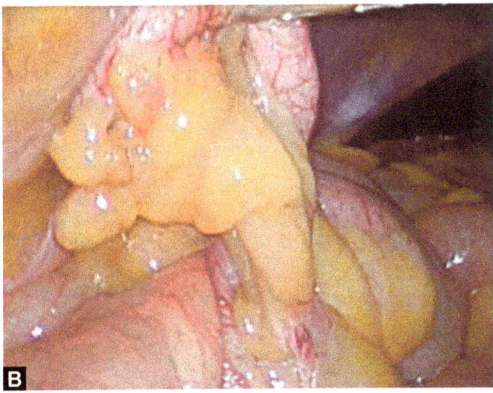

FIGS. 30A AND B: (A) Retrocecal appendix, base of appendix is visible; (B) Retrocecal appendix after dissecting out **(Video 5)**.

diagnose the appendicitis. One has to be very careful in history taking and examination to not to miss appendicitis.

PELVIC APPENDICITIS

It can produce diarrhea instead of constipation, if the inflamed appendix is in contact with rectum. If the inflamed appendix is in contact with the urinary bladder then it may cause frequency of micturition leading to the doubt of urinary tract infection **(Fig. 31)**.

> Per-rectal examination in males and bimanual examination in females by putting one hand over lower abdomen and finger in vagina done to not miss pelvic appendicitis.

Tenderness and abdominal muscle rigidity may altogether be absent and digital rectal examination may reveal tenderness in pouch of Douglas* (Rectovesical pouch).

The inflamed pelvic appendix may touch psoas muscle or internal obturator muscle and cause spasm of these muscle causing flexion of hip joint or flexion and internal rotation of thigh.

- *Post-ileal and pre-ileal appendicitis:* It causes diarrhea and one may miss appendicitis and diagnose as acute gastroenteritis. So, it is called as 'missed appendix'. Tenderness may be present just right side to umbilicus.
- *Sub-hepatic appendicitis:* The pain is present above RIF. It may mimic acute cholecystitis.

> **Key Point**
> Retrocecal appendicitis is the commonest appendicitis according to the anatomical position of appendix.

INVESTIGATIONS FOR APPENDICITIS

'Condemnation before investigation is the highest form of ignorance.'
—**Albert Einstein**

The acute appendicitis is diagnosed clinically only but investigations are done to avoid removal of normal appendix. Approximately 20% appendices removed on appendicectomy are found normal on histopathological examination. The most important criteria in diagnosis of acute appendicitis are given below.

> *Important preoperative investigations in acute appendicitis*:
> - Complete blood count
> - Urine analysis
> - Pregnancy test
> - Urea, creatinine and electrolytes
> - C-reactive protein
> - Radiography
> - Barium meal or enema
> - Ultrasound
> - Contrast-enhanced computerized tomography (CECT) scan of abdomen
> - Diagnostic laparoscopy
> - Alvarado scoring system
> - Nigam's Scoring System (NSS)

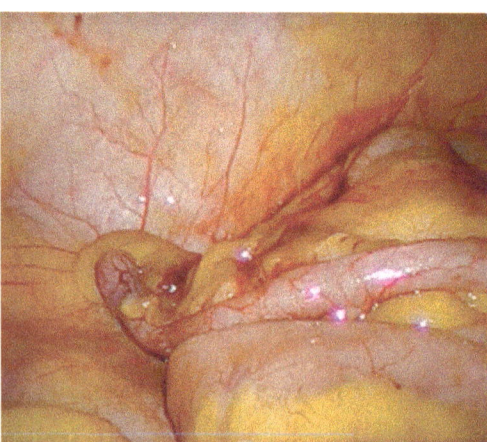

FIG. 31: Pelvic appendicitis **(Video 6)**.

---

*Pouch of Douglas is named after James Douglas (1675–1742), anatomist and male midwife, who practiced in London, England.

COMPLETE BLOOD COUNT

More than 90% of patients suffering with acute appendicitis have some leukocytosis. The total leukocyte count (TLC) is usually above 10,000/mm^3 (12,000–18,000/mm^3). There is shift toward left means polymorph nuclear cells predominance. In perforated appendicitis the count may be >18,000 mm^3. Serial WBC measurement improves the diagnostic accuracy, with a rising value over time commonly seen in the patients with appendicitis.[58]

> Appendicitis is the most important cause of acute abdomen in men under 30 years of age. When cardinal symptoms of sudden severe abdominal pain, tenderness at or near McBurney's point and muscular rigidity in RIF are found then diagnosis of appendicitis is considered in most of the cases. Anorexia, nausea, vomiting, tachycardia, elevated temperature, constipation, or diarrhea make the diagnosis more certain and presence of a tender lump in RIF confirms the diagnosis of appendicitis.

As a matter of fact the total number of the leukocytes is subject to fairly wide variations even under normal conditions, so that the conclusion drawn from an absolute count alone may prove entirely erroneous. While on one hand in the majority of individuals an absolute count from 5,000 to 7,500 is the rule, on the other hand in a lower state of nutrition than an average, lower values are also normally present (3,000–5,000), while higher figures (up to 10,000) may be found in unusually vigorous and well-nourished persons. It, thus, becomes clear that absolute count of 8,000–10,000 in a poorly developed and ill-nourished individual might really indicate a decided hyperleukocytosis. Reliance upon the absolute count alone may here give rise to disastrous consequences. High value, it is true, indicates in a general way that the disease is active, and increasing values—where repeated examinations are made—that the increase is progressive. Low count or falling values, on the other hand may indicate either that the disease is abating, or that the infection is unusually severe or that the perforation with general peritonitis has developed. In these cases again the differential leukocyte count will tell the true story. Eosinophil count is 'septic factor' in infective states such as appendicitis.

> Howard A Kelly said that my investigations into the occurrence of septic factor in appendicitis has led me to look upon this as one of the most constant features of the disease and as one of the utmost diagnostic importance. In its absence, I unhesitatingly rule out the diagnosis of an appendicitis of the common bacteriological type…… I have repeatedly seen instances in which a mass could be palpated in the RIF and in which no material increase in the total number of leukocytes was demonstrable, but I have yet to see a case in which an abscess existed and the differential count was normal.

URINE EXAMINATION

Dehydration is caused due to repeated vomiting. So the urine shows high specific gravity. Urine may also show RBCs and WBCs, if the appendix touches urinary bladder or ureter in pelvic or retrocecal appendicitis. If urine shows >20 WBC per high power field or shows >30 WBC per high power field, it indicates urinary tract infection (UTI). Bacteriuria in a catheterized patient is not generally seen with acute appendicitis.[59]

Failure to find blood or pus cells in the urine is not a certainty of exclusion of right renal or ureteric problem but the diagnosis of renal problem is less likely especially in presence of peritoneal signs.

PREGNANCY TEST

The negative pregnancy test will rule out RIF pain due to ectopic gestation.

BLOOD UREA, CREATININE AND ELECTROLYTES (SODIUM, POTASSIUM, AND CALCIUM)

Vomiting can cause raised blood urea and abnormal serum electrolytes. The estimation of urea, creatinine, and electrolytes also helps to assess the renal function of the patient which also helps the anesthetist for assessment for operation.

C-REACTIVE PROTEIN

C-reactive protein (CRP) estimation is found helpful in the diagnosis of acute appendicitis, CRP is produced by liver when infection occurs in any part of the body, it increases rapidly within first 12 hours and then within next 12 hours comes to normal level.

C-reactive protein levels above 1 mg/dL are found in acute appendicitis, very high level of CRP with leukocytosis indicates advance or gangrenous appendicitis. The high level of CRP in blood shows inflammation. CRP value comes to normal once infection is controlled.[28,60] It is not very useful. Clinically as it is non-specific and cannot distinguish between sites of infection.

RADIOGRAPHY

X-ray neither confirms acute appendicitis nor excludes it. It can be of benefit to exclude other pathology such as calculus in ureter. There is no classical sign of acute appendicitis on plain X-ray. Plain X-ray of abdomen is not a very important investigation in acute appendicitis except in perforation of appendix. Avoid doing radiographs if patient is pregnant. Acute appendicitis is quite common in young females so keep in mind the pregnancy when X-ray is advised. Following findings may help to support the diagnosis of acute appendicitis in association with clinical signs:

- *Sentinel loops of bowel:* These are seen as gas shadows due to localized ileus due to inflammation.
- *Calcified fecaliths:* Approximately 15% of cases of acute appendicitis show calcified fecaliths on X-ray. A fecalith shows laminated shadow. Presence of fecaliths in X-ray in RIF pain is suggestive of appendicitis.
- *Mass effect around the appendix:* The bowel loops are displaced away from appendicular lump.
- Presence of free gas under diaphragm is a sure sign of perforation of appendix but it is not always seen so absence of this sign does not rule out the diagnosis of appendicitis or perforation of appendix.
- Scoliosis of spine with concavity toward right side due to spasm of psoas muscle due to irritation by inflamed appendix is rarely seen on X-ray **(Fig. 32)**.
- Psoas muscle margin of right side are lost due to superimposed inflamed appendix.
- Retained barium from previous studies is to be noted. It is noted that inspissated barium from earlier barium enema or meal can rarely cause acute obstructive appendicitis.

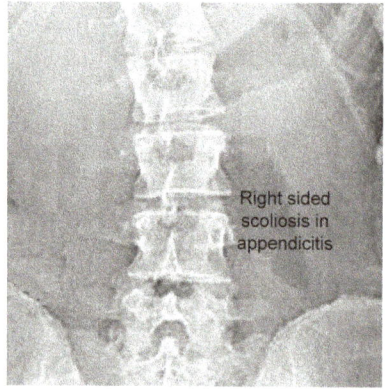

FIG. 32: Scoliosis towards right side in acute appendicitis.

- Blurring of preperitoneal fat on the flank is also an important sign on plain X-ray of abdomen.

Gas in appendix is not a sign specific for appendicitis and should not mandate laparotomy for appendicitis.[61]

> **Key Point**
> A perforated appendix rarely causes a pneumoperitoneum; presence of pneumoperitoneum confirms perforation but its absence does not rule out perforation of appendix.

BARIUM MEAL OR ENEMA

This investigation nowadays is not required due to early and easy availability of ultrasound and CT scan. Barium examination may show any of the following findings:
- Non-filling of appendix.
- Mucosal irregularity in terminal ileum.
- 'Reverse 3' sign of cecum due to indentation by inflamed and edematous appendix base is a typical radiological sign of acute appendicitis.
- Mass effect on colonic wall is seen in acute appendicitis.
- Mucosal wall characteristics can be seen which can differentiate appendicitis from inflammatory bowel disease.
- If the appendix fills on barium enema appendicitis is excluded on the other hand if the appendix is not filled, no determination can be made.[56] The appendix is not visualized on barium enema in 50% normal individuals. Barium enema may prove dangerous in acute appendicitis by causing perforation.

ULTRASOUND OF ABDOMEN (FIGS. 33A AND B)

Ultrasound cannot visualize a healthy normal appendix. It may not be very helpful in early acute appendicitis. It is more useful in excluding gynecological causes of RIF pain. Ultrasound is highly operator dependent that is the main limitation of ultrasound in diagnosis of acute appendicitis, frequently unable to visualize the normal appendix.[62]

> A blind ended tubular structure, easily compressible and <6 mm in diameter is the feature of a normal appendix and if it is found then the appendicitis is excluded from the diagnosis.

Ultrasound findings in acute appendicitis are:[48,63,64]
- Probe tenderness at McBurney's point.
- A blind-ending, tubular structure with thick wall, without peristalsis and non-compressible originating from cecum, is detected in RIF. It is seen especially when lumen is >6 mm diameter.
- Appendicolith may be present.

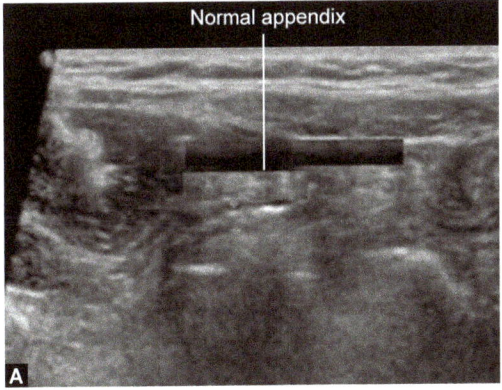
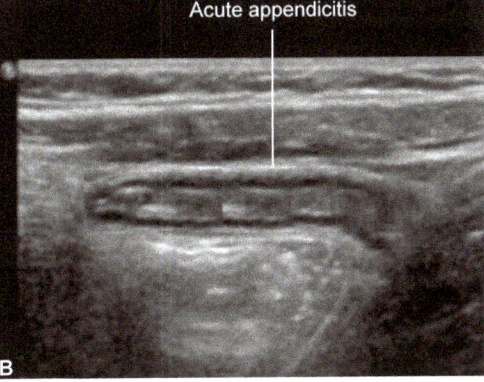

FIGS. 33A AND B: (A) Normal appendix; (B) Acute appendicitis.

- Intussusception
- Periappendicular fluid collection

If ultrasound of abdomen shows abscess cavity in an appendicular mass then drain the abscess.

Nowadays with better ultrasound machines and advanced probes the full-fledged acute appendicitis can be diagnosed in >90% of cases. In most of the hospitals, now ultrasound is used as a routine investigation in RIF pain. It is helpful in diagnosing appendicular lump and abscess.

Ultrasound can diagnose approximately 86% of appendicitis cases.[65] But the ultrasound is usually not used as a tool to diagnose acute appendicitis than to rule out other cause of such pain or when the diagnosis is uncertain or in female of child-bearing age. Tzanakis et al. proposed the use of ultrasound as it is more readily available than CT scan.[66]

Graded Compression Sonography

It is recommended as an accurate way to establish the diagnosis of appendicitis. The diameter of the appendix is measured in anteroposterior dimension with maximal compression. The presence of appendicolith establishes the diagnosis. Thickening of appendicular wall and periappendicular fluid are highly suggestive signs on ultrasound. The sonographic diagnosis of acute appendicitis has a specificity of 85–98%.[34,59,67]

Normal appendix demonstration on sonography is as easily compressible blind ending tubular structure 6 mm or less in diameter which excludes the diagnosis of acute appendicitis.

Transvaginal ultrasound alone or combination of transabdominal scan is a must in a female in reproductive age with RIF pain to diagnose acute appendicitis. It reveals pelvic pathology and fluid in pouch of Douglas.

Key Point
Ultrasound in diagnosing appendicitis has sensitivity of >85% and a specificity of >90%.[68,69] In experienced hands ultrasound has been reported to significantly lower the negative exploration rate.[70]

False Positive Ultrasound Scan
It occurs in the following conditions:
- Periappendicitis due to surrounding inflammation such as in Crohn's disease
- Dilated fallopian tube
- Inspissated stool looks like an appendicolith
- In obese patient, overlying fat may interfere with the compressibility.

False Negative Ultrasound Scan
It occurs in the following conditions:
- Appendicitis confined to its tip
- Retrocecal appendix
- Enlarged appendix may mimic loop of small bowel
- Perforated appendix may be compressible and taken as normal[71]

Advantages of Graded Compression Ultrasonography
- Reduced negative appendicectomies from 37 to 13%[72]
- Reduces preoperative time.
- Improves the diagnosis of acute appendicitis diagnosed on physical examination[73]

COMPUTED TOMOGRAPHY SCAN OF ABDOMEN

It is not used as a routine investigation.[74,75] Selective use of CT is required as standard approach. CT scan used in acute appendicitis can be focused and nonfocused or enhanced and nonenhanced. CECT of abdomen is a better option than NCCT (noncontrast CT). CT scan with oral contrast medium or rectal gastrografin enema may help in diagnosis of appendicitis.
- When patient scores 6 or <6 in Alvarado Scoring System.
- Particularly useful in elderly patients as it rules out intestinal obstruction, neoplasm, diverticulitis, and diagnoses acute appendicitis in absence of signs. CECT reduces the chances of removal of normal appendix.

Computed tomography scan can diagnose acute appendicitis in approximately 98% cases, i.e., 92–97% sensitivity, 85–94% specificity, 90–98% accuracy and 75–95% positive and 95–99% negative predictive values.[76-78] CT scan is good for patients who present late after 48 hours with appendicitis as mass or abscess.

Indications of Computed Tomography Scan in Acute Appendicitis

- Suspected case of acute appendicitis where the diagnosis is not confirmed by ultrasound and other investigations.[79,80]
- Appendicular abscess
- Pelvic abscess

Computed Tomography Findings in Acute Appendicitis (Fig. 34)

- Appendicolith
- Failure of appendix to fill with oral contrast
- Dilated appendix, diameter >6 mm
- Cecal wall thickening
- Probe tenderness
- Increased fat attenuation in RLQ
- Phlegmon in RLQ
- Abscess in RLQ or pelvis
- The wall of the inflamed appendix is circumferentially thickened and may appear as a 'halo' or 'target' CT findings of periappendiceal inflammation suggest appendicitis, these include[81]
  o Periappendiceal abscess
  o Fluid collection
  o Edema
  o Phlegmon

Periappendiceal inflammation is visualized as 'clouding of mesenteric fat' (dirty fat).[82]

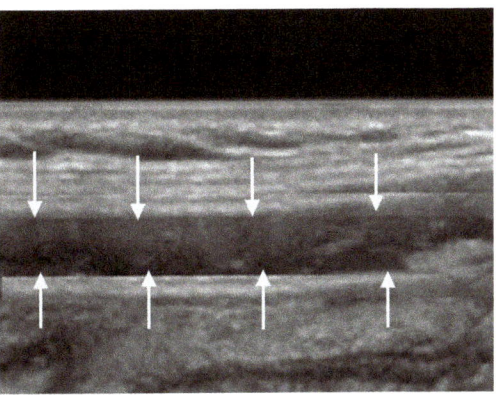

FIG. 34: CT scan of abdomen showing acute appendicitis.

Disadvantages of Computed Tomography Scan

- Expensive
- Radiation
- Cannot be used during pregnancy
- Some patients may develop allergy to dye used in CECT
- Some patients cannot take oral dye due to nausea and vomiting[70]
- Optimal CT technique requires complete small bowel opacification (CECT)[83]

Advantages of Computed Tomography Scan

- A study by Rao and colleagues showed that CT scan has reduced the incidence of negative appendectomies from 20 to 7%, it is confirmed by others too.[84,85]
- Decreased perforation rate from 22 to 14%.
- Established an alternative diagnosis in 50% cases
- Saved unnecessary appendicectomies
- Saved inpatient hospital stay days
- Lowered per patient cost.
- Improved image resolution to 0.5–1.0 cm range which has improved the accuracy of CT scanning[86,87]

DIAGNOSTIC LAPAROSCOPY

Diagnostic laparoscopy is particularly helpful in obese patients and females of child-bearing age to exclude acute gynecological pathology. It can help in 30–40% of negative appendicectomies, some surgeons routinely do diagnostic laparoscopy in all ovulating women with suspected acute appendicitis to avoid delay and negative appendicetomies.[88]

It is useful in following cases:
- Infants
- Elderly
- Female patients

If the findings are positive laparoscopic appendicectomy is done in same sitting.

SCORING SYSTEMS

Alvarado (MANTRELS) Scoring System

It is a system developed to diagnose acute appendicitis more precisely to avoid negative appendicectomies.

	Features	Score
Symptoms	Migrating RIF pain	1
	Anorexia	1
	Nausea, vomiting	1
Signs	Tenderness RIF	2
	Rebound tenderness	1
	Elevated temperature	1
Laboratory	Leukocytosis (>10 ×1,000 cells/mm³)	2
	Shift to left (segmental neutrophils) (>75%)	1
Total		10

Alfredo Alvarado, Contemporary Surgeon, Plantation, FL, USA, gave this scoring system which is most widely used globally. A score of 7 or more is strongly indicative of acute appendicitis.
- *Score <5*: Not sure of diagnosis of acute appendicitis
- *Score 5–6*: Compatible with acute appendicitis
- *Score 7–9*: Probably acute appendicitis
- *Score 10*: Confirmed acute appendicitis **(Fig. 35A)**.
- If score is 7 or more, admit the patient for urgent appendicectomy.
- If score is 5–6, further investigations are required to reach to a diagnosis.[23] Any patient with a score of <6 cannot have a perforated appendix.
- Alvarado scoring system is very effective in admission of suspected cases of acute appendicitis with score of 5 or 6.[89]

RIPASA Scoring System (Raja Isteri Pengiran Anak Saleha Appendicitis)

It is similar to Alvarado scoring system. It typically provides a quantitative value for a clinician's clinical score for appendicitis.

Nigam's Scoring System

It is invented to deal with drawbacks of Alvarado scoring system and improve accuracy.

Nigam's scoring system (NSS) has 17 scoring points. This scoring system can be divided into three parts, 6 and below 6, 7–10, and 11 and above. If NSS comes 6 or below, probably we are not dealing with acute appendicitis. If the score is between 7 and 10 probably diagnosis of appendicitis cannot be ruled out. If the score is 11 or more, we are dealing with a case of appendicitis. Higher the score after 11, severe is the inflammation, from acute appendicitis to impending perforation or gangrene. The scoring by NSS decides about the management of case also. Patients with score <6 are advised OPD treatment. Patients with score 7–10 are admitted to the hospital for observation and score 11 or above are operated. The diagnosis of acute appendicitis by NSS was compared with the ultrasonography findings, operation findings, and histopathological results.

We have to confirm the diagnosis of acute appendicitis before doing appendectomy otherwise there is chance of negative appendectomy **(Fig. 35B)**. NSS confirmed the diagnosis of acute appendicitis in all cases before appendectomy. The diagnosis was based on NSS which were compatible to the operative and histopathological finding in all cases. There was not a single case of negative appendectomy among 34 operated cases. The negative appendectomy rate was zero. Out of 34 patients diagnosed as appendicitis by NSS all patients underwent appendectomy and appendicitis was confirmed in all cases by operative and histopathological findings. Four patients were having perforation and these all patients had leukocytosis above 15,000 and tenderness in RIF was severe **(Figs. 36A and B)**.

Nigam's scoring system has better accuracy than Alvarado scoring system in diagnosing acute appendicitis (Nigam VK, Nigam S. Nigam's scoring system for acute appendicitis with high accuracy surpassing Alvarado scoring system. Int Surg J. 2022;9(4):835-40). NSS is an easy, economical, simple, accurate, fast, and dependable scoring system. NSS is best suited for small hospitals which lack advance investigative techniques such as ultrasound, CT scan, and magnetic resonance imaging (MRI).

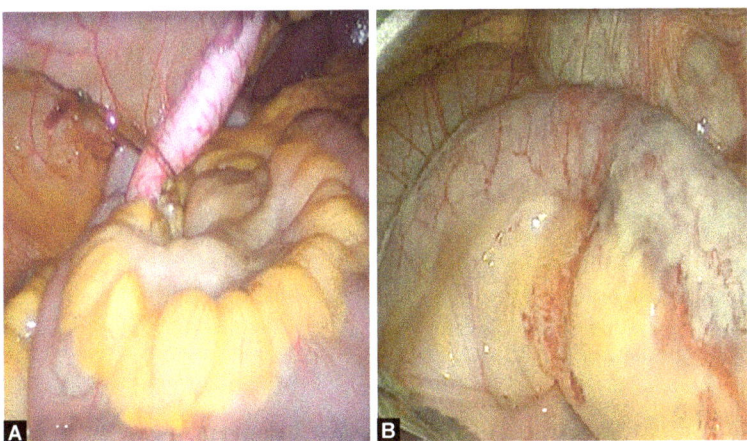

FIGS. 35A AND B: (A) Acute appendicitis—Alvarado score 10. (B) Perforated appendicitis—Nigam's scoring system score 15.

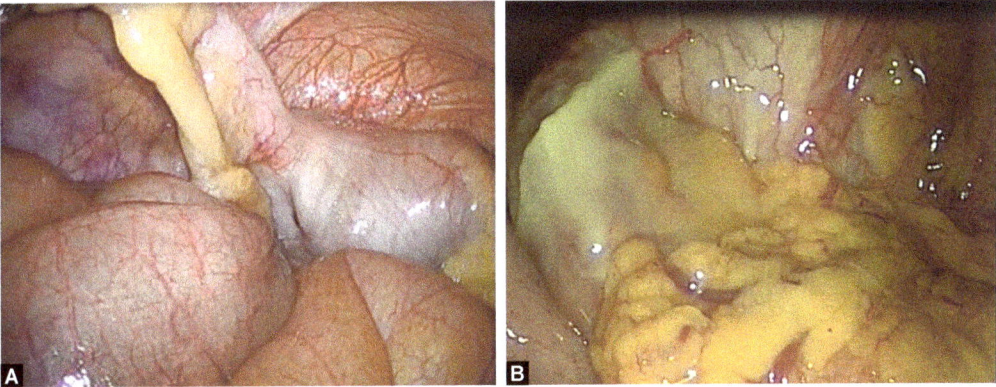

FIGS. 36A AND B: (A) Nigam's scoring system (NSS) – 12, (B) NSS – 15.

NUCLEAR MEDICINE INVESTIGATIONS

Two types of nuclear imaging are done for appendicitis diagnosis:[90-92]
1. Radiolabeled WBCs (Tc-99m WBC)
2. Immunoglobulin G (Tc-99m Igl)

The localization of Tc-99 labeled WBCs and Igl is done with the use of scintigraphy.

Their value lies only in cases with negative ultrasound and CT scan.

These are highly sensitive and highly specific but the procedure is time consuming and not widely available and not useful in emergency conditions.

VAGINAL EXAMINATION

Look for tenderness in movement of cervix if present then appendicitis is less likely, young women about the age of 20 years have highest incidence of normal appendix on operation and persistence of symptoms thereafter.[93]

> **Key Point**
>
> Blood count is the most important investigation in acute appendicitis as leukocytosis and or shift to left is found in >90% cases.

URINARY 5-HYDROXYINDO-LEACETIC ACID

Few studies have shown the estimation of urinary 5-hydroxyindoleacetic acid (U5-HIAA) can be of help in diagnosis of acute appendicitis due to presence of large amount of serotonin secreting cells in appendix. Level of U5-HIAA increases with the development of acute appendicitis and reduces with development of gangrene or necrosis.

> **Key Point**
>
> Appendicitis must be considered in the differential diagnosis of almost all cases of acute abdomen and must be excluded.[94]

DIAGNOSIS OF ACUTE APPENDICITIS

'The art of the practice of medicine is to be learnt only by experience, it's not by inheritance and it cannot be revealed.'
—**Sir William Osler**

One has to diagnose acute appendicitis in case of acute abdomen by excluding other causes.

> *Common causes of RIF pain*:
> - Acute gastroenteritis
> - Mesenteric lymphadenitis
> - Right ureteric colic
> - Ruptured ovarian follicle (Mittelschmerz)
> - Acute salpingitis
> - Ruptured ectopic pregnancy
> - Torsion of an ovarian cyst
> - Meckel's diverticulitis
> - Regional ileitis (Crohn's disease)
> - Acute pyelonephritis
> - Perforated duodenal ulcer
> - Acute cholecystitis
> - Acute pancreatitis
> - Acute intestinal obstruction

Surgeon's art of diagnosis and observation is nowhere challenged so much as in the diagnosis of appendicitis. History and clinical examination are the main criteria for diagnosis of acute appendicitis, more than any other parameter. The acute appendicitis is diagnosed solely by clinical examination. In doubt the surgeon must revisit the patient and examine again. The retrocecal and post-ileal appendicitis sometimes become puzzling and difficult to diagnose due to masked signs.

> When appendicitis appears in a classical form with typical sequential shifting pain, vomiting, and fever it is easily and promptly diagnosed and operated but when appendicitis appears in an atypical form it becomes a challenge to the surgeon to diagnose clinically.

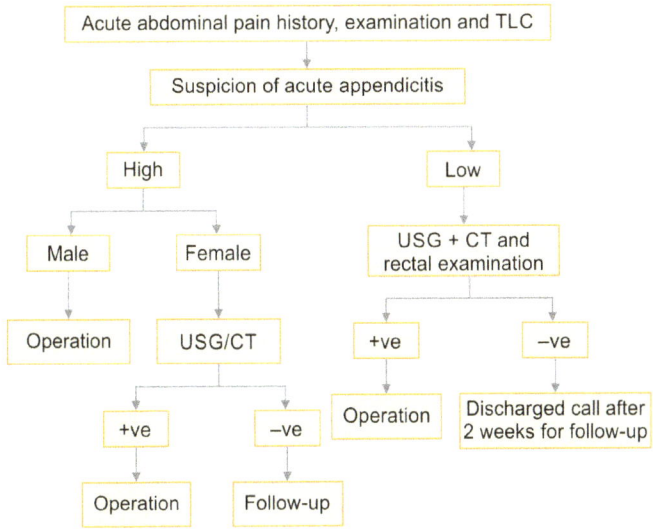

FLOWCHART 3: Algorithm for acute abdominal pain in relation to acute appendicitis.

It is better to remove a normal appendix than to delay diagnosis and end up with perforation. It is important to ask for pain, vomiting, and fever in detail **(Flowchart 3)**.

Following factors differentiate appendicitis from a non-surgical illness[95]
- Localized RLQ tenderness
- Rebound tenderness.
- Leukocytosis >11,500 cells/mL
- Neutrophil count >75%

It is seen that surgeon's misdiagnosis rate (the patient of normal appendices found at appendectomy) to be inversely related to perforation rate (the patient of perforated appendix found at appendectomy)[52] but some workers feel that perforated appendix patients have significantly longer prehospital delay.

Acute appendicitis is one of the most important members of the diseases of 'acute abdomen.'

The preoperative accuracy of diagnosis is accepted in between 85 and 90%. The commonest misdiagnosed cases are of acute mesenteric lymphadenitis. Diagnosis depends upon four factors, i.e., anatomic location of inflamed appendix, stage of the process (inflamed or ruptured), patients age, and sex.[96-100]

Symptoms of longer duration are major contributors to perforation. Perforation after presenting to surgical attention appears to be unknown.[27,28,52,60]

Obscured and masked forms of acute appendicitis: These patients do not have classical signs and symptoms of appendicitis. So, appendicitis is not suspected. A striking example is related with Treves, in which a middle aged gentleman, after being little out of sorts, was seized with pain in the hepatic region attended by a rigor and subsequent rise of temperature. The rigors were repeated, the fever became very high, jaundice supervened, and it became evident that the patient was suffering from pylephlebitis and liver abscess. No mischief could be detected, however, in any part of abdomen except about the liver. In 14 days he died, when the liver was found riddled with abscesses; the appendix, which was this organized and filled with pus, had evidently been the seat of long standing disease. (Appendicitis and Other Diseases of the Vermiform Appendix)

The increase in the use of diagnostic modalities such as abdominal ultrasonography and computed tomography do not appear to have improved the diagnostic accuracy of appendicitis at the population level.[15,101,102]

COMPUTER-ASSISTED DIAGNOSIS

By feeding symptoms and signs, various programs can give various differential and most probable diagnosis. It improves the diagnostic as well as clinical precision of surgeon.[103]

> **Key Point**
>
> The diagnosis of acute appendicitis is made primarily on the basis of history and the physical findings with additional assistance from laboratory and radiographic examinations.
>
> —Lally KP. Appendix. In: Townsend CM, David C. Sabiston Textbook of Surgery, volume 2, 17th edition. Amsterdam; Elsevier; 2004. p. 1384.

PROBLEMS OF ACUTE APPENDICITIS AT DIFFERENT AGE AND STAGE

> A child at the Johns Hopkins Hospital, aged 4 years, was seized after a hearty dinner with violent abdominal cramp, lasting some hours. She passed a comfortable night, however, and in the morning felt well, but her temperature was 104°F and pulse 160. At 10 am the abdominal pain returned and grew steadily worse: the abdomen seemed slightly swollen and tender, and the temperature was 105°F. A diagnosis of enterocolitis was made and an oil enema given. The next morning paroxysmal pain continued, referred by the child to the epigastric region. She lay with her knees drawn up. The abdomen was swollen and tender, especially in the right ileocecal and lumbar regions; the tongue was dry and coated, the temperature 104°F and the pulse 140, the leukocytes 32,000. Operation revealed a general septic peritonitis. The appendix showed an acute hemorrhagic inflammation with slight necrosis of the mucosa. Death occurred before the incision was closed.

In Infancy and Childhood (Figs. 37A and B)

The acute appendicitis is usually under-diagnosed. There are some special problems with younger age.

- Appendicitis is seen in neonates associated with aganglionosis and neonatal necrotizing enterocolitis[59]
- Infants and children are more sensitive to examination so it is not easy to do proper examination. Children <5 years of age have a negative appendicectomy rate of 25%, perforation rate of 45% where children >5 years of age have rates of negative appendectomy and perforation 10% and 20% respectively.[104,105]

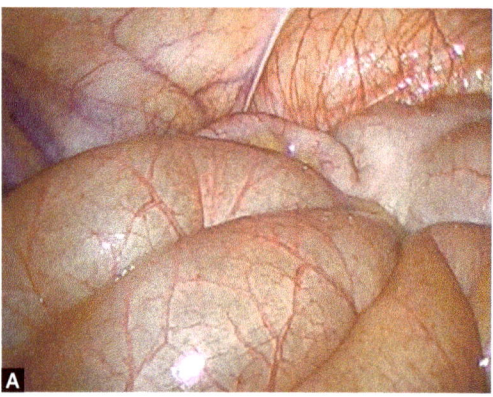 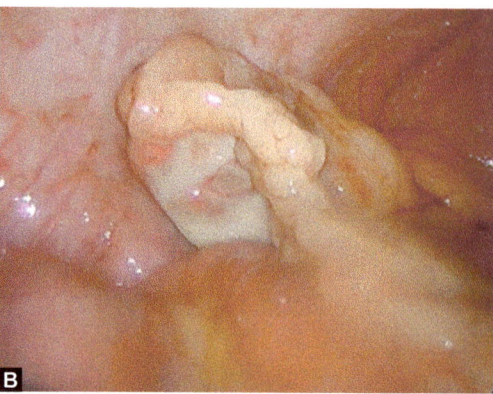

FIGS. 37A AND B: Acute appendicitis and perforated appendix in a children.

- Most of infants and children are uncooperative due to apprehension.
- Infants especially cannot complain correctly.
- Clinician has to win the confidence of the infant and child before proceeding for examination.

Differences between the appendix of the child and adult:
- Size of the appendix
- Thickness of appendicular walls
- Ceco-appendicular junction

Appendix in children is larger than in adults as compared to size of body and GIT.

Coats of the walls of the appendix are more delicate than in adults.

Ceco-appendicular junction is often funnel shaped when cecum and appendix are in same line. Valves at cecal junction of appendix do not close as in adults, this makes fecal contents easier to enter into the lumen of appendix and render its expulsion also easy.

- The omentum is not well developed in infants and children. Omentum is like a 'Bib' in child but an 'Apron' in adult. So appendicular lump does not develop and perforation occurs earlier **(Fig. 38)**.
- Eliciting tenderness in infants and children is not an easy task and you cannot do without it also. So palpate the abdomen of child with his own hand. The child will try not to touch the tender area or he will pull the hand.
- Constitutional disturbances are more in children.
- Temperature and pulse are high.
- There is complete dislike for food.
- There is diarrhea and vomiting instead of constipation so it mimics acute gastroenteritis and this is the main confusing factor in diagnosis of acute appendicitis at this age.
- 'Hunger Sign' if the child is being hungry then for sure he is not suffering with acute appendicitis (AA).
- In early stage the bowel sounds may be absent.
- Appendicular lump is rarely seen due to short omentum and poor inflammatory response.
- Early perforation is quite common in children so diagnosis at very early stage is essential to avoid perforation. Diagnosis is often delayed in children and infants.
- Vomiting is a common feature of appendicitis in children. It is rare to find acute appendicitis in children without vomiting.
- Approximately there are 80% chances of perforation with 50% mortality in infancy when acute appendicitis develops.
- Child should be asked to stand on right leg and hip. If he can probably he is not having acute appendicitis.

Perforation of appendix occurs so frequently in children that one has to follow the rule that 'Every child having RIF pain with diarrhea and vomiting should be suspected as suffering with acute appendicitis unless proved otherwise'.

In children the worms such as pinworms and roundworms have been considered one of the etiological factors. Sometimes deworming relieves from mild appendicitis symptoms.

- The mortality in infants and children due to acute appendicitis is more than adults. It is due to:

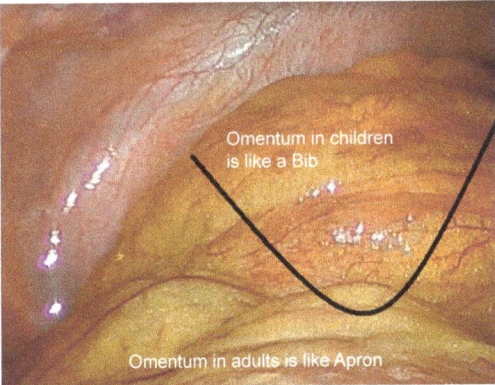

FIG. 38: Size of omentum in an adult and a child.

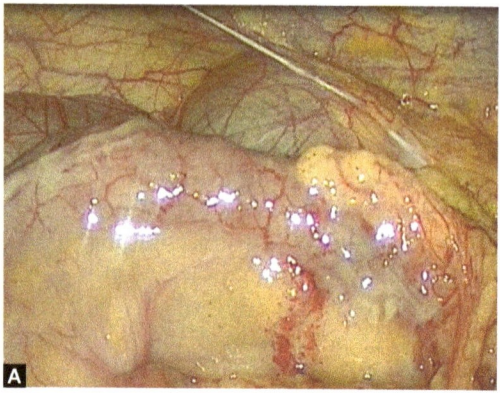
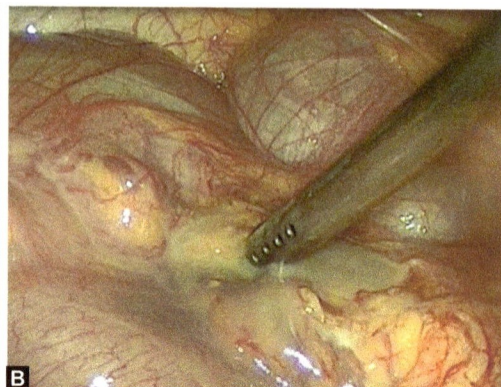

FIGS. 39A AND B: Early appendicular perforation and purulent peritonitis in 78 years old male.

- Omentum is underdeveloped so it cannot reach RIF and so cannot seal and limit or wall off the infection.
- Difficulty in diagnosis due to its resemblance to enteritis.
- Diagnostic laparoscopy is of great help for children as laparoscopy is effective form of treatment in children.[98]

Trauma
Blows, falls, and exertions in children occur due to running and playing, can also be considered as one of the etiological factors of appendicitis.

Rectal examination in children must not be omitted. The adult finger is longer for a child's rectum and this can reach high in pelvis avoiding not finding pelvic appendicitis.

Acute Appendicitis in Old Age

There are some special situations in old age due to these acute appendicitis in old age has become a serious problem.
- A total of 5–10% cases of acute appendicitis occur in old age, lower than in younger patients but the morbidity and mortality is higher due to more rapid progression to perforation. In patients older than 80 years of age, perforation rates of 49% and mortality rates of 21% have been reported,[99] some workers have reported perforation as high as 50%.[106,107]
- The clinical signs are not well marked at this age.
- The abdomen is lax due to muscle wasting or weakness, so the muscle guard or rigidity is not prominent.
- There is atherosclerosis in appendicular artery at this age and is responsible for rapid development of gangrene and perforation **(Figs. 39A and B)**.

> Although people older than 70 years constitute only 5–10% patients with appendicitis, morbidity, and mortality within this age group is disproportionately elevated. These patients may have significant comorbidities, which with atypical and delayed presentations contribute to an incidence of perforation as high as 70%.
>
> —Hardin DM Jr. Acute appendicitis: review and update. Am Fam Physician. 1999;60(7):2027-34.
>
> —Yamini D, Vargas H, Bongard F, Klein S, Stamos MJ. Perforated appendicitis: is it truly a surgical urgency? Am Surg. 1998;64(10):970-5.

- The distension of abdomen, lack of rigidity, vomiting, and constipation make the picture mimic acute intestinal obstruction. Sometimes this may lead to introduction of enema which can perforate the appendix in acute appendicitis.
- Recently it is observed that the incidence of acute appendicitis is decreasing in young adults and increasing in old age in spite of recent advances in imaging and laparoscopy.[108]

- Mortality rate in old age >65 years of age is 4.6%.
- Gangrene and perforation occurs more frequently in old age due to poor vascularity.
- Mortality is high due to:
  - Early gangrene and perforation
  - Delayed diagnosis
  - Associated old age medical diseases

Acute Appendicitis in Pregnancy

- Acute appendicitis is the most common extra-uterine disease requiring operation during pregnancy; incidence is one in 2,000 pregnancies.
- Acute appendicitis occurs most commonly in first and second trimester.
- In normal pregnancy TLC may be between 15,000 and 20,000 and in acute appendicitis it can go higher, in 10% cases it may be normal.
- There is a chance of abortion if appendicectomy is done but one has to weigh the risk.
- Mortality increases considerably by appendicectomy in third trimester.
- In first trimester the nausea and vomiting of appendicitis is taken wrongly as morning sickness which delays the diagnosis and treatment but nausea and vomiting after first trimester must raise doubt of acute appendicitis.
- Rebound tenderness and muscle guarding are less marked due to lax abdomen.
- Marked leukocytosis and ultrasonography may help to reach the diagnosis.
- Mortality in both mother and fetus increases with trimester and delay in diagnosis.[109] In third trimester fetus mortality rate is 20% whereas maternal mortality rate is 9%. RB Parker was of the view that after 6 months the mortality is 20%—10 times greater than in first 3 months.[110]

> The relationship between the disease of the appendix and disease of the pelvic organs in women may be either accidental or casual; and the most obvious classification of disease of the appendix from this point of view is following:
> - Cases in which the disease of appendix is primary and the pelvic affection is secondary, that is to say, consequent on the lesion of appendix.
> - Cases in which the gynecological affection, whether it is tubal, uterine, or ovarian, is primary, and the disease of appendix is secondary.
> - Cases in which the disease of the pelvic organs and the disease of the appendix are independent of each other.
>
> —Howard H Kelly

- Laparoscopic surgery becomes technically difficult after 26 weeks of pregnancy.
- Appendicectomy is the treatment of choice in all trimester of pregnancy as soon as it is diagnosed.
- The enlarged uterus causes upward displacement of cecum and appendix during second and third trimesters of pregnancy which may cause confusion in diagnosing appendicitis with acute cholecystitis.
- Visceral and parietal peritoneum are separated due to enlarged uterus so somatic component of pain decreases.
- Sometimes necrobiosis of uterine fibroids or concealed accidental hemorrhage may cause similar pain as of acute appendicitis.
- Careful history and positive Rovsing sign help to diagnose acute appendicitis.
- Put the patient in supine position and mark the most tender spot with a marker and then put the patient in left lateral position. In acute appendicitis the maximum tender spot will not shift but in a uterine pathology it will shift.

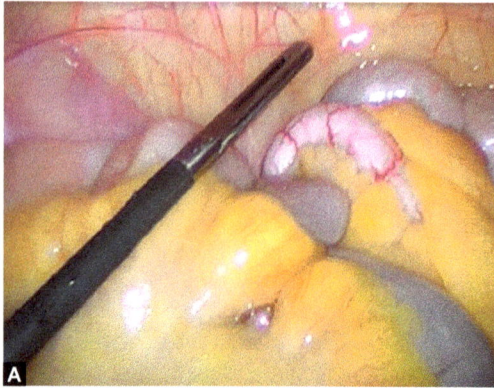 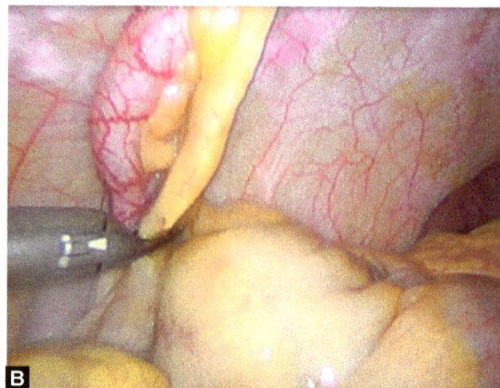

FIGS. 40A AND B: Acute catarrhal appendicitis in a young female patient of 27 years of age.

- Pyelitis, pyelonephritis, and cystitis are common during pregnancy. Pyelitis or pyelonephritis may mimic acute appendicitis. So one should keep in mind these conditions during pregnancy.

> As a rule, the appendix is merely adherent by its distal portion but more or less extensive pathological changes in its wall are frequently formed. The appendix in women, as we have said, frequently occupies the pelvic position and is in contact with the upper portion of the right broad ligament. In such cases perisalpingitis readily involves the peritoneal surface of the appendix.
> (Appendicitis and Other Diseases of the Vermiform Appendix)

- Appendicectomy during pregnancy carries 10–15% risk of premature labor and it increases to 30% in presence of perforation.[47]
- Intrauterine fetal death occurs in 3–5% cases of acute appendicitis and 35% in perforation of gangrenous appendix.[100,111,112]
- Acute appendicitis is evenly distributed among all trimesters but maximum incidence of perforation occurs during third trimester.

Appendicitis in Young Females

A lot of gynecological problems mimic acute appendicitis so every young female going for appendicectomy must undergo gynecological examination by a gynecologist and lower abdominal and pelvic and endovaginal ultrasound to avoid negative appendicectomies **(Figs. 40A and B)**.[78]

Acute Appendicitis in Obese

- Obesity makes it difficult to elicit the signs to diagnose acute appendicitis and so the diagnosis is delayed.
- Acute appendicitis in a female patient is dealt with differently **(Flowchart 4)**.
- Technical difficulties in obesity make laparoscopic appendicectomy a better option than open appendicectomy. So diagnostic laparoscopy should be done if confirmed, appendicectomy is done.

APPENDICITIS IN PATIENTS WITH HUMAN IMMUNODEFICIENCY VIRUS INFECTION

- Incidence of acute appendicitis in general population is 0.1–0.2% whereas in human immunodeficiency virus (HIV) infected patients is 0.5%.[113,114]
- HIV patient will demonstrate a relative leukocytosis and not absolute leukocytosis.[115]
- The risk of perforation in cases of HIV infected patients is higher, 43% were found having perforation on laparotomy,[116] the perforation is also associated with low clusters of differentiation (CD4) count.

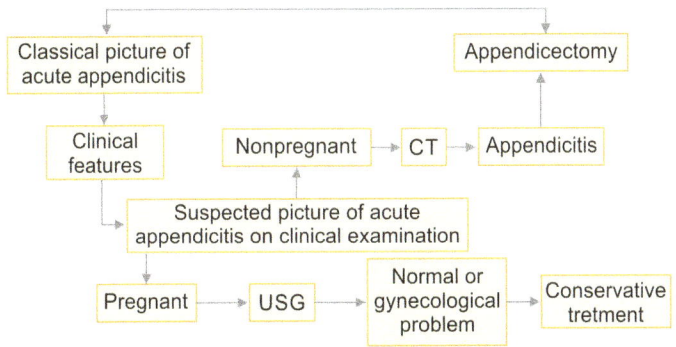

FLOWCHART 4: Clinical algorithm in a female patient of acute appendicitis.

- RLQ pain in HIV infection patients may be found associated with opportunistic infection and must be looked for, i.e., cytomegalovirus (CMV), Kaposi's sarcoma, tuberculosis, lymphoma, and other infective colitis.[117] This broad differential diagnosis often results in delay in diagnosis and late presentation to surgical evaluation at which time perforation may be more likely.[114,118]
- Postoperative morbidity rate is higher in HIV-infected patients with perforation and hospital stay is also prolonged.

STUMP APPENDICITIS

It is defined as 'appendicitis in the remaining appendicular stump after appendectomy.' Surgeons must also remember that a previous appendectomy does not definitely exclude the diagnosis of appendicitis, as 'stump appendicitis,' although rare but has been described.[119] RLQ tenderness is always present.

> Surgeon must also remember that a previous appendectomy does not definitely exclude the diagnosis of appendicitis, as 'Stump appendicitis'... Although rare, has been described.
> —Mangi AA, Berger DL. Stump appendicitis. Am Surg. 2000;66(8):739-41.

ASYMPTOMATIC APPENDICOLITH

As the more sensitive methods of investigation are more widely used like CT scan, more and asymptomatic appendicoliths will be diagnosed. Appendicolith may be present in normal appendix and acute appendicitis is also found without appendicolith so the appendicolith is not pathognomonic of acute appendicitis. Lowe and associates[120] studied CT scan of children with suspected appendicitis and compared with CT scan of children with abdominal trauma. Six (14%) of 44 patients with suspected appendicitis had an appendicolith but proved not having appendicitis and 2 (3%) of the 74 trauma patients had appendicolith. So appendicectomy for symptomless or asymptomatic appendicolith cannot be recommended.[121]

One must bear in mind the various 'standards' and less common sites of the appendix. Acute appendicitis has been seen in appendices trapped in inguinal, femoral and even in umbilical hernias.[122]

> **Key Point**
> Shifting pain and signs of local peritoneal irritation are two hallmarks of accurate diagnosis of appendicitis.

DIFFERENTIAL DIAGNOSIS OF ACUTE APPENDICITIS

'Think of uncommon manifestation of common conditions rather than common manifestations of uncommon conditions.'
—Matz R

Differential diagnosis is a process of differentiating between the conditions which show similar signs and symptoms so mimic the real disease. The process is based on symptoms, signs, laboratory results, history, and physical examination etc. The aim of differential diagnosis (DDx) is to arrive at correct diagnosis by excluding other provisional diagnoses. Similarly acute appendicitis is diagnosed in a suspected case.

> The frequent possibility of error in the diagnosis of appendicitis is shown by the large number of cases…illustrating the various lesions of the pelvis and abdomen which have been mistaken for appendicitis.
> —JM Spillissy. Ann Surg. 1902;35:758.

IN CHILDREN

Acute Mesenteric Lymphadenitis

- It is most commonly confused disease with acute appendicitis in children.
- Recent history of upper respiratory tract infection is present.
- The pain is colicky in nature, which lasts for few minutes.
- Vomiting is less marked than in acute appendicitis.
- Cervical lymph nodes may be enlarged.
- Shifting tenderness may be present if child is placed in left lateral position.
- True muscle rigidity is rare.
- Relative lymphocytosis may be present.
- It is a self-limiting disease.

- If the diagnosis is in doubt then urgent exploration is safest action.

Acute Gastroenteritis

- It usually presents as intestinal colic with vomiting and diarrhea.
- Tenderness is less localized and even may be no tenderness at all.
- Other members of family are also affected at the same time.
- Laboratory values may be normal.
- In viral gastroenteritis stool is watery and profuse.
- In typhoid fever diagnosis is made by prostration, maculopapular rash, leukopenia, and culture of *Salmonella typhi* from stool and blood, 1% patient develop terminal ileum perforation requiring urgent surgical interference.

Meckel's Diverticulitis (Fig. 41)

- Johann Friedrich Meckel* described the diverticulum in 1809.
- Clinically it cannot be differentiated from acute appendicitis.
- Sometimes pain in Meckel's diverticulitis is more central or to left than in acute appendicitis.
- There may be intermittent lower gastrointestinal bleeding.

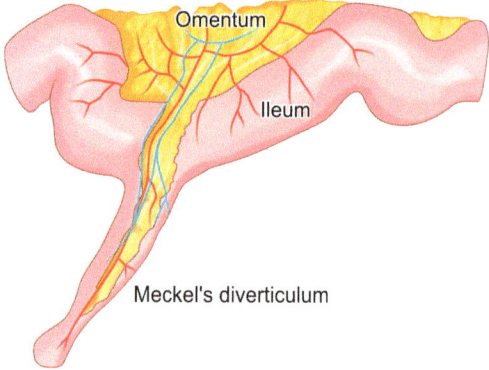

FIG. 41: Meckel's diverticulum.

---

*Johann Friedrich Meckel (1781–1833), Professor of Anatomy and Surgery, Halle, Germany.

Rule of 2 of Meckel's diverticulum
Meckel's diverticulum occurs in 2% children at the age of 2 years, it usually measures 2 inches in size, it arises at about 2 feet distance from ileocecal junction, can have two types of tissues, i.e., gastric and pancreatic, and it has a gender ratio of 1:2 in females and males.

Intussusception

- The intussusception is commonest at the age of 18 months whereas acute appendicitis is rare before the age of 2 years **(Fig. 42)**.

In children:
- Acute mesenteric lymphadenitis
- Acute gastroenteritis
- Meckel's diverticulitis
- Intussusception
- Henoch–Schönlein purpura
- Lobar pneumonia

In adult male:
- Ureteric colic
- Regional enteritis
- Perforated duodenal ulcer
- Torsion of testis
- Acute pancreatitis
- Rectus sheath hematoma
- Right-sided acute pyelonephritis
- Amebic typhlitis
- Yersinia ileitis

In adult female:
- Mittelschmerz (mid-cycle follicular cyst rupture)
- Pelvic inflammatory disease (PID) including salpingitis and salpingo-oophoritis
- Pyelonephritis
- Ectopic pregnancy
- Torsion or rupture of ovarian cyst
- Endometriosis
- Gallstone colic

In elderly:
- Diverticulitis
- Acute intestinal obstruction
- Carcinoma of colon

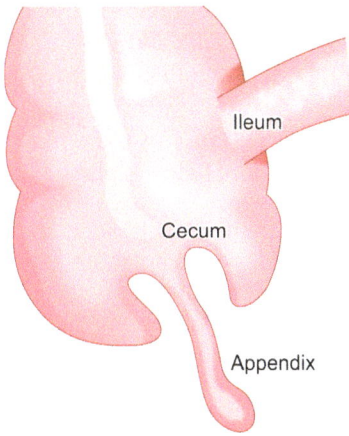

FIG. 42: Intussusception of appendix into cecum.

- Torsion of appendix epiploicae or epiploic appendicitis
- Mesenteric infarction
- Leaking aortic aneurysm

Rare differential diagnosis
'Distension, rigidity, vomiting, pain are actors abdominal which often deign, to act on behalf of the chest, spine or brain or general ills of which typhoid's the main.'

From '*The Acute Abdomen in Rhyme*' by 'Zeta' (Sir Zachary Cope)

- Amoebic typhlitis
- Spinal conditions:
  ○ Tuberculosis of spine
  ○ Metastatic carcinoma
  ○ Multiple myeloma
  ○ Osteoporotic vertebral collapse
- Preherpetic pain in right 10th and 11th dorsal nerves
- Tabetic crises
- Abdominal crises of:
  ○ Porphyria
  ○ Diabetes mellitus
- Leukemic ileocecal syndrome
- Primary peritonitis
- Sigmoid diverticulitis
- Carcinoma of cecum

- A sausage-shaped lump is palpable in lower abdomen, usually in right side and RLQ feels empty.

- It occurs in well-nourished child.
- Colicky pain occurs and child doubles up but in between colics the child appears well.
- After several hours of pain stool mixed with mucus and blood is passed.

If the intussusceptions is large as the bowel enters the distal bowel, it can be seen or felt at anus. Rectal examination may detect a polyp-like mass in the rectum. So, the rectal examination in acute abdomen in children must not be omitted. In intussusceptions the invagination may be partial or complete or appendix with cecum can invaginate into the colon.

Henoch–Schönlein Purpura

- Henoch* described this form of purpura in 1886. Johann Lucas Schönlein** described this form of purpura in 1837.
- Preceded by sore throat or respiratory infection.
- Abdominal pain can be very severe.
- Ecchymotic rash on external surfaces of limbs and buttocks.
- Microscopic hematuria is common.
- Platelet count and bleeding time are normal.
- Joint pain and nephritis may be present.

Lobar Pneumonia

- Pain of pleurisy and lobar pneumonia at right base may mimic acute appendicitis pain.
- There is minimal or absent abdominal tenderness and muscle guarding.
- Pleural friction—rub or altered breath sounds are present.
- There is marked pyrexia.
- X-ray of chest is diagnostic.

Abnormal symptoms in cases of pneumonia are not very common but also not very uncommon.

JL Morris of Boston has given a picture of such cases, so completely and clear that nothing is wanting and he warns us that 'The abdomen has been twice opened in children by well-known Boston surgeons of appendicitis, when the trouble was lobar pneumonia.'
—JL Morris (Annal Gyn Paed.1900;13:143).

IN ADULT MALE

Typhoid and tuberculosis of intestine can cause ulceration and perforation of intestine can sometimes resemble appendicitis and other times appendicitis can be mistaken for typhoid and tuberculosis.

Ureteric Colic

- If stone is lodged in ureter near the site of appendix it mimics acute appendicitis.
- Pain radiates from loin to groin.
- Cough test is negative but positive in acute appendicitis.
- Urine examination will reveal RBCs.
- Ultrasound, CT scan, and intravenous urography (IVU) are diagnostic.

Regional Enteritis (Regional Ileitis or Crohn's Disease)

- History of abdominal cramps, diarrhea, and weight loss.
- Doughy vague tender lump in RIF with fever, RLQ pain, and leukocytosis is present.
- Mesenteric lymph node may be palpable.
- Small bowel barium enema will show 'string sign of Kantor.'
- Pain is very severe, much more than what happens in acute appendicitis.

Perforated Duodenal Ulcer

- The duodenal perforation sometimes may mimic acute appendicitis when the duodenal contents, pass along the paracolic gutter to the RIF and especially

---

*Eduard Heinrich Henoch (1820–1910), Professor of Diseases of Children, Berlin, Germany.
**Johann Lucas Schönlein (1793–1864), Physician, Charity Hospital, Berlin, Germany.

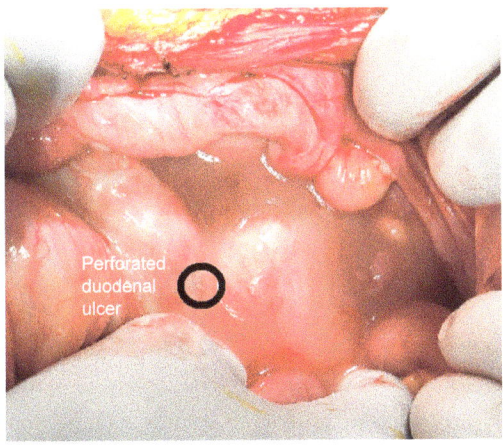

FIG. 43: Perforation of duodenal ulcer.

when perforation seals and upper abdominal features are reduced **(Fig. 43)**.
- There always is a past history of dyspepsia.
- Sudden onset of pain which starts in epigastrium and settles in RIF whereas in acute appendicitis pain starts in umbilical area.
- Pain in perforated duodenal ulcer is much more intense than in acute appendicitis.
- In perforated duodenal ulcer rigidity in epigastrium and right hypochondrium is present.
- In erect X-ray chest shows gas under diaphragm in 70% patients which is diagnostic of perforated duodenal ulcer.

Torsion of Testis
- Torsion of undescended testis causes similar pain but scrotum is found empty.
- Occurs usually in a young adult male.
- Scrotal examination is diagnostic.
- Color Doppler or an ultrasound of scrotum will confirm the diagnosis.

Acute Pancreatitis
- Epigastric pain which radiates to back by penetrating directly to back.
- Referred pain of acute appendicitis in epigastrium is of much less severity.
- High level of serum amylase, >1000 IU is diagnostic of acute pancreatitis.
- History of alcohol intake or gallbladder disease is present.

Rectus Sheath Hematoma
- It is due to rupture of inferior epigastric artery usually after a violent attack of cough or strenuous exercise.[123]
- It is a rare entity.
- Acute pain and tenderness in RIF after an episode of strenuous physical exercise.
- Localized pain without gastrointestinal upset is the rule.
- Elderly patient on anticoagulant therapy may get it after a minor and trivial trauma.

Right-sided Acute Pyelonephritis
- There is increased frequency of micturition
- The tenderness in loin is accompanied with fever, rigors, bacteriuria, and pyuria.
- It is difficult to differentiate between acute pyelonephritis and acute appendicitis during pregnancy as appendix is lifted up by uterus and comes at level of kidney.

Amebic Typhlitis
- It is characterized by diarrhea and blood mixed mucus.
- There is tenderness at 'Manson-Bahr amebic point' in LIF, Sir Philip Manson-Bahr gave this point corresponding to McBurney's point in LIF. In amebiasis there are two tender spots, one over cecum at McBurney's point in RIF and other over sigmoid colon over Manson-Bahr* point in LIF **(Fig. 44)**.

---
*Eduard Heinrich Henoch (1820–1910), Professor of Diseases of Children, Berlin, Germany.

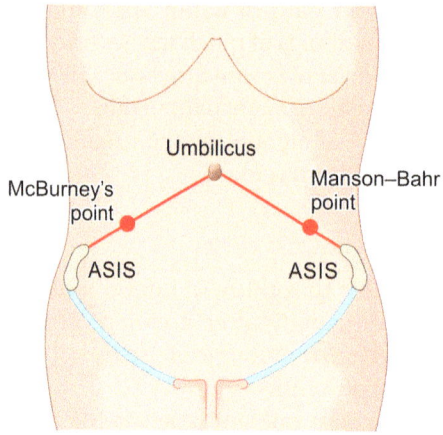

FIG. 44: McBurney's point and Manson–Bahr point.

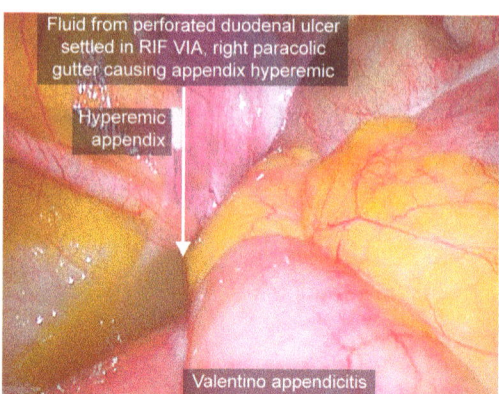

FIG. 45: Valentino appendix.

> The following incident took place in 1989. Mohammed Abdul-Al-Awadh, 43 years old, was brought to the emergency ward of Aden Refinery Company Hospital in Aden, Yemen, suffering from severe lower abdominal pain along with vomiting and fever for about 24 hours. He narrated a typical history of migratory pain. This led to a diagnosis of acute appendicitis, which a clinical and ultrasound examination later confirmed.
>
> Appendectomy was performed and the appendix was found to be mildly inflamed with some fluid around it. However, the patient did not improve after surgery and continue to exhibit the same distressing symptoms as before. In fact, his condition deteriorated. Re-operation was done and, to our surprise it was discovered that a perforated duodenal ulcer was responsible for the mild inflammation of the appendix and the fluid gathered around it. The patient recovered and was discharged in good condition.
>
> —40 Minutes with God

Valentino Appendix

It is also called as valentino syndrome or valentino appendicitis. In perforated duodenal ulcer the contents and bile from the ulcer hole pass down through right paracholic gutter in RIF causing local peritonitis and hyperaemia of appendix, resembling appendicitis. Clinical features resemble acute appendicitis, as happened in this case. It is named after a famous film director Rudolph Valentino, who suffered like this. In 1926, Valentino collapsed in a New York City hotel, and underwent surgery for persumed appendicitis at New York Polytechnic Hospital. At the time he was found to have a perforated ulcer. Postoperatively, he developed peritonitis, multiple organ system dysfunction and died several days later (Valentino looses battle with death: Greatest of screen lovers fought valiantly for life. The Plattsburgh Sentinel. 1926;1) **(Fig. 45)**.

Yersinia Ileitis (Pseudoappendicitis)

- About 6% cases of acute mesenteric lymphadenitis and 5% cases of acute appendicitis are caused by Yersinia infection.
- It is a condition which mimics acute appendicitis. It is caused by Yersinia pseudotuberculosis organism. The terminal ileum looks red, edematous, and inflamed.
- It subsides by itself.
- It does not require any treatment.

IN ADULT FEMALE

Inflammatory diseases of the right uterine adnexa more frequently mimic appendicitis than other parts. Some genital tract ailments in a female of child-bearing age mimic acute appendicitis. A careful history of menstrual cycle, vaginal discharge, and pregnancy may help to reach to diagnosis.

After expulsion of fetus uterus suddenly contracts and it can cause rupture of appendicular or periappendicular abscess leading to a grave situation.

> In the 5th or the 6th month of pregnancy, a typical appendicitis developed, that soon subsided with a disappearance of all symptoms. The pregnancy went on the term, and a normal delivery followed, but to 2 days later the patient died from peritonitis. Autopsy showed that the contraction of the uterus had caused rupture of an abscess.
> —Mauret (Zait. f. Gyn. No. 94. p. 1359)

Mittelschmerz

The typical mid cycle lower abdominal or pelvic pain is indicative of Mittelschmerz. It is the rupture of mid cycle follicular cyst with bleeding. Mittelschmerz name is given to this condition as pain occurs at the midpoint of menstrual cycle.
- Usually no GIT symptoms
- Patient is not looking sick or toxic.
- Pregnancy test is negative.
- Usually not much signs present.
- Leukocytosis and fever are absent or minimal.
- Diagnostic laparoscopy may be required.

Pelvic Inflammatory Disease

It is a common condition and includes following conditions:
- Salpingitis
- Endometriosis
- Tubo-ovarian sepsis
- Every young female should be suspected of pelvic inflammatory disease (PID) in lower abdominal pain. It is very common.
- History of purulent vaginal discharge, dysmenorrhea and burning pain during micturition are important features.
- Anorexia, nausea, and vomiting are absent.
- Pain is felt on both sides and lower than in appendicitis.
- The pain is typically bilateral.
- Pain starts within 7 days of menstruation and stays for >2 days.
- On vaginal examination the cervical and bilateral adnexa are found tender.
- Transvaginal ultrasound is of help in reaching diagnosis.
- Diagnostic laparoscopy may be of help to diagnose it in difficult situations.
- Thorough examination and keeping in mind PID can reduce negative appendectomies.

Pyelonephritis

- Patients of pyelonephritis have dull pain in lumbar region.
- Patients usually have high fever associated with rigors.

Ectopic Pregnancy

- Right-sided tubal pregnancy or right-sided ruptured tubal ectopic mimics the acute appendicitis.
- There is no shifting of pain from umbilicus to RIF.
- Usually a history of missed period is present.
- Urinary pregnancy test may be positive but usually patient does not show that she is pregnant.
- Severe pain on movement of cervix on vaginal examination.
- A mass with increased level of chorionic gonadotrophins.
- Culdocentesis revealing blood and decidual tissue is diagnostic.
- Pelvic ultrasound is a must for ectopic and is diagnostic. It may show tubal abnormality.
- Ruptured ectopic with hemoperitoneum is difficult to miss as patient may be in

- shock with severe pain, which will not subside till operation is done.
- There may be paraumbilical ecchymosis or discoloration (Cullen's sign).

> Rupture of the gallbladder occurring suddenly without previous evidence of any disease of the gallbladder has been mistaken for acute perforative appendicitis. Several examples of this mistake are recorded. A man of 45 years of age, who, while lifting a heavy weight was seized with severe epigastric pain and collapsed. A diagnosis of appendicitis was made. The next he had but a slight rise of temperature; his pulse was 120 beats/minute; his face was anxious; the pain was localized over McBurney's point and a tenderness well marked. The right rectus muscle was rigid. When the abdomen was opened a quart or more of bile gushed out, and the attack was found to be due rupture of enlarged distended gallbladder.
> —GM Pond. Med Rec. April, 1898, p 585.

Torsion of an Ovarian Cyst

- Torsion or hemorrhage in ovarian cyst may cause sudden sever pain in abdomen.
- Low grade fever with vomiting may be present.
- A mass is felt in RIF if cyst is big.
- Pelvic ultrasound and CT scan are diagnostic.

Endometriosis

Endometriosis in RQL can mimic AA as the endometrial tissue can get deposited over right ovary, right fallopian tube, and the appendix.

Gallstone Colic

Gallstone colic can mimic acute appendicitis but the pain will be located in or near right hypochondrium and may be radiating to back whereas the acute appendicitis pain is in RIF...

> A very interesting case is related…in which, after the appendix had been extirpated at an operation for acute perforative appendicitis, a severe hemorrhage suddenly welled up from the depth of the pelvis. Investigation of the case of this accident revealed a fresh rupture of an ectopic pregnancy on the left side, a 1 month's fetus being found.
> —Summa (St. Loius Cour. of Med., 1900, p. 434).

IN ELDERLY

> Appendix in old age progressively atrophies. Usually the appendix is shorter than in adult. The frequency of appendicitis becomes less in old age; it becomes rare after 80. Due to laxity of abdominal walls in old age guarding and rigidity are reduced but pus collection increases than in adults. It is often seen that there is no correlation between clinical and operative findings, it is commonly noted in very old, very young, and pregnant patients.

Diverticulitis

Diverticulitis develops due to inflammation of colonic diverticulum. CT scan is diagnostic investigation for diverticulitis.

Acute Intestinal Obstruction

- Acute appendicitis is uncommon in elderly and intestinal obstruction is common.
- The diagnosis of intestinal obstruction is easy as X-ray abdomen and ultrasound are diagnostic.
- Early decision for surgery is important.

Carcinoma of Colon

Acute appendicitis can be a sign of cancer of colon as the growth may obstruct the lumen of appendix.

CHAPTER 6 Diseases of Appendix

> **Key Point**
> It is often seen that there is no correlation between clinical and operative findings, it is commonly noted in very old, very young, and in pregnancy.

Torsion of Appendix Epiploica or Epiploic Appendicitis[111]

It is an infarction of an appendix epiploica due to its torsion. Appendices epiploicae are small peritoneal sacs filled with fat and are attached with colon. Pain may be mild or severe, lasts for few days.
- Site of pain is the colon area.
- There is no anorexia, sequence of symptoms, and shifting pain of appendicitis.
- Patient does not look ill.
- Nausea and vomiting are uncommon.
- Recurrence of pain occurs.
- Local signs of tenderness and rebound tenderness are present.

Mesenteric Infraction

It causes interruption of the blood supply to varying portions of the small intestine. Mortality is approximately 50%. Early diagnosis and surgical treatment are of utmost importance. In case where acute mesenteric ischemia (AMI) is suspected urgent computed tomography angiography (CTA) should be performed.

Leaking Aortic Aneurysm

It causes sudden and severe pain in abdomen and 80% patients die before reaching hospital.

> **Key Point**
> Appendices epiploicae are present in colon but absent in rectum.

RARE DIFFERENTIAL DIAGNOSIS

Amebic Typhlitis

Amebic typhlitis can present as appendicitis as it is the inflammation of cecum which harbors appendix.

Spinal Conditions

- Tuberculosis of spine or Pott's spine is a common condition. It causes nerve root compression which may appear as appendicitis pain if T10 or T11 are affected.
- Lumbar spine rigidity may be present.
- Movement aggravates pain.
- No intestinal symptoms

Preherpetic Pain

- Preherpetic pain especially of 10th and 11th dorsal nerves, which occurs over same area of appendicitis.
- There is marked hyperesthesia.
- Pain is not shifting.
- There is no muscle rigidity or guarding.
- Herpetic eruption will develop after few hours.

Tabetic Crisis

It is rare nowadays.

Abdominal Crisis of Diabetes Mellitus

- History of diabetes mellitus
- No abdominal rigidity
- Abdominal crisis of porphyria
- Severe attacks of intestinal colic occur.
- Urine is of orange color, which changes to high color when exposed to sunlight.
- It is precipitated by barbiturates.

Leukemic Ileocecal Syndrome

- It is rare.
- It occurs in immunosuppressive patient.
- Gram-negative septicemia (clostridium septicum) occurs.

Primary Peritonitis[112]

It occurs in fallowing conditions:
- Nephrotic syndrome
- Cirrhosis
- Immunosuppression

It is diagnosed by peritoneal aspiration showing only Gram-positive cocci.

Sigmoid Diverticulitis

- It has almost identical findings such as appendicitis on left side but if sigmoid colon loop is big and lies right to the midline then it becomes clinically impossible to differentiate acute sigmoid diverticulitis from acute appendicitis.
- CT scan of abdomen is of value to differentiate acute sigmoid diverticulitis from acute appendicitis.
- Ultrasound is not of much value.

Carcinoma of Cecum

- Sometimes carcinoma of cecum may mimic acute appendicitis, especially when it is perforated.
- History of change of bowel habits and anemia with a palpable mass are diagnostic of carcinoma of cecum.
- Contrast CT scan is important diagnostic tool.

Key Point

Whatever is the patient's age and sex, in acute abdominal pain, acute appendicitis must be in your list of differential diagnosis.

COMPLICATIONS OF APPENDICITIS

'Lesser the indication for surgery greater the complications.'
—**Anonymous**

In 1886, Fitz reported the associated mortality rate of appendicitis to be 67% without surgical therapy.[3] Currently the morality rate of acute appendicitis is reported to be <1%.[124] The elderly patients have a higher rate of complications.[108]

Complications of appendicitis:
- Perforation of appendix
- General peritonitis
- Appendicular abscess
- Appendicular lump or mass
- Septicemia
- Portal pyemia
- Infertility
- Recurrent appendicitis
- Obliteration of the appendix
- Intestinal obstruction
- Appendicular cysts
- Vascular infections as complications of appendicitis

PERFORATION OF APPENDIX

'The appendix having been perforated by ulceration occasioned by the lodgment of fecal concretions in its cavity, extravasation takes place, and inflammation of more severe and serious kind... nature sometimes succeeds in limiting the inflammation—but—at other times diffused over the whole abdomen—and quickly proves fatal.'
—**Thomas Hodgkin, 1836**

Urgent appendicectomy is the treatment of choice for acute appendicitis which prevents the risk of perforation. Average rate of perforation of appendix in acute appendicitis is 25.8%. Children younger than 5 years and patients older than 65 years have highest rate of perforation (45% and 51% respectively). Nonoperative treatment exposes the patient for perforation.[77]

Perforation usually occurs due to increased intraluminal pressure, which occurs in obstructive appendicitis. Patient having nonobstructive appendicitis rarely gets perforation, if at all, it is late. Perforation is uncommon within first 12 hours.

Longer duration of pre-hospital delay is the major contributor to perforation. Perforation after presenting to surgical attention appears to be less common.

—Hail DA et al. (Arch Surg 1997; 132:153-157).

—Pittman-Waller VA, Myers JG, Stewart RM, Dent DL, Page CP, Gray GA, et al. Appendicitis: why so complicated? Analysis of 5755 consecutive appendectomies. Am Surg. 2000;66(6):548-54.

CHAPTER 6 Diseases of Appendix

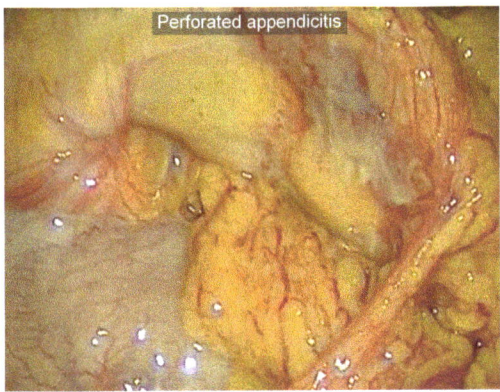

FIG. 46: Perforated appendix.

The accuracy in diagnosing acute appendicitis does not change the rate of perforation. Surprisingly the diagnosis accuracy diminishes but appendicectomy rate increases. Usually perforated appendix is brought from home, it is rare to happen in admitted hospital patient. Hospital admitted patient can be diagnosed after some time if he/she is not diagnosed early.

> When appendix perforates then septic matter which enters the peritoneal cavity is of small quantity. At first the exudates becomes serofibrinous and soon becomes purulent. Intestine surface looses shine and loops of intestine glue together by thin, weak, fibrinous adhesions and are covered with flakes of fibrins.

Overall about 20% of all patient with acute appendicitis have perforation at the time of operation. At the extremes of age (<5 years and >60 years) the rate of perforation is to the region of 60% **(Fig. 46)**.[125]

Site of Perforation (Figs. 47A and B)

- Tip of appendix
- Anti-mesenteric border of appendix—this is the most frequent site of perforation.
- At the site of obstruction—it is not a very early complication of appendicitis. Usually does not occur before 24 hours. It occurs after 2nd day. The antibiotics are not to replace appendicectomy, meaning they are no substitutes for appendicectomy, instead antibiotics try to suppress symptoms cause delay in diagnosis and this leads to perforation. The perforation leads to:
  - Generalized peritonitis
  - Intraperitoneal abscess

Perforated appendix usually does not cause pneumoperitoneum as the gas liberated is not much and is absorbed quickly.

> **Key Point**
> Perforated appendix rarely causes pneumoperitoneum.

Promoting factors of general peritonitis due to perforation of appendix are:
- Extremes of age—too young or too aged.
- Diabetes mellitus
- Poor nutritional state of the patient
- Other debilitating conditions
- Immunosuppression
- Previous abdominal surgery—which reduces the ability of greater omentum to wall off the infection.
- Pelvic appendix—it hangs freely in pelvis without protection.
- Obstruction of appendix lumen, e.g., finding a fecalith in the lumen of appendix on exploratory laparotomy for any other reason is an indication of appendicectomy to prevent future acute appendicitis and generalized peritonitis.

When to Suspect Perforation?

Perforation of appendix in a case of acute appendicitis should be suspected in the following conditions:
- Fever higher than 102°F
- WBC count >18,000/mm^3
- Sudden increase of pain in RIF with localized rebound tenderness
- Generalized peritonitis

When to Suspect General Peritonitis?

When perforation of appendix leads to general peritonitis you will find:
- Patient looks toxic
- Tenderness all over abdomen

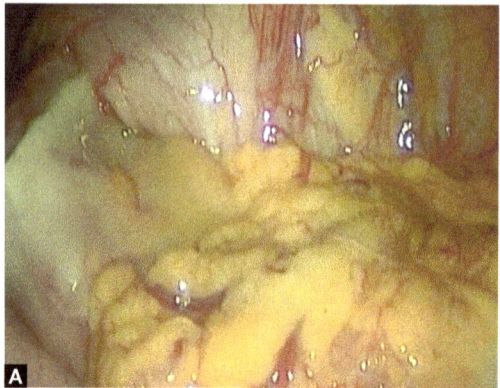 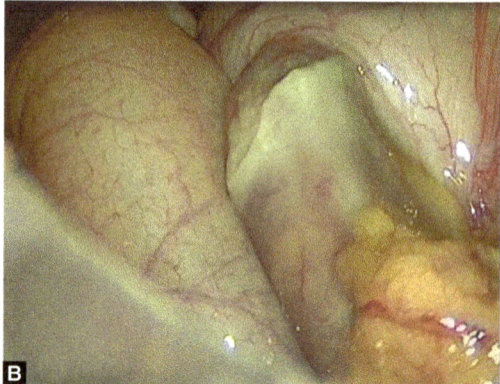

FIGS. 47A AND B: (A) Perforated appendix with purulent peritonitis; (B) Perforated appendix with peritonitis and flakes of fibrin **(Video 3)**.

- Initial board like rigidity of abdomen later distension of abdomen
- Vomiting
- Absolute constipation
- High fever
- No bowel sounds, silent abdomen

Treatment

- *If it presents as small abscess*: Incision and drainage is done extraperitoneally and after 6-week interval appendicectomy is advised.
- *If generalized peritonitis is present*: Laparotomy is done. Appendicectomy is done if appendix is easily accessible.
- *If appendix is inaccessible*: It appendix is found inaccessible and could not be removed then interval appendicectomy is recommended after 6 weeks.

GENERAL PERITONITIS

It develops after perforation of appendix, when the protective phenomenon of body tries to seal it off from other parts of peritoneal cavity by omentum and loops of small bowel, fails. The pain, fever, tenderness, and rigidity increase. At this stage or later the abdomen should be opened, midline or right paramedian incision. Peritoneal lavage by normal saline should be performed.

Some researchers believe that as per exudate in peritoneal cavity after perforation of appendix following types of peritonitis can happen:
- Acute fibrinous peritonitis
- Acute serofibrinous peritonitis
- Acute fibrinopurulent peritonitis
- Acute purulent peritonitis
- Acute dry or septic peritonitis

> This is now an accepted fact that the appendix is the most common source of localized peritonitis in RIF and general peritonitis. A perforated appendix can cause localized peritonitis, generalized peritonitis, phlebitis, liver abscesses, and septicemia. Generalized peritonitis sometimes present in the early stage of acute appendicitis. In other cases, it starts from RIF and then becomes generalized. Out of 50 cases observed at the John's Hopkins Hospital, three showed symptoms of peritonitis from the beginning, 20 within the first 48 hours and the reminder in from 2–5 days. Whether arising early or late, the onset of general peritonitis symptoms are usually abrupt—beginning with intense radiating abdominal pain. (Appendicitis and Other Diseases of the Vermiform Appendix)

> The most significant evidence of nature's ability to limit infection and protect is seen in case of appendicitis. In case of acute appendicitis with advance infection the omentum gravitates here and surrounds the appendix to avoid spread of infection, that is why the omentum is called, 'abdomen policeman.'

APPENDICULAR ABSCESS

First reported case of appendicular abscess was reported in 1848 and operated by Henry Hancock, Surgeon, Charing Cross Hospital, London. There is tender mass in RIF with high fever which may be associated with chills. Ultrasound and CT scan are diagnostic **(Figs. 48A and B)**.

> *Causes of appendicular abscess:*
> - Appendicular mass does not resolve with OSR and converts to abscess.
> - Acute appendicitis leads to abscess formation.

Appendicular abscess should be drained. If easily appendicectomy can be performed, do it, otherwise do not do blind dissection. Interval appendicectomy is done after 6–8 weeks. Usually the appendicular abscess develops from appendicular mass which fails to resolve **(Figs. 49A to C)**.

Important features of appendicular abscess are:
- Hot and tender mass in RIF.
- High pyrexia with chills and rigors
- High TLC (>14,000)
- Increase in size of appendicular mass
- Shift to left, polymorphs increase
- Tachycardia

> *Sub-phrenic abscess*
> It may occur between diaphragm and liver which is the commonest site for a sub-phrenic abscess. It may occur in one of the three following ways:
> 1. As a part of general systemic infection
> 2. As a localized abscess from general purulent appendicitis
> 3. Direct extension from infected appendix by lymphatics
>
> Sub-phrenic abscess may occur even after recovery from acute appendicitis.

Indications of Operation in Appendicular Abscess

- When an appendicular mass fails to reduce in size after 5th day of Ochsner-Sherren regimen (OSR).
- When temperature goes beyond 100°F in spite of IV antibiotics. Incision is placed

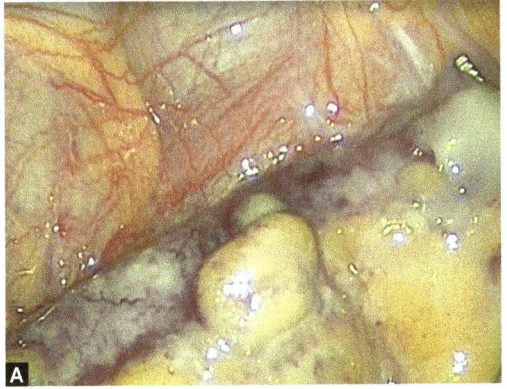
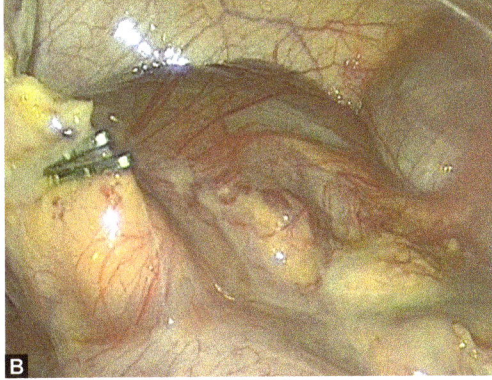

FIGS. 48A AND B: Acute purulent peritonitis **(Video 1)**.

CHAPTER 6 Diseases of Appendix

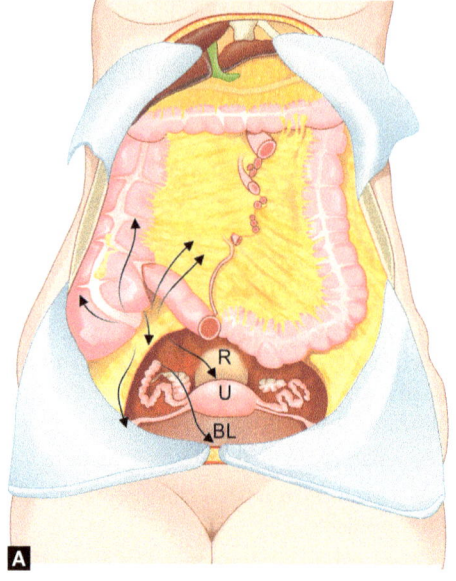
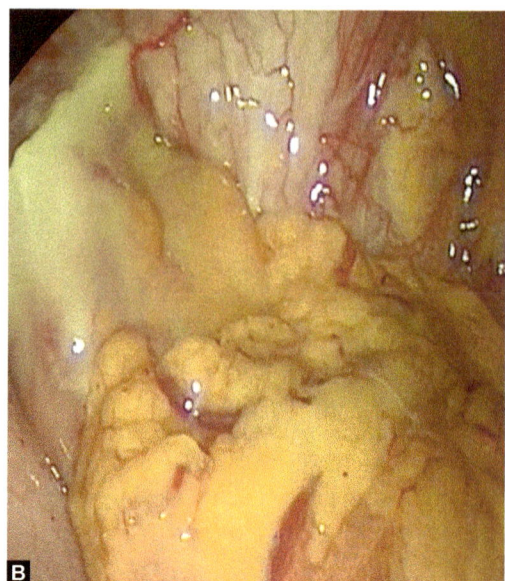
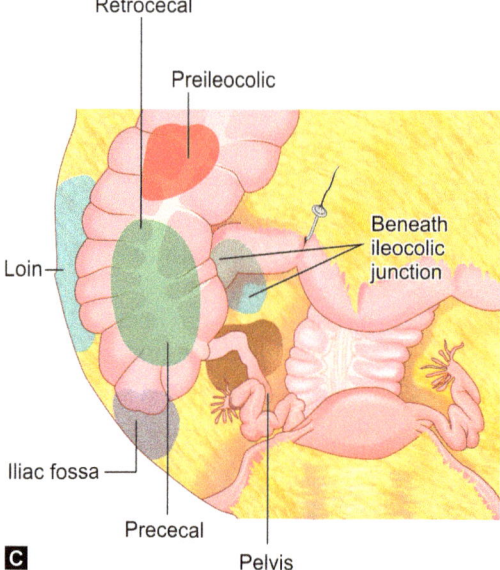

FIGS. 49A TO C: Locations of appendicular abscess and its spread.

Courtesy: Kelly HA. Appendicitis and Others Diseases of the Vermiform Appendix. Philadelphia: JB Lippincott Company.

medial to right ASIS, muscle fibers are separated. Peritoneum is pushed medially and finger is passed gently and pus comes out, the septas are broken by finger. A rubber drain is put.

Warning

Remember two points when dealing with an appendicular abscess:
1. Do not explore to look for inflamed appendix as it is both difficult and dangerous.

CHAPTER 6 Diseases of Appendix

2. Interval appendicectomy is advised but defer it, if patient gets symptoms again then do appendicectomy. Patients may not have symptoms again as appendix might have been destroyed by infection.

Usually appendicectomy is not done when drainage of abscess is done. Appendicular abscess develop due to:
- When appendicular mass fails to resolves and forms abscess.
- As a complication of appendicectomy

Site of appendicular abscess:
- Commonest site is lateral part of RIF (retrocecal appendicitis)
- In pelvis (pelvic appendicitis)

A digital rectal examination (DRE) in a man and vaginal examination in a married women must not be omitted. When the inflamed appendix is situated in the pelvis then bimanual examination, a finger in rectum and one hand over lower abdomen must be tried.

Ultrasound and CT diagnose the appendicular abscess and they are also used for guided drainage of abscess. The location of appendiceal abscess depends upon the position of cecum, position, and length of appendix. The most common site is RIF and the second most common site is pelvis. If abscess develops in a retrocecal appendix the chances of peritonitis diminish.

Fate of an appendicular abscess:
- Rupture of an abscess
- Resolution of abscess by absorption
- Surgical drainage

Rupture of Appendicular Abscess

Appendicular abscess can rupture and can cause:
- Fistulae between:
  - Appendix and urinary bladder
  - Appendix and small bowel
  - Appendix and sigmoid colon
  - Appendix and rectum
- Intraperitoneal residual abscesses:
  - Pelvic abscess
  - In between coil of small bowel
  - Paracolic abscess
  - Sub-diaphragmatic abscess
  - Sub-hepatic abscess

Resolution of appendicular abscess
Appendicular abscess can resolute in following ways:
- Resolution by rupture of an abscess—it produces tissue necrosis due to pressure and abscess wall give way at a point of least resistance.
- Resolution by absorption of its contents—it may be partial or complete. Sometimes only the liquid part of abscess gets absorbed and solid part forms a mass.

Role of Interval Appendicectomy after Appendicular Abscess

In most of the cases of appendicular abscess, the appendix is destroyed by necrosis and gangrene so appendicectomy should be performed only if symptoms recur, otherwise you may not be able to find appendix.

APPENDICULAR LUMP OR MASS (PHLEGMON) (FIGS. 50A AND B)

Appendicular mass can develop in any case of acute appendicitis if appendectomy is not done.

A total of 2-5% patients with appendicitis present with a palpable mass in RLQ.[126] Usually appendicular mass develops on 3rd day from start of the attack of acute appendicitis. When infection goes beyond the wall of appendix or appendix becomes gangrenous then small bowel loops and omentum come near appendix and try to limit the spread of infection. The omentum that is why called as 'policeman of abdomen.' It is nature's attempt to limit and prevent spreading infection causing generalized peritonitis.

If an appendicular mass develops in a patient whose age is 50 years or above, CECT abdomen must be done after resolution of the appendicular mass to rule out malignancy.

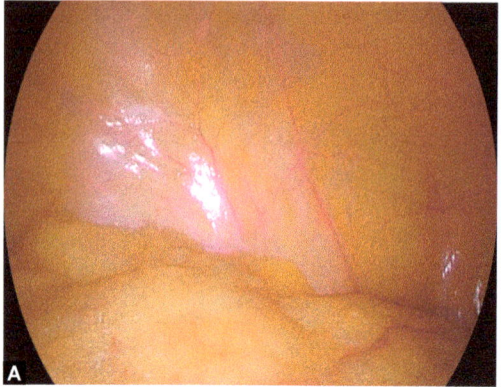 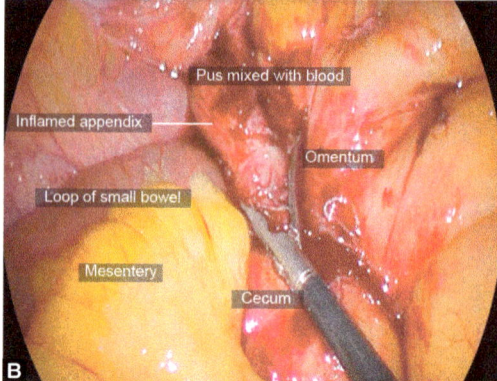

FIGS. 50A AND B: Appendicular lump and constituents **(Videos 7 and 8)**.

Constituents of Appendicular Lump

An appendicular lump consists of:
- Inflamed appendix in the center of lump
- Cecum
- Loops of small bowel
- Omentum
- May be some pus, usually there is no pus. There is a tender lump in RIF. Usually the appendicular mass resolves after conservative treatment.

Appendicular mass is a tender, firm, well-circumscribed localized mass, and smooth lump. It is non-mobile, does not move with respiration, and is resonant on percussion **(Fig. 51)**.

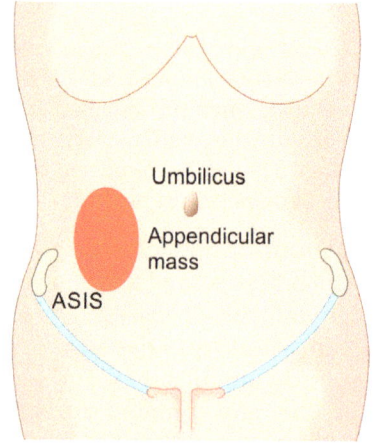

FIG. 51: Appendicular mass.

Post-appendicectomy Pyrexia

What to look in post-appendicectomy pyrexia?
- Wound for infection. Look for hyperemia, cellulitis, or pus discharge.
- Examine lungs for atelectasis or pneumonia.
- Examine legs to rule out DVT.
- DRE to rule out pelvic abscess.
- Keep in mind intraperitoneal abscess, i.e., 'when pus is somewhere, pus is nowhere, and pus is under diaphragm'. Remember this saying so you will not forget to examine the extra RIF sites of pus collection: Extra RIF sites of pus are—
  - Sub diaphragmatic abscess
  - Sub hepatic abscess
  - Paracolic abscess
  - Interloop small bowel abscess
  - Pelvic abscess
  - Abscess at operative site

CHAPTER 6 Diseases of Appendix

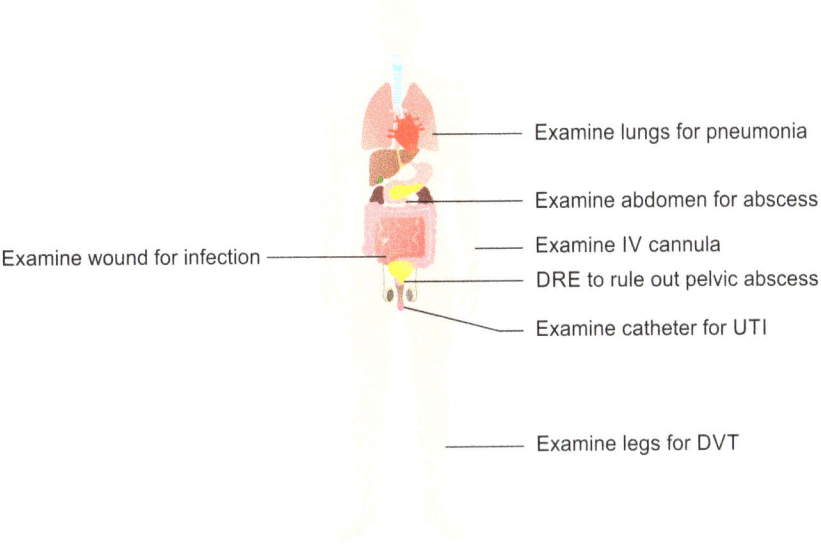

FIG. 52: Post-appendicectomy pyrexia.

- See IV cannula site for thrombophlebitis, change it every 3rd day.
- Catheter for UTI. UTI is one of the main causes of post-appendicectomy pyrexia as organism colonizes here and causes inflammation.
- Examine eyes—for jaundice—as pyrexia may be due to hepatitis.
- Examine urine for pyelonephritis.
- In child look tonsils for tonsillitis and ear for otitis media **(Fig. 52)**.

Mortality from Appendicitis

- Mortality from appendicitis is reducing. It was 9.9 deaths per 100,000 in 1939 and 0.2 per 100,000 in 1986.
- In ruptured appendix mortality increases up to 3%—a 50-fold increase, in elderly it goes up to 15%.[127]

'Acute appendicitis indicates silently that 'Don't mess with me' (don't delay the treatment) otherwise I will really mess with your health and even life.'
—**Vinod Kumar Nigam**

Main cause of mortality in appendicitis is 'burst appendix' usually due to delay in diagnosis or operation. There is a list of celebrities who died of appendicitis and its complications:

Juan Carreño, Óscar Catacora, Noah Caton, Paul Sentell, Herbert B Shonk, Sidney Howe Short etc.

Source: https://en.wikipedia.org/wiki/Category:Deaths_from_appendicitis.

Causes of Mortality

- Uncontrolled sepsis, i.e., septicemia, peritonitis, and intraperitoneal abscess
- Pulmonary embolism

Differential Diagnosis of Appendicular Mass (Fig. 53)

Differential diagnosis of appendicular mass:
- Carcinoma of cecum
- Ileocecal hyperplastic tuberculosis
- Crohn's disease
- Actinomycosis
- Ovarian carcinoma
- Ilial lymphadenitis
- Parametritis
- Amebic typhlitis
- Twisted ovarian cyst

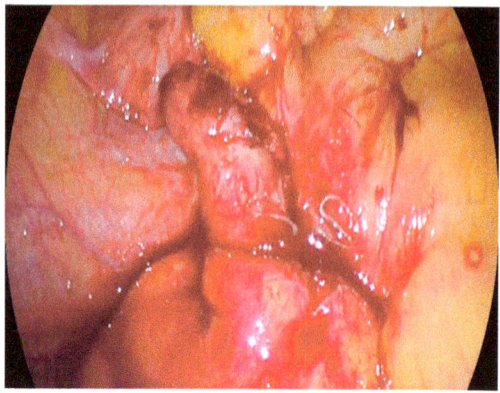

FIG. 53: Appendicular lump on exploration **(Video 8)**.

Treatment

The regimen of treatment is called 'Ochsner-Sherren regimen.'*

Principle of Ochsner–Sherren Regimen

The inflammatory process of acute appendicitis is localized. Appendicular mass formation is nature's protective phenomenon. The operative search for the appendix may prove difficult and dangerous due to edema of cecum and surrounding tissue, a fecal fistula can develop.

Ochsner-Sherren regimen is a preparation for operation and not a postponement of appendicectomy.

> *Ochsner–Sherren regimen:*
> - Bed rest
> - Nil orally
> - Nasogastric aspiration
> - Observation chart for pulse/temperature/size of mass
> - IV fluids
> - IV antibiotic

The OSR consists of:
- Bed rest
- Head end of bed is kept 30° up.

- Patient is kept nil orally. Gradually orally water started 30 mL hourly then 60 mL. First oral fluids are given then gradually semisolids and then solids are started in 3-4 days.
- Observation chart is maintained. Pulse and temperature recorded 4 hourly.
- Daily abdomen examined and reexamined
  o Limits of the lump is marked with a skin marker to see whether lump increases or decreases.
- Intake output chart is maintained.
- Hourly nasogastric aspiration by Ryle's* tube is done. Aspirate is collected, measured, color noted, and shown to surgeon.
- IV fluid intake record is kept.
- IV antibiotics—a third generation Cephalosporin and Metronidazole are given targeting aerobic, Gram-negative and anaerobic organisms.[93,128]
- After 48 hours clinical improvement should be seen.
- Oral hygiene is maintained by 8 hourly mouth washes.
- Deterioration in condition after 48 hours indicates development of peritonitis.
- If patient has not passed stool for 4-5 days then glycerin suppository is given.
- Desire for food occurs on 4th-5th day which is good sign.
- Usually an appendicular mass takes 2-6 weeks to resolve.

Contraindications of Ochsner–Sherren Regimen

- When one cannot make definite diagnosis between acute appendicitis and any other cause of acute abdomen which needs urgent operation, e.g., rupture of ectopic gestation.
- Infection is still limited to appendix and appendicectomy can be done.

---

*John Alfred Ryle (1889–1950), Professor of Physics, The University of Cambridge and Professor of Social Medicine, The University of Oxford, England; developed Ryle's tube in 1921.

- When the patient is an infant or child, perforation occurs early.
- If patient is >60 years of age when perforation and peritonitis occur without much sign.

Fate of Appendicular Lump
- Resolution or
- Appendicular abscess
- In 9-15% cases of appendicular lump OSR fails requiring operative intervention. Percutaneous or operative drainage of abscess is not considered as failure.[129] 40% patients require appendicectomy before the planned time of interval appendicectomy, 6-10 weeks.[130]

Future Plan
Interval appendicectomy is advised after complete resolution of appendicular mass. The full resolution of appendicular mass takes 6-8 weeks. So interval appendicectomy should be done after 6-8 weeks.

How You Assess Improvement by Ochsner-Sherren Regimen?
- Pain is diminishing and localizing.
- The size of lump is reducing.
- Temperature becoming normal
- Pulse rate returning to normal
- No vomiting and nasogastric aspiration is reducing in quantity. Patient is discharged only when he/she is taking normal diet and passing normal stools.

When to Stop Ochsner-Sherren Regimen?
- Rising pulse rate
- Increasing and spreading abdominal pain
- Increase in size of appendicular mass
- Increase in nasogastric aspiration amount or vomiting
- Diarrhea with infection, mucus in stool
  - This shows that patient is not getting controlled by nature and treatment anymore and peritonitis is setting in so urgent operation is required.

SEPTICEMIA
It can occur at any stage of acute appendicitis but commonly seen in perforation and peritonitis.

PORTAL PYAEMIA OR SUPPURATIVE PYLEPHLEBITIS AND PYEMIC ABSCESSES
Pus emboli from suppurative appendicitis enter tributaries of mesenteric vein reach liver causing multiple abscesses. These are caused by *E. coli* present with high fever and jaundice. Now it is not commonly seen due to good antibiotics **(Fig. 54)**.

> - Portal pyemia is a rare entity now. It is a form of septic portal system thrombosis and causes septicemia which is a dangerous entity and that is why carries a poor prognosis. It is common in immunosuppressed patients.
> - Portal pyemia causes tender and enlarged liver with jaundice.
> - It is treated by IV fluids and antibiotics.

Abscess can also develop due to portal pyemia in kidneys, lungs, brain, spleen etc. Pyrexia accompanies with chills, rigors, fever, and excessive sweating. Fever is intermittent with periods of a pyrexia. It may even run for months.

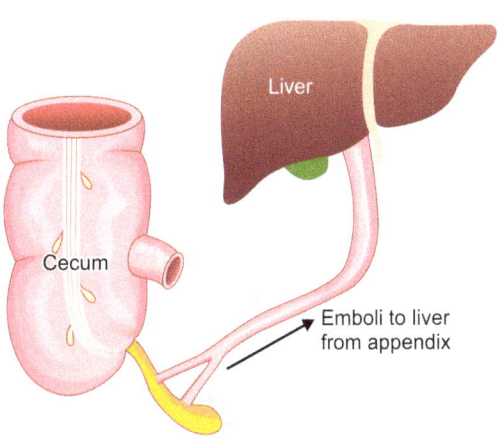

FIG. 54: Emboli from appendix reached liver via portal vein.

INFERTILITY

In a young girl perforated appendix can cause frozen pelvis, due to extensive chronic inflammation in pelvis leading to infertility.[131-134]

RECURRENT APPENDICITIS

See page 31.

OBLITERATION OF THE APPENDIX

Obliterated appendix appears as thick and rigid or it may become a thin fibrous strand or band. Whole appendix may be obliterated or only tip gets affected resulting in clubbed appearance. If the middle of the appendix is affected and atrophies then appendix appears as a dumbbell. The color of the appendix becomes pale in obliteration of appendix, but if only tip is involved then the rest of the appendix is pink as normal appendix. On cross section, the appendicular wall consists only of two layers, outer muscular layer and inner or central layer of fibrous tissue.

> Some researchers feel that obliteration of the appendix is not due to an inflammatory process, but is an involution process in a functionless appendix. Others believe it is due to a chronic inflammatory process forming fibrous tissue causing gradually complete obliteration of appendix lumen.

INTESTINAL OBSTRUCTION

Usually intestinal obstruction develops as a late complication of the acute appendicitis. It develops when patient recovers fully from attack of acute appendicitis, it may also develop in course of chronic appendicitis. The cause of intestinal obstruction is usually bands, or sharp flexure and adhesions developed due to earlier attack.

APPENDICULAR CYSTS

Retention cysts of appendix are produced in appendicitis if a portion of the lumen of appendix distal to the obstruction remains patent the normal secretion is accumulated and a retention cyst develops. Sometimes the appendicular luminal tube is occluded at more than one site then multiple cysts develop. Usually the contents of the retention cysts are clear.

> J Herb describes a case in which a globular cyst, 23 cm in circumference projected from middle of the appendix on the side opposite the mesenteric border, while in one case of Ribbert ………a cluster of cysts formed. (Appendicitis and Others Diseases of the Vermiform Appendix)

VASCULAR INFECTIONS AS COMPLICATION OF APPENDICITIS

Infection can spread far by circulation from infected appendix and can cause following complications:
- Thrombotic and embolic processes
- Erosion hemorrhage can occur in stomach and intestine in acute appendicitis.
- Gangrene by embolus blocking an artery.
- Lymphatic spread can lead to sub-phrenic abscess, or lymphadenitis.

Key Point
To avoid the complications of acute appendicitis in doubtful uncertain cases admit the patient and re-examine and re-evaluate the patient without feeling embarrassed or ashamed of not diagnosing at first instance.

CHAPTER 6 Diseases of Appendix

TREATMENT OF ACUTE APPENDICITIS

'The surgical student should be aware of the surgical consequences of the past, the tactics of the present and the strategy of immediate future.'
—Ian Aird

GENERAL PRINCIPLES

The goal of the treatment of acute appendicitis is three fold:
1. Early diagnosis
2. Urgent appendicectomy
3. Prevention of complications

Urgent appendicectomy is the golden rule—it is done by open, the conventional or by laparoscopic method.

The aim of doing appendicectomy is to prevent the complications of appendicitis so there should not be delay in removing the inflamed appendix.

On the other hand, the normal appendix should not be removed unnecessarily. Early diagnosis and early appendicectomy reduces incidence of complications, morbidity, and mortality.

The discomfort and risk associated with operation of appendicitis cannot be compared with discomfort and risk (morbidity and mortality) associated with perforation of appendix and peritonitis.

Appendicectomy is the treatment of choice for acute appendicitis.

Appendicectomy can be performed by two methods.
1. Open or conventional appendicectomy
2. Laparoscopic appendicectomy

Key Point

Urgent appendicectomy is the treatment of acute appendicitis but a delay of few hours with antibiotics in an admitted case is accepted.

PROGNOSIS OF ACUTE APPENDICITIS

'We know a great deal more about the causes of physical disease than we know about the causes of physical health.'
—M Scott Peck

- If appendicectomy is done properly and early then recovery is fast and patient goes home without any long term effects.
- The mortality in uncomplicated cases of acute appendicitis is <0.1%.
- The mortality in perforated appendix with peritonitis is <1%.
- The mortality in perforated appendix in elderly patients is up to 15–20%.
- The mortality rate of acute appendicitis is nowadays falling due to:
  ○ Early diagnosis
  ○ Early appendicectomy when the infection is limited to the appendix
  ○ Increasing awareness of the public.

SOME GOLDEN RULES IN ACUTE APPENDICITIS

'Happy is the one who has no serious consequences of his erroneous diagnosis to regret.'
—Marsh

- Rectal examination must be done in every patient of RIF pain.
- Gynecological examination is a must for every child-bearing age female especially 13–25 years suffering with RIF pain.
- There is no harm in removing a normal appendix but there is big harm in not removing inflamed appendix.
- Always examine external genitals in a young male with RIF pain.
- Take decision immediately and not to postpone it for next morning as hours matter in acute appendicitis not days.

- When you go for a ward round always examine the pulse of patient yourself.

> Are the symptoms, both general and local, subsiding; are they becoming more severe; or are they apparently stationary? If after 24 hours the patient is seemed to be getting worse instead of better, complications may usually be expected. If after 36–48 hours there is continuous high fever and a corresponding rapid pulse, suppuration or general infection is strongly suggested. A rapidly increasing pulse rate, especially when out of proportion to fever, is one of the most urgent symptoms, usually signifying gangrene or perforation with beginning peritoneal infection or general septicemia.
>
> —Harold A Kelly

ROLE OF ANTIBIOTICS IN RIGHT ILIAC FOSSA PAIN

'Some remedies are worse than the disease.'
—**Publilius Syrus**

- Do not give antibiotics blindly in RIF pain unless correct diagnosis is made. Antibiotic may mask the symptoms and signs of inflammation then diagnosis will be more difficult. Antibiotics may 'half treat' or 'partial treat' and it will remain a chronic problem.
- Pus of the abscess will become sterilized and it will be acting as a foreign body and an irritant causing pain.
- Remember pus cannot be absorbed by antibiotics, it has to be removed.
- Pelvic abscess can cause frozen pelvis if treated with antibiotics without drainage.
- Infertility is noted in females after pelvic abscess, especially when antibiotics are used for long without removing pus.
- In acute appendicitis, 'triple regimen' includes ampicillin, aminoglycoside, and metronidazole, was started 40 years back and is still in use. In every case of acute appendicitis we do not require this combination. In uncomplicated and simple appendicectomy antibiotics may not be required >1-2 days.

SOME IMPORTANT AND PRACTICAL HINTS TO THE BEGINNERS

'As a general rule, the most successful man in life is the man, who has the best information.'
—**Benjamin Disraeli**

- Do not rely solely on laboratory investigations, e.g., TLC and urine examination which can be normal.
- If you cannot diagnose for sure and have doubt then do not commit but reexamine the patient.
- Laparoscopy may be helpful in both diagnosis and treatment.
- Ultrasound of abdomen cannot diagnose 100% in early stage of acute appendicitis and it may be deceptive. So depend more upon signs and symptoms than on ultrasound. A normal ultrasound is not a contraindication for appendicectomy.
- Localized abscess can be aspirated by CT guidance under local anesthesia which reduces the morbidity.
- Do not try medical therapy, e.g., antibiotics, once you have made the diagnosis of appendicitis always advise urgent appendicectomy.
- With laparoscopy, several time-honored rituals have been proven unnecessary. Josef E Fischer, Editor of Master of Surgery, says 'We currently do not oversee the appendiceal stump or cauterize the mucosa after using a stapler.'[135,136]
- If you cannot decide, call some more experienced surgeon, remember your timely decision can prevent your patient's morbidity and mortality.
- Various studies have shown that during pregnancy laparoscopic appendectomy

can be done with low incidence of fetal loss.[137,138] But it should be done with caution.[139] Open approach should be used after first trimester.[140]

> Site of incision is very important in appendicitis operation. If the incision is not in right site then searching the appendix between the loops of small intestine can frustrate you.

SOLUTION

- Incision should not be >3 cm medial to ASIS.
- Give more importance to the situation of the appendix than cosmetic reason.
- Do not hesitate to enlarge the incision if you require more space.
- Do not hesitate to open the rectus sheath medially if you feel the space is less and a lot of retraction is required. The junction of internal oblique muscle and rectus sheath is the thinnest part so incise here.
- The best way to gain more space is to enlarge the incision by cutting deep muscles in the line of skin incision and converting a muscle splitting to muscle cutting, incision and catch the bleeders.[136]

OTHER CONDITIONS OF APPENDIX

- Mucocele of appendix
- Pyocele of appendix or empyema of appendix
- Intussusception of appendix
- Diverticulum of appendix
- Cyst of appendix

MUCOCELE OF APPENDIX

Mucocele of appendix is a retention cyst of appendix. It is of four types:
1. Retention cyst
2. Mucosal hyperplasia
3. Cystadenoma
4. Cystadenocarcinoma

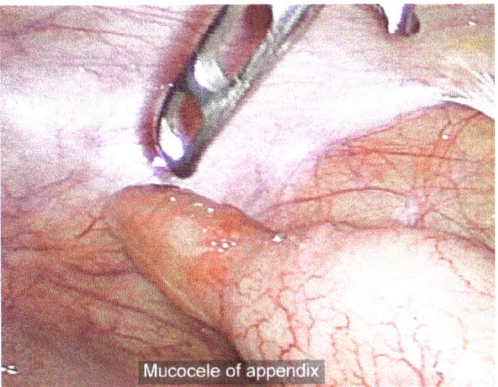

FIG. 55: Mucocele of appendix.

Sometimes obstruction of lumen of appendix happens without development of infection, it leads to mucocele of appendix as mucus secretion continues in spite of obstruction of the lumen of appendix. The mucus gets collected in appendix. It should be differentiated from cystadenocarcinoma of appendix **(Fig. 55)**.

The symptoms of mucocele of appendix are like mild recurrent appendicitis. If infection occurs then it turns to empyema of the appendix. It is diagnosed by ultrasound and CT scan.

Treatment of mucocele of appendix is appendicectomy.

Malignant Mucocele

It is a mucous papillary adenocarcinoma grade I of appendix.

PYOCELE OF APPENDIX OR EMPYEMA OF APPENDIX

- Distention of appendix with pus is called 'empyema or pyocele' of appendix.
- Mucocele of appendix may convert to empyema due to infection and pus formation.
- Rupture of empyema of appendix causes generalized peritonitis.
- Treatment of empyema of appendix is appendicectomy.

INTUSSUSCEPTION OF APPENDIX

It is a rare condition and usually occurs in children. It is diagnosed only when operation is done for acute appendicitis.

Clinical Features

Its symptoms are of subacute appendicitis.

Complications

- Appendicocecal or appendiculo-cecocolic intussusception.
- Appendix may slough out and treated as agenesis of appendix later on.

Treatment: Appendicectomy

Diverticulum of Appendix

It is a rare entity.

Diverticulum of appendix is of two types **(Fig. 56)**
1. Congenital or true diverticulum.
   - It has all the layers of wall of appendix.
2. Acquired or false diverticulum

It has only mucus membrane and no muscle layer. It occurs due to rise of pressure inside the lumen of appendix as in mucocele. The mucosa is pushed out of weak spots in muscle layer, 'Hiatus muscularis.'

Diverticula of appendix can also occur by external traction by adhesions. When the lumen of appendix gets blocked at a place cystic distension of appendix occurs which follows development of diverticulum. It is more common when the muscular walls of the appendix are weakened. Appendicular diverticula may be single or multiple. Most of the diverticula in an appendix developed between the folds of mesoappendix. Diverticula of appendix can occur at any site in appendix, but commonly found at the tip of the appendix.

TUMORS OF APPENDIX

'We often make progress by reading the work of the great men of the past.'
—Charles H Mayo (1865–1939)

Tumors of appendix:
- Benign tumors:
  - Lymphoma
  - Fibroma
  - Myxoma
  - Angioma
  - Myoma
  - Endometriosis
- Malignant tumors:
  - Carcinoid tumor
  - Adenocarcinoma
  - Pseudomyxoma peritonei

These are extremely rare tumors.

Mostly the tumors of appendix are malignant, benign tumors are rarer than malignant tumors.

Key Point

If a perforated appendix is found during laparoscopy continue and complete appendicectomy laparoscopically.

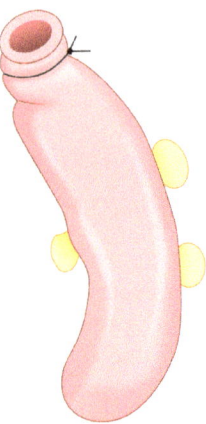

FIG. 56: Diverticula of appendix.

BENIGN TUMORS OF APPENDIX

Following benign tumors of appendix are reported but are extremely rare.
- Lymphoma
- Fibroma
- Myxoma
- Angioma
- Myoma
- Endometriosis

Endometriosis

Endometriosis of appendix is not an extremely rare entity. It causes pain in RIF which becomes monthly and is associated with melena.

Treatment: Appendicectomy

MALIGNANT TUMORS OF APPENDIX

- Carcinoid tumor or argentaffinoma of appendix
- Adenocarcinoma of appendix
- Pseudomyxoma peritonei

Carcinoid Tumor or Argentaffinoma of Appendix

It is found one case in 400 appendix specimens subjected for histopathology after appendicectomy in acute appendicitis. One study has shown mean age of carcinoid of appendix 42.2 years and predominance in females.[141]

Origin
- Kulchitsky cells of crypts of Lieberkühn (Johann Nathanael Lieberkühn, 1711–1756, physician and anatomist, Berlin, Germany).
- It is the commonest tumor of appendix.
- Most common site of carcinoid tumor is appendix.

Site
- It can be found at tip, base, or body of appendix.
- Most commonly it is found near tip of appendix, (70% cases).

Pathology
- It is yellow, firm and small tumor.
- It is situated between mucosa and peritoneal coat of appendix.
- Tumor cells are typically arranged in small nests.
- Carcinoid tumor of appendix very rarely gives metastasis, only in 2% cases. One unique carcinoid tumor is 'Goblet cell carcinoid' (adenocarcinoma). The histological behavior of tumor is between carcinoid tumor and adenocarcinoma of appendix.
- This tumor arises from argentaffin or enterochromaffin cells. Argentaffin cells are present among the cells lining the wall of appendix. The cytoplasmic granules of these cells stain black with silver salts so called 'Argentaffin' and brown with chromium salts so called 'Enterochromaffin' cells. They are classified as a type of APUD cells.

Treatment

The malignant potential of the tumor is related to its size.
- Appendicectomy is the treatment of choice if the tumor is <2 cm in size.
- Right hemicolectomy is done if:
  - Tumor is >2 cm in size
  - Cecal wall is involved.
  - Regional lymph nodes are enlarged.

Carcinoid Syndrome

It is due to chemicals in carcinoid tumor. These chemicals are:
- 5-HT (5-hydroxytryptamine or serotonin)
- 5-hydroxytryptophan
- 5-HIAA

- Histamine
- Kallikrein
- Bradykinin

Clinical Features of Carcinoid Syndrome

Carcinoid tumors which metastasize to liver are sometimes associated with a symptom complex called carcinoid syndrome which is characterized by mnemonic (Mn)—DABAR.
D – Diarrhea
A – Attack of bronchial asthma due to histamine.
B – Increased borborygmi
A – Attack of flushing of face is induced by alcohol.
R – Reddish blue hue (cyanosis) due to histamine.

Carcinoid syndrome is rarely associated with appendix carcinoid unless widespread metastases are present, which occurs in 2.9% of cases. Symptoms due to carcinoid are rare although tumor can obstruct the appendix lumen and result in acute appendicitis.[142-144]

Adenocarcinoma of Appendix

The most common presentation of carcinoma of appendix is acute appendicitis.
- It is a very rare tumor.
- Usually the tumors are diagnosed late.
- Neoplasm occurs is three major histologic subtypes.[145]
  - Mucinous adenocarcinoma
  - Colonic adenocarcinoma
  - Adenocarcinoid
- Mucus secreting adenocarcinoma of appendix can rupture and disseminate malignant cells in peritoneal cavity and cause pseudomyxoma peritonei.
- 10% patients have dissemination at the time of operation.

Malignant mucocele: It is a mucus secreting papillary adenocarcinoma where appendix gets distended with mucoid secretion.

Treatment
- Right hemicolectomy.
- If pseudomyxoma peritonei then resection of involved peritoneum is also done and then chemotherapy is given.

Pseudomyxoma Peritonei

Recent studies suggest that appendix is the site of origin for most of the cases of pseudomyxoma and not ovary.

Mucin-secreting adenoma (mucinous cyst adenoma) and adenocarcinoma (mucinous cyst adenocarcinoma) invade through the wall of appendix and produce intraperitoneal seedlings and spread to whole peritoneal cavity. Abdomen is filled with yellow-colored jelly. It is a locally malignant condition. It does not give extraperitoneal metastasis. Diagnosis is made by ultrasound and CT scan. It is three times more common in females than males.

Treatment

Debulking surgery is done with appendicectomy. The jelly is scoped out. Recurrence is common but takes years to develop.[47,146] Resection of peritoneum and intraperitoneal chemotherapy helps some patients.

> **Key Point**
> Computed tomography scan is a must after resolution of an appendicular mass in a patient >50 years of age so not to miss a tumor of appendix or cecum which are mostly malignant.

VIDEOS

Video 1: Acute on Chronic Appendicitis—Spiral Appendix
Video 2: Adhesions due to Previous Attacks of Appendicitis
Video 3: Purulent Appendicitis with Perforation

Video 4: Acutely Inflamed Appendix
Video 5: Retrocecal Appendicitis—Exploration
Video 6: Subcecal Appendicitis
Video 7: Appendicular Lump—Base of Appendix Detached
Video 8: Appendicular Lump—Exploration

REFERENCES

1. Fitz RH. Persistent omphalo – mesenteric remains: their importance in the causation of intestinal duplication, cyst formation, and obstruction. Am J Med Sci. 1884;88:30.
2. Skandalakis JE, Gray SW, Ricketts R. The colon and rectum. In: Skandalakis JE, Gray SW (Ed): Embryology for Surgeons. Baltimore: Williams and Wilkins; 1994. p. 242.
3. Buschard K, Kjaeldgaard A. Investigation and analysis of the position, fixation, length and embryology of the vermiform appendix. Acta Chir Scand. 1973;139:293.
4. Ajmani ML, Ajmani K. The position, length and arterial supply of vermiform appendix. Anat Anz. 1983;153:369.
5. Fayez JA, Toy NJ, Flanagan TM. The appendix as the cause of chronic lower abdominal pain. Am J Obstet Gynecol. 195;172:122-23.
6. Jaffe BM, Berger DH. Schwartz's Principles of surgery, 8th edition. New York: McGraw Hill; 2005. p. 1133.
7. Cooperman M. Complications of appendectomy. Surg Clin North Am. 1983;63:1233.
8. Paterson – Brown S, Thomson BNJ. The Acute Abdomen and Peritoneal Cavity Surgical Studies, 3rd edition. Amsterdam: Elsevier; 2005. p. 584.
9. Fernel J. Universa medicina. In: Major RH (Ed). Classic Descriptions of Disease, 3rd edition. Springfield, IL: CC Thomas; 1945. pp. 646-8.
10. Kelly HA. Appendicitis and Others Diseases of the Vermiform Appendix. Philadelphia: J. B. Lippincott Company; 1905. p. 68.
11. Graffeo CS, Counselman FL. Appendicitis. Emerg Med Clin North Am. 1996;14:653-71.
12. Kelly HA. Appendicitis and Others Diseases of the Vermiform Appendix. Philadelphia: J. B. Lippincott Company; 1905; 25.
13. Fitz RH. Perforating inflammation of the vermiform appendix, with special reference to its early diagnosis and treatment. Trans Assoc Am Physicians. 1886;1:107-44.
14. Seal A. Appendicitis: a historical review. Can J Surg. 1981;24:427-33.
15. Flum DR, Morris A, Koepsell T, Dellinger EP. Has misdiagnosis of appendicitis decreased over time? A population-based analysis. JAMA. 2001;286:1748-53.
16. Kelly HA. Appendicitis and Others Diseases of the Vermiform Appendix. Philadelphia: J. B. Lippincott Company; 1905; 56
17. Kelly HA. Appendicitis and Others Diseases of the Vermiform Appendix. Philadelphia: J. B. Lippincott Company; 1905; 57
18. Kelly HA. Appendicitis and Others Diseases of the Vermiform Appendix. Philadelphia: J. B. Lippincott Company; 1905; 58
19. Kelly HA. Appendicitis and Others Diseases of the Vermiform Appendix. Philadelphia: J. B. Lippincott Company; 1905; 59
20. Kelly HA. Appendicitis and Others Diseases of the Vermiform Appendix. Philadelphia: J. B. Lippincott Company; 1905; 60-61.
21. Kelly HA. Appendicitis and Others Diseases of the Vermiform Appendix. Philadelphia: J. B. Lippincott Company; 1905; 66-67.
22. Tail L. Surgical treatment of typhlitis. Birmingham Med Vev. 1890;27:26-34.
23. Owen TD, Williams H, Stiff G, Jenkinson LR, Rees BI. Evaluation of the Alvarado score in acute appendicitis. J R Soc Med. 1992;85:87-9.
24. Mann CV, Russell RCG, Williams NS. Bailey and Love's Short Practice of Surgery, 22nd edition. United Kingdom: Chapman and Hall; 1995. p. 832.
25. Kelly HA. Appendicitis and Others Diseases of the Vermiform Appendix. Philadelphia: J. B. Lippincott Company; 1905; 139-140.
26. Hale DA, Molloy M, Pearl RH, Schutt DC, Jaques DP. Appendectomy: A Contemporary appraisal. Ann Surg. 1997;225(3):252-61.
27. Wangensteen OH, Buirge RE, Dennis C, Ritchie WP. Studies in the etiology of acute appendicitis: the significance of the structure and function of the vermiform appendix in the genesis of appendicitis. Ann Surg. 1937;106:910-42.
28. Wangensteen OH, Dennis C. Experimental proof of the obstructive origin of appendicitis in man. Ann Surg. 1939;110:629-47.
29. Jeffery RB, Fainig FC, Townsend RC. Acute appendicitis; Sonographic Criteria based on 250 cases. Radiology. 1987;163:11-14,
30. Kokoska ER, Silen ML, Tracy TF Jr., Dillon PA, Kennedy DJ, Cradock TV, et al. The impact of intraoperative culture on treatment and outcome in children with perforated appendicitis. J Pediatr Surg. 1999;34:749.
31. Baron EJ, Bennion R, Thompson J, Strong C, Summanen P, McTeague M, et al. A microbiological comparison between acute and complicated appendicitis. Clin Infect Dis. 1992;14:227-231.

32. Bennion RS, Baron EJ, Thompson JE, Downes J, Summanen P, Talan DA, et al. The bacteriology of gangrenous and perforated appendicitis revisited. Ann Surg. 1990;211:165-71.
33. Altemeier WA. The bacterial flora of acute perforated appendicitis with peritonitis. Ann Surg. 1938;107:517-28.
34. Bilik R, Burnweit C, Shandling B. Is abdominal cavity culture of any value in appendicitis? Am J Surg. 1998;175:267-70.
35. Singh JP, Mariadson JG. Role of the faecolith in modern-day appendicitis. Ann R Coll Surg Engl. 2013; 95:48-51.
36. Teixeira PG, Demetriades D. Appendicitis: changing perspectives. Adv Surg. 2013;47:119-40.
37. Farmer DL. Clinical practice guidelines for paediatric complicated appendicitis: the value in discipline. JAMA Surg. 2016;151(5):e160193.
38. D`Souza N, Nugent K. Appendicitis. Am Fam Physician. 2016;93:142-3.
39. Harkin AH, Moove EE. Abernathy's Surgical Secrets, 5th edition. Amsterdam: Elsevier; 2004. pp. 139-41.
40. Petroianu A. (2012). Acute appendicitis: propedeutics and diagnosis. Inflammatory diseases. [online] Available from https://cdn.intechopen.com/pdfs/28061/InTech-Acute_appendicitis_propedeutics_and_diagnosis.pdf. [Last accessed January, 2024].
41. Petroianu A, Alberti LR, Zac RI. Faecal loading in the cecum as a new radiological sign of acute appendicitis. World J Gastroenterol. 2005;11: 4230-32.
42. Petroianu A, Alberti LR, Zac RI. Assessment of the persistence of fecal loading in the cecum in presence of acute appendicitis. Int J Surg. 2007;5:11-6.
43. 115.Rautio M, Saxen H, Siitonen A, Nikku R, Jousimies-Somer H. Bacteriology of histopathologically defined appendicitis in children. Pediatr Infect Dis J. 2000;19:1078-83.
44. Miranda R, Johnston AD, O'Leary JP. Incidental appendectomy: Frequency of pathologic abnormalities. Am Surg. 1980;46(3):355-7.
45. Soffer D, Zait S, Klausner J, Kluger Y. Peritoneal cultures and antibiotic treatment in patients with perforated appendicitis. Eur J Surg. 2001;167: 214-6.
46. Lemieur TP, Rodriguez JL, Jacobs DM, Bennett ME, West MA. Wound management in perforated appendicitis. Am Surg 1999;65:339-443.
47. Fisher KS, Ross DS. Guidelines for therapeutic decision in incidental appendectomy. Surg Gynecol Obstet 1990;171:95-98.
48. Franke C, Bohner H, Yang Q, Ohmann C, Röher HD. World J Surg. 1999;23:141-6.
49. Irvin TT. Abdominal pain: a surgical audit of 1190 emergency admissions. Br J Surg. 1989;76:1121-5.
50. Flum DR, Koepsell T. The clinical and economic correlates of misdiagnosed appendicitis: Nationwide analysis. Arch Surg. 2002;137:799.
51. Jaffe BM, Berger DH. Schwartz's Principles of surgery, 8th edition. New York: McGraw Hill; 2005. p. 1120.
52. Burkitt DP. The aetiology of appendicitis. Br J Surg. 1971;58:695-9.
53. Butler C. Surgical pathology of acute appendicitis. Hum Pathol. 1981;12:870.
54. Hinson FL, Ambrose NS. Pseudomyxoma Peritonei. Br J Surg. 1998;85:1332.
55. Fischer JE. Appendicitis and appendiceal abscess, Editors comment, mastery of surgery, 5th edition. Philadelphia: Lippincott Williams and Wilkins; 2007. p. 1439.
56. Mosdell DM, Morris DM, Fry DE. Peritoneal cultures and antibiotic therapy in pediatric perforated appendicitis. Am J Surg. 1994;167:313.
57. Dunning PG, Goddman MD. The incidence and value of rectal examination in children with suspected appendicitis. Ann R, Coll Surg Engl. 1991;73:233-4.
58. Finlay DJ, Doherty GM, et al. Acute Abdominal pain and appendicitis, The Washington Manual of surgery. Philadelphia: Lippincott Williams and Wilkins; 2002. p. 592.
59. Schwartz SI. Appendix. In: Schwartz SI, Shires GT, Spencer FC (Eds). Principles of surgery, 5th edition, Volume 2. New York: McGraw Hill; 1989. p. 1135.
60. Teacher I, Landa B, Cohen M, Kabnick LS, Wise L. Scoring system to aid in diagnoses of appendicitis. Ann Surg. 1983;198:753-9.
61. Shaffer HA, Harrison RB. CAS in the appendix: A sometimes significant but nonspecific diagnostic sign. Arch Surg. 1979;114:587-9.
62. Pittman-Waller VA, Myers JG, Stewart RM, Dent DL, Page CP, Gray GA, et al. appendicitis: why so complicated? Analysis of 5755 consecutive appendectomies. Am Surg. 2000;66:548-54.
63. Puylaert JBCM, Rutgers PH, Lalisang RI, de Vries BC, van der Werf SD, Dörr JP, et al: N Engl J Med. 1987;317:666-9.
64. Roosevelt GE, Reynolds SL. Acad Emerg Med. 1998;5:1071-75.
65. Hale DA, Jaques DP, Molloy M, Pearl RH, Schutt DC, d'Avis JC. Appendectomy. Improving care through quality improvement. Arch Surg. 1997;132:153-7.
66. Randen AV, Lameris W, Wouter H, et al. A comparison of the Accuracy of Ultrasound and Computed Tomography in common diagnoses causing acute abdominal pain. Eur Radiol. 2011;21(7):1535-45.

67. Berry J, Malt RA. Appendicitis near its centenary. Ann Surg. 1984;200:567.
68. Chen SC, Chem KM, Wong SM, Chang KJ. Abdominal sonography screening of clinically diagnosed suspected appendicitis before surgery. World J Surg. 1998;22:449-52.
69. Puylaert JBCM. Acute appendicitis: US evaluation using graded compression. Radiology. 1986;158:355-60.
70. Puig S, Hormann M, Rebhandl W, Felder-Puig R, Prokop M, Paya K. US as a primary diagnostic tool in relation to negative appendectomy: Six years' experience. Radiology. 2003;226:101-4.
71. Bower RJ, Bell MJ, Ternberg JL. Diagnostic value of the white blood count and neutrophil percentage in the evaluation of abdominal pain in children. Surg Gynecol Obstet. 1981;152:424-6.
72. Smith DE, Kirchmer NA, Stewart DR. Use of the barium enema in the diagnosis of acute appendicitis and its complications. Am J Surg. 1979;138:829.
73. Douglas CD, Macpherson NE, Davidson PM, Gani JS. Randomised controlled trial of Ultrasonography in diagnosis of acute appendicitis, incorporating the Alvarado score. Brit Med J. 2000;321(7266):919-22.
74. Balthazar EJ, Rofsky NM, Zucker R. Appendicitis: The impact of computed tomography imaging on negative appendectomy and perforation rates. Am J Gastroenterol. 1998;93:768-71.
75. Weyrant MJ, Eachempati SR, Maluccio MN, Spigland N, Hydo LJ, Barie PS. The use of computed tomography for the diagnosis of acute appendicitis in children does not influence the overall rate of negative appendectomy or perforation. Surg Infect. 2001;2:19-23.
76. Funaki B, Grosskreutz SR, Funaki CN. Using unenhanced helical CT with enteric contrast material for suspected appendicitis in patients treated at a community hospital. Am J Roentgenol. 1998;171:997.
77. Raman SS, Lu DSK, Kadell BM, Vodopich DJ, Sayre J, Cryer H. Accuracy of nonfocused helical CT for the diagnosis of acute appendicitis: A 5-years review. Am J Roentgenol. 2002;178:1319-25.
78. Stroman DL, Bayouth CV, Kuhn JA, Westmoreland M, Jones RC, Fisher TL, et al. The role of computed tomography in the diagnosis of acute appendicitis. Am J Surg. 1999;178:485-9.
79. Raptopoulos V, Katsou G, Rosen MP, Siewert B, Goldberg SN, Kruskal JB. Acute appendicitis: Effect of increased use of CT on selecting patients earlier. Radiology. 2003;226:521-6.
80. Wilson EB, Cole JC, Nipper ML, Cooney DR, Smith RW. Computed tomography and Ultrasonography in the diagnosis of appendicitis. Arch Surg. 2001;136(6):670-5.
81. Urban BA, Fishman EK. Targeted helical CT of the acute abdomen: Appendicitis, diverticulitis, and small bowel obstruction. Semin Ultrasound CT MR. 2000;21:20-39.
82. Lally KP. Appendix. In: Townsend CM, David C. Sabiston Textbook of surgery, volume 2, 17th edition. Amsterdam; Elsevier; 2004. p. 1384.
83. Rao PM, Rhea JT, Novelline RA, Mostafavi AA, Lawrason JN, McCabe CJ. Helical computed tomography combined with contrast material administered only through the colon for imaging of suspected appendicitis. AJR Am J Roentgenol. 1997;169:1275-80.
84. Bendeck SE, Nino-Murcia M, Berry GJ, Jeffrey RB Jr. Imaging for suspected appendicitis: Negative appendectomy and perforation rates. Radiology. 2002;225:131-6.
85. Naoum JJ, Mileshi WJ, Daller JA, Gomez GA, Gore DC, Kimbrough TD, et al. The use of abdominal computed tomography scan decreases the frequency of misdiagnosis in cases of suspected appendicitis. Am J Surg. 2002;184:587-90.
86. Fuchs JR, Schlamberg JS, Shorteeve MJ, Schuler JG. Impact of abdominal CT imaging on the management of appendicitis: An update. J Surg Res. 2002;106(1):131-6.
87. Rao PM, Rhea JT, Rattner DW, Venus LG, Novelline RA. Introduction of appendiceal CT: Impact on negative appendectomy and appendiceal perforation rates. Ann Surg. 1999;229(3):344-9.
88. McCusker ME, Cote TR, Clegg LX, Sobin LH. Primary malignant neoplasms of the appendix: A population – based study from the Surveillance, Epidemiology and Results program, 1973 – 1998. Cancer. 2002;94:3307-12.
89. Chan MYP, Tan C, Chiu MT, et al. Surg JR Coll Surg Edinblrel. 2003;1:39-41.
90. Kipper SL Rypins EB, Evans DG, Thakur ML, Smith TD, Rhodes B. Neutrophil-specific 99mmTc-labeled anti-CD15 Monoclonal antibody imaging for diagnosis of equivocal appendicitis. J Nucl Med. 2000;41:449-55.
91. Typins EB, Kpper SL. 99mmTc-hexamethylpropyleneaurine scan for diagnosing acute appendicitis in children. Ann Surg. 1997;63:878-81.
92. Wong DW, Vasinrapec P, Spieth ME, Cook RE, Ansari AN, Jones M Jr, et al. Rapid detection of acute appendicitis with 99mmTc-labeled intact polyvalent human immune globulin. J Am Coll Surg. 1997;185:534-43.
93. Nitecki S, Assalia A, Schein M. Contemporary management of the appendiceal mass. Br J Surg. 1993;80:88-20.
94. Silen W. Cop's Early Diagnosis of the Acute Abdomen, 20th edition. New York: Oxford University Press; 2000.

95. Deans GT, Spence RA. Neoplastic lesions of the appendix. Br J Surg. 1995;82:299.
96. Bongard F, landers DV, Lewis F. Differential diagnosis of appendicitis and pelvic inflammatory disease. A prospective analysis. Am J Surg. 1985;150:90.
97. Jepsen OB, Korner B, Lauritsen KB, Hancke AB, Andersen L, Henrichsen S, et al. Yersinia enterocolitica infection in patients with acute surgical abdominal disease. A Prospective study. Scand J Infect Dis. 1976;8:189-94.
98. Knight PJ, Vassy LE. Specific diseases mimicking appendicitis in childhood. Arch Surg. 1981;116: 744.
99. McDonald JC. Nonspecific mesenteric lymphadenitis: Collective review. Surg Gynecol Obstet. 1963;116:409.
100. Morrison JD. Yersinia and viruses in acute non-specific abdominal pain and appendicitis. Br J Surg. 1981;68:284.
101. Rao PM, Rhea JT, Novelline RA, Mostafavi AA, McCabe treatment of patients and use of hospital resources. N Engl J Med. 1998;338:141-6.
102. Urbach DR. Appendectomy, controversies in Laparoscopic surgery. Berlin/Heidelberg: Springer, Springer International Edition; 2006. p. 375.
103. Ellis BW. Hamilton Baileys Emergency Surgery, 13th edition. London: Hodder Arnold; 2006. p. 401.
104. McBurney C. The incision made in the abdominal wall in cases of appendicitis. Ann Surg. 1994;20:38.
105. Seem K. Endoscopic appendectomy. Endoscopy. 1983;15:59.
106. Hardin D. Acute appendicitis: review and update. Am Fam Physician. 1999;60:2027-36.
107. Yamini D, Hernan V, Bongard F, Klein S, Stamos MJ. Perforated appendicitis: is it truly a surgical urgency? Am Surg. 1998;64:970-5.
108. Hui TT, Major KM, Avital I, Hiatt JR, Margulies DR. Outcome of elderly patients with appendicitis. Arch Surg. 2002;137:995-1000.
109. Al-Mulhim AA. Acute appendicitis in pregnancy: A review of 52 cases. Int Surg. 1996;81:295-7.
110. Mann CV, Russell RCG, Williams NS. Bailey and Love's Short Practice of Surgery, 22nd edition. UK: Chapman and Hall; 1995. p. 833.
111. Jaffe BM, Berger DH. Schwartz's Principles of Surgery, 8th edition. New York: McGraw Hill; 2005. p 1127.
112. Jaffe BM, Berger DH. Schwartz's Principles of Surgery, 8th edition. New York: McGraw Hill; 2005, p 1128.
113. Wells SB, Beaton HL. Appendiceal disease in HIV – infected homosexual men. AIDS Reader Sept/Oct: 173, 1991.
114. Flum DR, Steinberg SD, Sarkis AY, Wallack MK. Appendicitis in patients with acquired immunodeficiency syndrome. J Am Coll Surg. 1997;184:481-6.
115. Mueller GP, Williams RA. Surgical infections in Aids patients Am J Surg. 1995;169(5A Suppl):34S.
116. Bova R, Meagher A: Appendicitis in HIV – Positive patients. Aust N Z J Surg. 1998;68:337-9.
117. Lowy AM, Barie PS. Laparotomy in patients infected with human immunodeficiency virus: Indications and outcome. Br J Surg. 1994;81:942.
118. Whitney TM, Macho JR, Russell TR, Bossart KJ, Heer FW, Schecter WP. Appendicitis in acquired immunodeficiency syndrome. Am J Surg. 1992;164:467-70.
119. Mangi AA, Berger DL. Stump appendicitis. Am Surg. 2000;66:739-41.
120. Lowe LH, Penney MW, Scheker LE, Perez R Jr, Stein SM, Heller RM, et al. Appendicolith revealed on CT in children with suspected appendicitis: how specific is it in the diagnosis of appendicitis? AJR Am J Roentgenol. 2000;175:981-4.
121. Smink DS, Soybel DI. Appendix and Appendictomy, Maingots Abdominal operations, 11th edition. New York: McGraw Hill; 2007. p. 607.
122. Prown SP. Acute Appendicitis, Hamilton Bailey's Emergency surgery, 13th edition. London: Hodder Arnold; 2006. p. 401.
123. Burnand KG, Young AE, Lucas J. The New Aivd's companion in Surgical studies, 3rd edition. Amsterdam: Elsevier; 2005. p. 582.
124. Lewis F. Appendix. In: Davis JH (Ed). Clinical Surgery, 1st edition, Volume 1. St. Louis: Mosby; 1987. p. 1581.
125. Cuschievi A, Steele RJC, Moossa AR. Essential Surgical Practice, 4th edition. London: Hodder Arnold; 2002; p. 563.
126. Jordan JS, Kovalcik PJ, Schwab CW. Appendicitis with a palpable mass. Ann Surg. 1981;193:227-9.
127. Encohsson L, Hellberg A, Rudberg C, Fenyö G, Gudbjartsson T, Kullman E, et al. Laparoscopic vs. open appendectomy in overweight patients. Surg Endosc. 2001;15:387-92.
128. Gillick J, Velayudham M, Puri P. Conservative management of appendix mass in children. Br J Surg. 2001;88:1539-42.
129. Sauerland S, Lefering R, Neugebauer EA. Laparoscopic versus open surgery for suspected appendicitis. Cochrane Database Syst Rev. 2002;(1):CD001546,
130. Scott-Conner CE. Laparoscopic gastrointestinal surgery. Med Clin North Am. 2002;86:1401.
131. Andersson R, Lambe M, Bergstrom R. Fertility patterns after appendicectomy: Historical cohort study, BMJ. 1999;318:963-7.

132. Urbach DR, Cohen MM. Is perforation of the appendix a risk factor for tubal infertility and ectopic pregnancy? An appraisal of the evidence. Can J Surg. 1999;42:101-8.
133. Mueller BA, Daling JR, Moore DE, Weiss NS, Spadoni LR, Stadel BV, et al. Appendectomy and the risk of tubal infertility. N Engl J Med. 1986;315:1506-8.
134. Puri P, McGuinness EP, Guiney EJ. Fertility following perforated appendicitis in girls. J Pediatr Surg. 1989;24:547-9.
135. Jones DB. Laparoscopic Appendectomy, mastery of surgery, 5th edition. Philadelphia: Lippincott Williams and Wilkins; 2007. p. 1439.
136. Paterson–Brown S. Acute Appendicitis Hamilton Baileys Emergency Surgery, 13th edition. London: Hodder Arnold; 2006. p. 403.
137. Ortega AE, Hunter JG, Peters JH, Swanstrom LL, Schirmer B. Laparoscopic Appendectomy Study Group. A prospective, randomized comparison of laparoscopic appendectomy with open appendectomy. Am J Surg. 1995;169:208-12;discussion 212-3.
138. Urbach DR. Appendectomy, controversies in Laparoscopic surgery. Berlin/Heidelberg: Springer, Springer International Edition; 2006. p. 380.
139. De Perrot M, Jenny AM, Kohlik M, Morel P. Laparoscopic appendectomy during pregnancy. Surg Laparosc Endosc Percutan Tech. 2000;10:368-71.
140. Friedman JD, Ramsey PS, Ramin KD, Berry C. Pneumoamnion and pregnancy loss after second-trimester laparoscopic surgery. Obstet Gynecol. 2002;99(3):512-3.
141. Sandor A, Modlin IM. A retrospective analysis of 1570 appendiceal carcinoids. Am J Gastroenterol. 1998;93:422-8.
142. Leardi S, Delmonaco S, Ventura T, Chiominto A, De Rubeis G, Simi M.. Recurrent abdominal pain and 'chronic appendicitis.' Minerva Chir. 2000;55:39.
143. Mussack T, Schmidbauer S, Nerlich A, Schmidt W, Hallfeldt KK. Chronic appendicitis as an independent clinical entity. Chirurg. 2002;73:710-5.
144. Wang HT, Sax HC. Incidental appendectomy in the era of managed care and laparoscopy. J Am Coll Surg. 2001;192:182.
145. Sugimoto T, Edwards D. Incidence and costs of incidental appendectomy as a preventive measure. Am J public Health. 1987;77:471.
146. Connor SJ, Hanna GB, Firzelle FA. Appendiceal tumors: Retrospective clinicopathologic analysis of appendiceal tumors from 7970 appendectomies. Dis Colon Rectum. 1998;41:75.

CHAPTER 7

Operative Surgery of Appendix

*'It takes 5 years to learn when to operate and
25 years to learn when not to.'*
—Anonymous

INTRODUCTION

Since the first appendicectomy done by Claudius Amyand in 1735 on a boy, it is the treatment of choice for appendicitis. Appendicitis is a common problem and the gold standard treatment of appendicitis is appendicectomy. There is a possibility of developing complications in inflamed appendix if there is a delay in appendicectomy. Complications can be serious like perforation of the appendix and general peritonitis and therefore, the appendicectomy for inflamed appendicectomy is considered as medical emergency. The delay in diagnosis and treatment of appendicitis is at all costs must be avoided to not to put the life of the patient in danger. Emergency appendicectomy is one of the most commonly performed emergency surgery all over the world. Appendicectomy can be performed by open or conventional method or endoscopically by laparoscopic method. Usually the appendicectomy whether done by laparoscopic method or open is a safe operation. Appendicectomy usually does not cause any problem in future life. One can live normally with no appendix.

> **Things to remember:**
> - Appendicectomy is surgical removal of vermiform appendix.
> - Appendicectomy is usually performed as an emergency operation.
> - Delay in appendicectomy is to be avoided to prevent complications such as perforation of appendix and general peritonitis.

ANATOMY OF RIGHT ILIAC FOSSA IN RELATION TO APPENDIX SURGERY

The anterior abdominal wall has following features.

Skin

The skin of anterior abdominal wall has enormous capacity of stretching as during pregnancy.

Superficial Fascia

It has two layers below the level of umbilicus and one layer above the umbilicus.
The two layers of superficial fascia are:
1. *Camper's fascia* superficial fatty layer
2. *Scarpa's fascia* deep membranous layer

Cutaneous Nerves

Cutaneous nerves are derived from lower five intercostal nerves, subcostal nerve, and iliohypogastric nerve.

Cutaneous Arteries

These are branches of arteries that accompany nerves:
- Superior epigastric artery
- Inferior epigastric artery
- Lower intercostal arteries

Cutaneous Veins

- Accompany arteries
- Veins radiate from umbilicus, veins above umbilicus drain to superior vena cava and vein from below umbilicus drain to inferior vein cava.

MUSCLES OF ANTERIOR ABDOMINAL WALL

There are four muscles on either side of midline:
1. External oblique muscle
2. Internal oblique muscle
3. Transversus abdominis muscle
4. Rectus abdominis muscle

External Oblique Muscle (Figs. 1A and B)

- It originates from lower eight ribs.
- It inserts in xiphoid process, linea alba, pubic symphysis, pubic crest, and pectineal line.

Direction of Fibers

- Medially
- Downward
- Forward:
  - Fleshy fibers of muscle are laterally present and tough and whitish aponeurosis is situated medially. The junction of fleshy fibers and aponeurosis of external oblique muscle is approximately medial to a line drawn down from tip of 9th costal cartilage, medial to this line is aponeurosis and lateral is fleshy muscle fibers.

Internal Oblique Muscle

- It originates from inguinal ligament, iliac crest, and thoracolumbar fascia.
- It inserts as aponeurosis to lower four costal cartilages, xiphoid process, linea alba, pubic crest, and pectineal line.

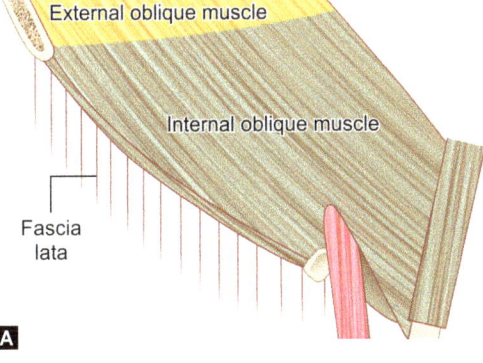
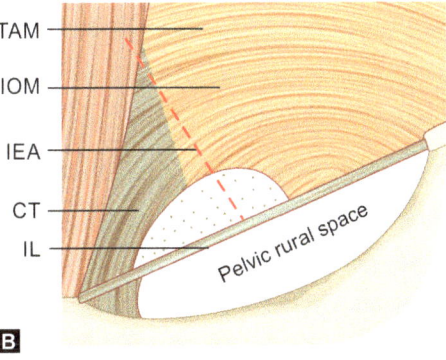

FIGS. 1A AND B: Muscles of anterior abdominal wall—external oblique muscle (EOM), internal oblique muscle (IOM), transversus abdominis muscle (TAM), rectus abdominis muscle (RAM), inferior epigastric artery (IEA). (CT: conjoint tendon; IL: inguinal ligament)

Direction of Fibers

- Medially
- Upward
- Forward
- Aponeurosis of internal oblique muscle is in medial part. Internal oblique aponeurosis takes part in formation of rectus sheath. It forms two layers, anterior and posterior, above the point midway between umbilicus and pubic symphysis, below this point it forms only anterior layer. The posterior layer of internal oblique aponeurosis ends at a point midway between umbilicus and pubic symphysis and is called 'arcuate line' or 'fold of Douglas' or 'linea semilunaris'.

Transversus Abdominis Muscle

- Originates from inguinal ligament, iliac crest, thoracolumbar fascia, and lower six costal cartilages.
- Inserts at xiphoid process, linea alba, pubic crest, and pectineal line.

Direction of Fibers

- Medially
- Horizontally
- Forward
- The neurovascular plane of anterior abdominal wall lies between internal oblique and transversus abdominis muscle. Various nerves and vessels run in this plane so while splitting or cutting this muscle take care of nerves and blood vessels sometimes bleeding from here can be annoying **(Fig. 2)**.

Rectus Abdominis Muscle (Figs. 3A and B)

- Rectus abdominis muscle runs vertically, originating as two heads from pubic crest and anterior pubic ligament.

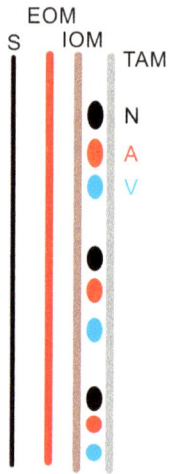

FIG. 2: Location of neurovascular bundle in abdominal wall.
(A: artery; EOM: external oblique muscle; IOM: internal oblique muscle; N: nerve; S: skin; TAM: transversus abdominis muscle; V: vein)

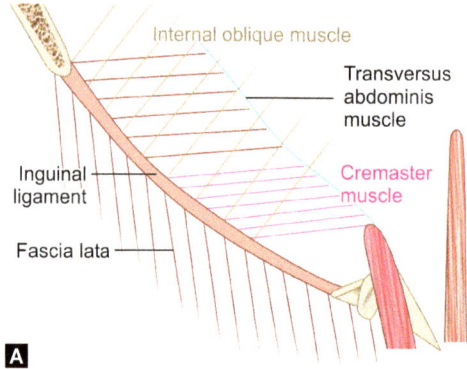
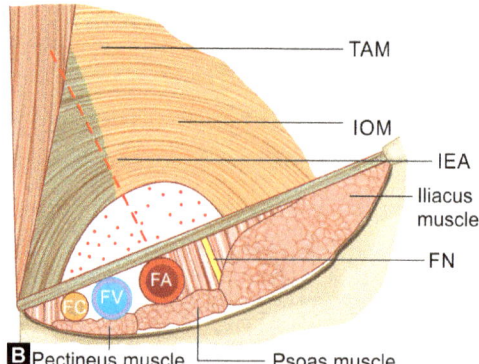

FIGS. 3A AND B: Muscles of anterior abdominal wall—external oblique muscle, internal oblique muscle, transversus abdominis muscle, rectus abdominis muscle, and inferior epigastric artery.
(FC: femoral canal; FV: femoral vein; FA: femoral artery; FN: femoral nerve; IEA: inferior epigastric artery; IOM: internal oblique muscle; TAM: transversus abdominis muscle)

- Inserts at xiphoid process and 7th, 6th, and 5th costal cartilages.
- There are three tendinous intersections in rectus abdominis muscle which divide the muscle in smaller parts at three levels:
  i. Xiphoid process
  ii. Umbilicus
  iii. Between xiphoid process and umbilicus
- Fascia transversalis lines the transversus abdominis muscle and is separated from peritoneum by connective tissue.

INFERIOR EPIGASTRIC ARTERY

- It arises from external iliac artery, it runs upward and medially in extraperitoneal connective tissue, reaches rectus sheath, and divides in upper and lower branch.

> Important point to remember is that neurovascular bundle runs between internal oblique and transversus abdominal muscle. Iliohypogastric nerve pierces internal oblique muscle about 2.5 cm in front of anterior superior iliac spine (ASIS) and then runs medially and forwards and pierces external oblique fascia 2.5 cm above inguinal ligament. This nerve can be damaged in big incision for appendicectomy and can cause right inguinal hernia.

- Ilioinguinal nerve pierces internal oblique muscle and runs below iliohypogastric nerve and external oblique muscle and runs with spermatic cord in inguinal canal and emerges from superficial inguinal ring.

PREOPERATIVE PREPARATION FOR APPENDICECTOMY

> In general every general practitioner should think of appendicitis in a patient with abdominal pain, fever, nausea, and vomiting. It can be confirmed by referring the patient to a surgeon. This is the way to give the patient benefit of doubt and avoid complications.

- Shaving of the part is done in ward before surgery. It is done from nipples to midthigh level. Nowadays shaving one night before operation is avoided if possible to reduce chance of postoperative infection as skin abrasions will act as ports of entry for bacteria and will give time to multiply.
- Patient is told to pass urine before going to operation theater (OT).
- Nil per os (NPO = Nil Per Oral, nothing by mouth)—a 6-hour fasting is required but in emergency, appendicectomy can be done in a shorter essential period for preoperative preparation.
- Intravenous fluid is to be given to avoid dehydration and to maintain normal urinary output.
- Antibiotics, intravenous antibiotics have been shown to reduce significantly the incidence of postoperative wound infection and intra-abdominal abscess formation.[1] Antibiotics should be administered 30 minutes prior to incision to achieve required tissue level of antibiotics. Antibiotics alone have been used in rare situations such as with sailors on long submarine tours[2] and long distance travelers. Intravenous antibiotics given to cover gram negative and anaerobic organisms, the commonly used such antibiotics are:
  ○ Cephalosporin
  ○ Metronidazole
  ○ Amikacin or other aminoglycoside
- Some doctors prefer a 1 gm metronidazole suppository before operation.
- Nasogastric tube should be introduced if you suspect perforation or peritonitis or patient is profusely vomiting.
- If patient has fever then cold sponging is done to reduce temperature.
- Preanesthetic medicines are given according to anesthetist's advice.

CHAPTER 7 Operative Surgery of Appendix

- Patient's anxiety and apprehension are reduced by properly explaining about the anesthesia and operative procedure.
- An indwelling Foley's catheter is passed in patient with generalized peritonitis.

> **Key Point**
>
> It is extremely dangerous to give a large enema or a purgative to a patient of acute abdomen. It is better to do per-rectal examination and put one or two glycerin suppositories in rectum cautiously.

APPENDICECTOMY OR APPENDECTOMY

'As long as the abdomen is open you control it. Once closed, it controls you.'
—**Moshe Schein**

APPENDICECTOMY

- In 1736 Claudius Amyand (1685–1740, Surgeon, St. George's Hospital, London, England) successfully removed an acutely inflamed appendix from the hernial sac of a boy.

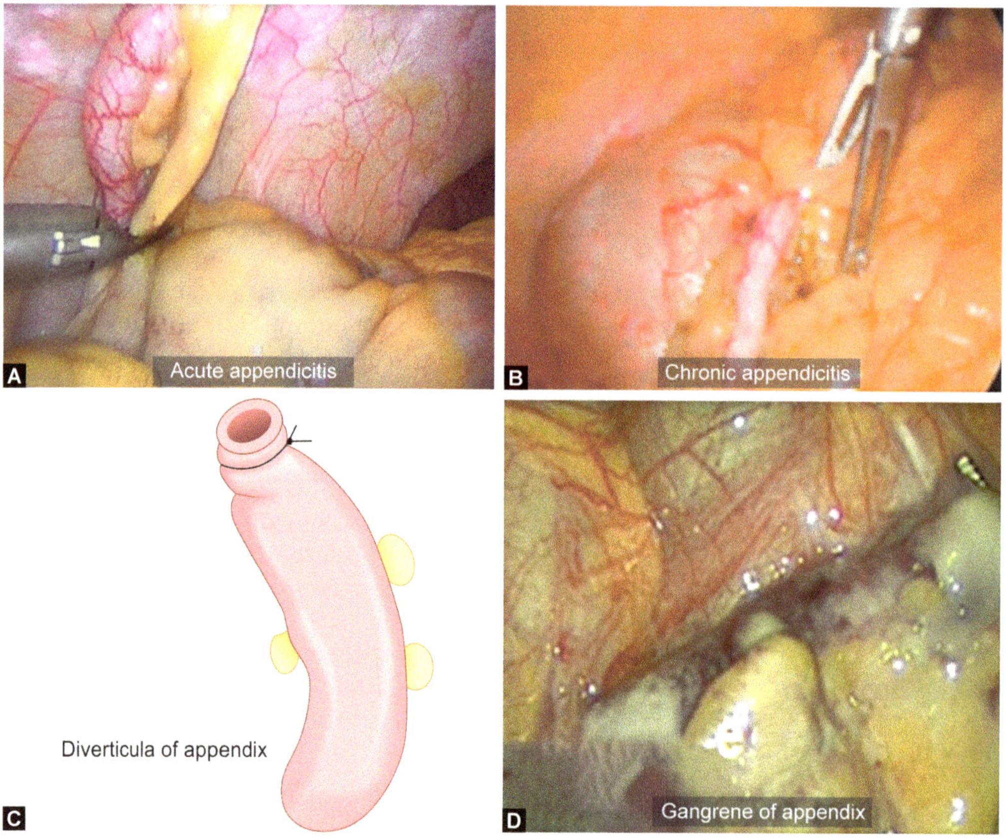

FIGS. 4A TO D: Common indications of appendicectomy.

Appendicitis is the most common indication of appendicectomy, including its complicated entities **(Figs. 4A to D)**.

- Lawson Tait (1845–1899, Surgeon, Hospital for Diseases of Women, Birmingham, England) was first surgeon to perform first planned appendicectomy in May 1880 but he did not report it till 1890.
- Thomas Morton (1835–1903, Surgeon, Philadelphia, PA, USA) was the first to diagnose appendicitis, drain the abscess, remove the appendix, and publish in 1887.

DEFINITION

Removal of appendix is called appendicectomy or appendectomy (in British English it is called appendicectomy and in American English appendectomy)

Types of appendicectomy:
- *Appendicectomy*:
  - Open or conventional appendicectomy
  - Laparoscopic appendicectomy
- Interval appendicectomy
- Incidental appendicectomy
- Retrograde appendicectomy
- Inversion appendicectomy

INDICATIONS OF APPENDICECTOMY

- Acute appendicitis
- *Appendicular tumor*:
  - Carcinoma of appendix involving only mucosa but not the base of appendix
  - Small carcinoid tumor <2 cm in size and at body or tip of appendix
- Subacute appendicitis
- Chronic appendicitis
- Recurrent appendicitis
- Interval appendicectomy after appendicular mass

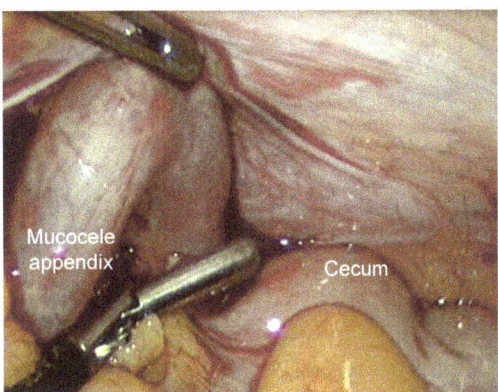

FIG. 5: Mucocele of appendix.

- Mucocele of appendix **(Fig. 5)**.
- Empyema of appendix
- Endometriosis of appendix
- Diverticulum of appendix—the acquired diverticulum of appendix perforates early if appendicitis develops.

OPEN OR CONVENTIONAL APPENDICECTOMY

Anesthesia

- Usually the anesthetist decides during pre-anesthesia checkup (PAC) about kind of anesthesia is required.
- General anesthesia is preferred.
- Spinal anesthesia is also used.
- Local anesthesia with sedation and intravenous (IV) analgesics can be tried in very sick patient with other serious systemic ailments and or where other forms of anesthesia are contraindicated.

Key Point
Reexamine the abdomen of anaesthetized patient, you may palpate a mass which was not palpable before, make it a habit.

Position: Supine

OPERATION SITE PREPARATION

- Skin is prepared with methylated spirit and the 10% povidone-iodine solution.
- Spirit absorbs the moisture and evaporates making skin dry. By evaporating it reduces the temperature of skin and then acts as an antiseptic.
- Povidone-iodine solution acts as bactericidal in a very short time contact with skin, almost in 15 seconds it gives its effect.
- *EUA (examination under anesthesia):* The whole abdomen is palpated after giving general anesthesia. If there is a lump it will be felt. Size of mass is noticed which helps to decide about appropriate incision.

STEPS OF APPENDICECTOMY

Steps of Open Appendicectomy

- Incision
- Identification and isolation of appendix
- Cutting of mesoappendix
- Removal of appendix
- Inspection of operative site, cecum, terminal ileum, and pelvic organs
- Closure of wound

INCISIONS (FIGS. 6A AND B)

'Surgery is like love making, must be done gently with adequate exposure.'
—Anonymous

Common incisions for appendicectomy:
- Gridiron incision (McBurney's incision)
- Lanz or crease incision
- Rutherford Morison's muscle cutting incision
- Lower right paramedical incision
- Lower midline incision
- Medial muscle cutting incision (Fowler–Weir approach)
- Battle's pararectus incision
- Rockey–Davis incision

Antibiotics should be administered 30 minutes prior to incision to achieve adequate tissue levels. Intravenous antibiotics have been shown to reduce significantly the incidents of postoperative wound infection and intra-abdominal abscess.

—Andersen BR
[Cochrane Database Syst Rev. 2003;(2):CD001439]

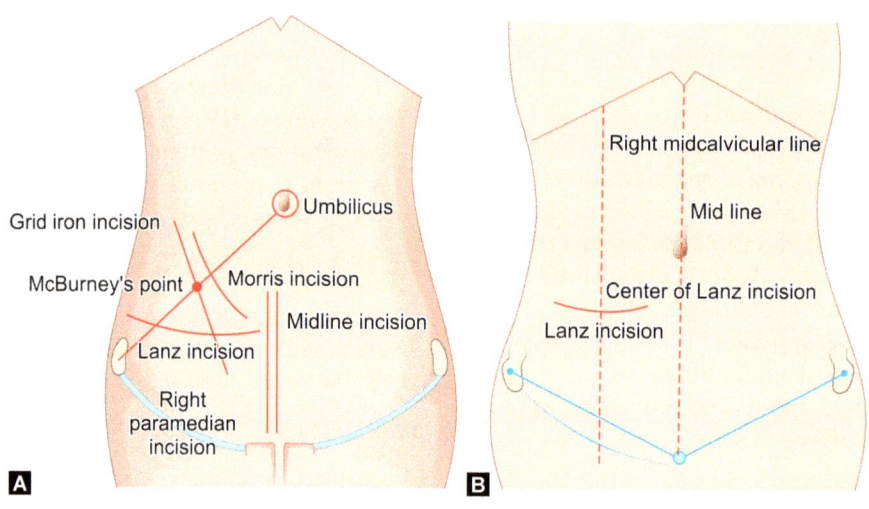

FIGS. 6A AND B: Incisions used for appendicectomy.

The most commonly used incision in appendicectomy is gridiron incision. Gridiron is a frame of cross-beams. It is used to support a ship during repairs.

GRIDIRON INCISION

First described by Lewis Linn McArthur (1858–1934, Surgeon, St. Luke's Hospital, Chicago, IL, USA) it is also called McBurney's gridiron incision **(Fig. 6C)**.

Principle: It is a muscle splitting incision. It is used to cause rapid healing and least damage to anatomy of anterior abdominal wall.

The incision made in the abdominal wall in cases of appendicitis with a description of a new method of operating (McBurney C. Ann Surg. 1894;20:38-43).

Advantages of Gridiron Incision

- No nerve injury
- It heals fast
- Lowest mortality rate
- No muscle damage
- Less time consuming compared to muscle cutting incisions.

Disadvantages of Gridiron Incision

- Cosmetically not very good
- Medial extension of the incision can damage inferior epigastric vessels.

Steps of Gridiron Incision

- Center of gridiron incision lies at McBurney's point and is perpendicular to the line joining ASIS and umbilicus.
- It is a 5–7 cm-long incision.
- It can also be adjusted by moving up or down as surgeon feels according to the position of cecum and appendix.
- Skin, superficial fascia, Camper's fascia, and Scarpa's fascia are divided in the line of incision.
- In subcutaneous layer a branch of superficial circumflex artery is caught and cauterized or ligated.
- The external oblique aponeurosis is divided in the line of its fibers which is in same line as the incision. The external oblique fibers are kept separated by retraction with the Czerney's retractors **(Fig. 7)**.
- A Mayo's scissors or artery forceps is inserted and opened between the fibers of internal oblique muscle and transversus abdominis muscle, which splits the fibers of muscles. Now two index fingers are introduced and pulled apart to enlarge the space.
- Now the peritoneum is visible.
- Peritoneum is exposed by retraction.

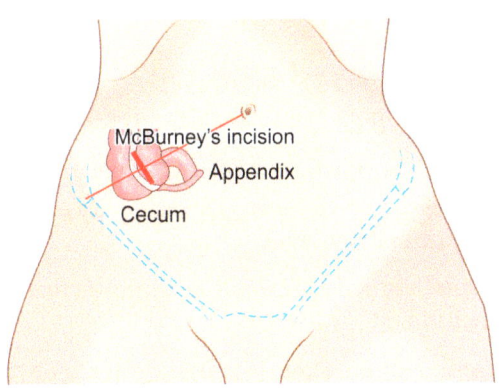

FIG. 6C: McBurney's gridiron incision.

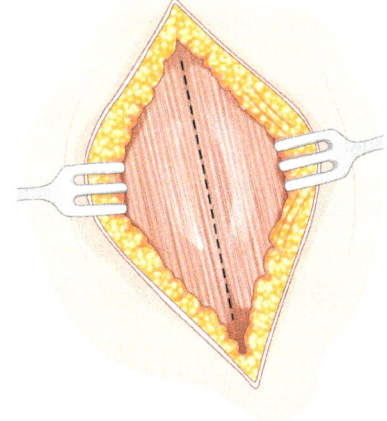

FIG. 7: Division of external oblique aponeurosis.

- Two Langenbeck's retractors are inserted deep to the muscles and the peritoneum is exposed. Peritoneum is incised between two artery forceps. First the peritoneum is picked up by surgeon by an artery forceps. The peritoneum is now picked up by the assistant by an artery forceps in front of surgeon's artery forceps. Now surgeon leaves the peritoneum and again catches the fold of peritoneum to avoid injury to the underlying bowel. Now surgeon feels the fold of peritoneum between his thumb and index finger to confirm that bowel is not caught between artery forceps. Now he cuts the peritoneum fold with a knife. Do not cut by scissors as scissors can cut bowel within peritoneum fold.
- As soon as the peritoneum is opened air sucks in and intestinal loops fall back then the small cut is extended with scissors.
- Gridiron incision can be converted to Rutherford Morison incision and can be extended up or down by cutting the muscle fibers if the exposure is not sufficient.

Closure of Incision

- The closure is done in layers.
- First the peritoneum and fascia transversalis are sutured with 2/0 Vicryl.
- Secondly the fibers of internal oblique and transversus abdominis are sutured together.
- Thirdly aponeurotic layer of external oblique is sutured.
- Fourthly the subcutaneous tissue and skin are approximated by staples or 3/0 prolene or subcuticular sutures. Even in advance appendicitis or perforation, primary closure is cost effective and without high risk of wound infection, with proper use of antibiotics.[3,4]

LANZ OR CREASE INCISION

Otto Lanz (1865–1935, Surgeon, Amsterdam, the Netherlands) started this incision.

Principle: It is a cosmetic incision as it is a transverse incision in the skin crease, i.e., Langer's lines, which heals well and gives the scar in skin crease.

Steps

- Incision is made approximately 2 cm below the level of umbilicus in right iliac fossa (RIF).
- Its center lies in mid-clavicular mid-inguinal line.
- Further exploration is like gridiron incision. It can be made much lower in skin crease so as to hide the scar with swimming suit.
- It is a 5–7 cm-long incision.

Advantages of Lanz Incision

- It is a cosmetic incision and leaves better scar.
- It can be extended medially or laterally when required.
- The exposure is better.

Disadvantages of Lanz Incision

- You have to open rectus sheath on its lateral border for extending the incision medially.
- One cannot deal with high or subhepatic appendix by extending the incision. This incision has to be closed and a new appropriate incision is to be applied.
- Medial extension of the incision can damage inferior epigastric vessels.

RUTHERFORD MORISON'S MUSCLE CUTTING INCISION

James Rutherford Morison (1853–1939, Professor of Surgery, Durham, England) describes it first time.

Principle: It is an oblique muscle cutting incision.

Details of incision: It starts at McBurney's point and goes up laterally.

- It cuts external oblique aponeurosis, internal oblique and transverses abdominis muscle in same line.
- Further steps are like gridiron incision.

Indications of Rutherford Morison's Incision

- Appendicectomy
- To expose ureter
- To expose external iliac vessels.

Disadvantages of Rutherford Morison's Incision

- Chances of postoperative hernia are more due to nerve injury and local muscle cutting.
- Incisional hernia is also seen if wound is not well repaired.
- More chances of wound infection than other incisions due to more bleeding.
- Chances of postoperative hematoma are more.

Lower Midline or Right Paramedian Incision

- A lower midline incision is preferred over lower right paramedian incision.
- *Indication:* It is used when in doubt about diagnosis of perforation and peritonitis.

Advantages of Lower Midline Incision

Midline incision is easy to extend upward if there is perforated duodenal ulcer.
- It gives good access to pelvic cavity as well as abdominal cavity.
- Easy to close.
- Less damaging to the tissues so early healing.

Advantages of Right Paramedian Incision

- It gives good access to pelvic organs.
- It can be extended up if perforated duodenal ulcer is present.

Disadvantages of Lower Midline or Right Paramedian Incision

- Lot of retraction is required to expose appendix and cecum. It gives poor access in retrocecal appendicitis.
- Chances of postoperative hematoma and infection are more with this incision as it behaves as trapdoor for infection.
- It can contaminate the peritoneal cavity.

Steps

Right paramedian incision is made:
- 2.5 cm right to midline
- 2.5 cm below umbilicus
- 2.5 cm above pubic symphysis
- Skin, subcutaneous tissue, Camper's fascia, and fascia of Scarpa are incised in line of incision.
- The anterior rectus sheath is cut in same line.
- The right rectus muscle is retracted laterally to avoid injury to nerves of rectus muscle as they come from lateral side.
- Branches of inferior epigastric vessels are ligated.
- Posterior rectus sheath up to arcuate line and peritoneum are incised between two artery forceps.

FOWLER–WEIR APPROACH

Similar to Battle's incisions but muscles are cut medially over rectus muscle.
- Not used nowadays.

BATTLE'S PARARECTAL INCISION

(William Henry Battle, 1855–1936, started this incision, Battle WH modified incision for removal of the vermiform appendix. Br Med J. 1895;2:1360.)

It is not used nowadays.

Indication of Battle's pararectal incision:
- Appendicectomy
- Gynecologic operations

Procedure
- Made on lateral and lower part of right rectus muscle.
- Skin, subcutaneous tissue, and anterior rectus sheath are divided in same line.
- Rectus muscle retracted medially.
- Posterior rectus sheath above arcuate line incised.
- Peritoneum opened between two artery forceps and the opening is increased above and below by scissors.

Disadvantages
- More chances of wound infection.
- More chances of incisional hernia.
- Injury to intercostal nerves supplying rectus muscle.
- Not good access to appendix.

ROCKEY–DAVIS INCISION

It is similar to Lanz incision. It is a transverse muscle splitting incision. It is extended up to rectus sheath for better exposure.[5]

> **Key Point**
> The incision should be centered over point of maximal tenderness. In case of abscess incision should be placed laterally to do retroperitoneal drainage.

IDENTIFICATION OF CECUM

- One retractor is placed in medial side of the wound.
- If pus is present, take a swab for culture and sensitivity before removing it by suction.
- *Identify the cecum by:*
  - Anterior taenia coli
  - Its whitish pale in color whereas ileal loops are pinkish
  - Absence of appendices epiploicae

Delivering the Cecum and the Appendix

Hold the cecum with a swab by thumb and index finger and bring it out in wound by pulling it down and medially **(Fig. 8)**.

Identification and Isolation of Appendix

- Appendix is caught with a Babcock forceps near its tip encircling it and not crushing. Now it is pulled so as to see mesentery and base of appendix clearly.

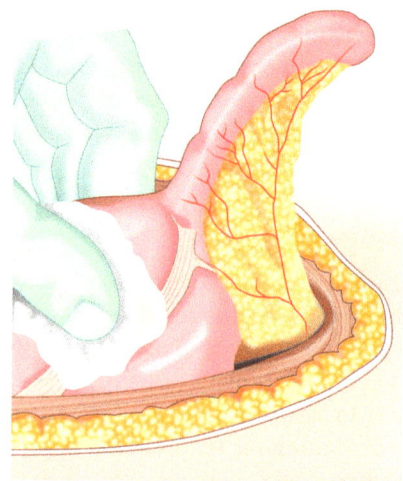

FIG. 8: Holding cecum with a gauze piece.

- The loops of ileum are returned back to peritoneal cavity.
- The abdominal pack is put around to wall off peritoneal cavity from the wound.
- One can easily reach cecum by following the peritoneal reflection from abdomen wall.
- Sometimes even sigmoid colon and transverse colon could be present in RIF. Transverse colon has omentum attached to it and sigmoid colon is identified by its mesocolon whereas cecum has no mesocolon or omentum.
- A word of caution—do not use cautery near bowel as thermal injury may cause necrosis later on which can form a fecal fistula.
- Right index finger is introduced into the wound to help in gentle delivery of appendix by hooking but must be done under vision. Now the cecum is given to assistant to hold.

> Surgeon must prepare himself or herself to how to deal with appendix. The appendix may be a typical one having infection only limited to itself or it may be adherent to some other organ or it is retrocecal or the inflammation has involved cecum also. Surgeon must familiarize himself/herself well with the normal and abnormal conditions of vascularization of appendix so as not to cause hemorrhage.

> **Key Point**
>
> *If the appendix is not found*: Search for other nearby infected organs such as Meckel's diverticulum, gynecological problem (salpingitis), appendix may be absent or autodigested by previous infection.

CUTTING OF MESOAPPENDIX (FIGS. 9A AND B)

- Mesoappendix is made tense by holding and pulling the appendix with Babcock forceps or mesoappendix is caught with curved artery forceps.
- One pointed and curved mosquito artery forceps is introduced in mesoappendix near its base near appendicular artery. The 4-0 Vicryl ligature is passed in this hole and appendicular artery is ligated. Gradually in the same manner whole mesoappendix is ligated close to the appendix.
- Accessory appendicular artery is also ligated.

> In most of the cases vessels are clearly divided at the base of the appendix and in such cases ligature can be applied high enough to have perfect control of all vessels. In some cases cecal artery also supplies base of the appendix. Here one has to be cautious against bleeding after amputation of appendix.

REMOVAL OF APPENDIX

Crush the base of appendix with a straight artery forceps which crushes only mucus membrane and muscle coat but does not crush the serosa. The crushed mucosa and muscle coat block the lumen. Ligate the appendix base at the crush site with 3/0 Vicryl.

When the Base of Appendix is Not Crushed?

- If appendix is gangrenous.
- If there is a perforation at the base of appendix.
- If base of appendix and cecum are edematous.

> Occasionally, in certain cases, the appendiceal inflammation extends to the base of the appendix or beyond to the cecum. The division of the appendix through inflamed, infected tissue leaves the potential for leakage of cecal contents with a residual abscess or fistula.
> —Poole GV (Am Surg. 1993;59:624-5)

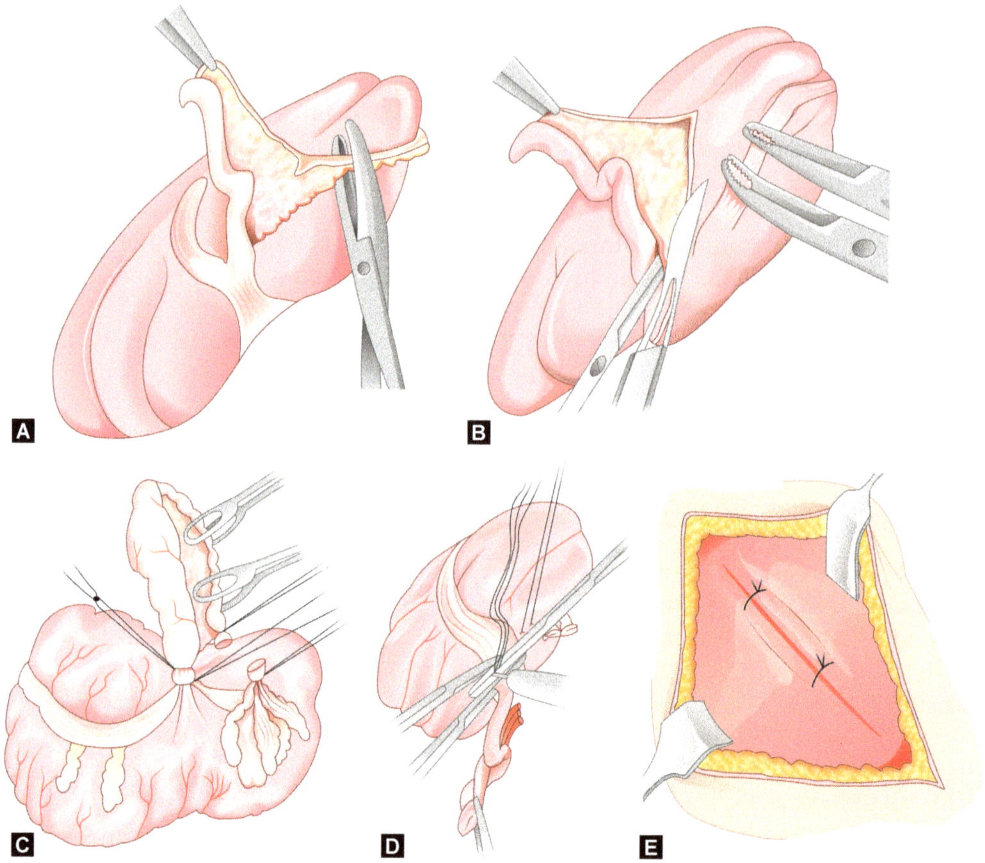

FIGS. 9A TO E: Various steps of open appendicectomy.

- A purse string suture or 'N' shape suture with 3/0 Vicryl is applied. It is applied on the wall of cecum around the base of appendix. Take care of not injuring any blood vessels while taking purse string suture as it may became a big hematoma in the wall of cecum. It is a seromucosal suture. Take taenia coli in it to give strength to this ligature **(Figs. 9 and 10)**.
- Clamp the base of the appendix with an artery forceps 5 mm away from ligature.
- Before putting the clamp on appendix milk the intervening portion of appendix between ligature and this artery forceps by sliding this artery

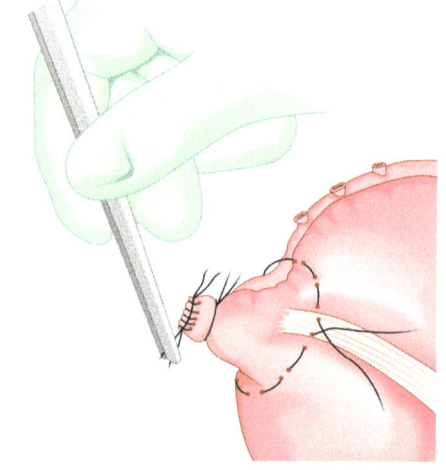

FIG. 10: Purse string suture and stump of appendix.

forceps, to avoid soiling of operation site when appendix is cut.
- Now the appendix is cut flushed with artery forceps by a knife.
- Place a swab behind the appendix base to avoid spillage.
- Cut the ligature of appendix stump.
- The cut stump of appendix is touched with phenol or betadine solution or spirit or cauterized by diathermy to avoid contamination.

Burying the Base of Appendix

Recent prospective studies show no advantages to appendical stump inversion.[6,7] Inversion may also have the deleterious effect of deforming the cecal wall which could be misinterpreted as a cecal mass on future contrast radiographs.[7] Furthermore, the long standing notion that stump inversion reduces postoperative adhesion was discredited by Strut and colleague.[8] Now the general opinion is to avoid the burying of the base of appendix (Fig. 11).

- Invaginate the stump with pursue string suture or 'figure of Z or N' suture by holding the stump base near knot of purse string suture with a straight toothless dissecting forceps while pushing the stump of appendix in cecum the purse string suture is tied then cut this ligature 5 mm from knot.[9]

> **Key Point**
>
> If the appendix is found not inflamed. Then look for:
> - Meckel's diverticulum
> - Perforated duodenal ulcer, bile trickling down from paracolic gutter
> - Gynecological cause

INSPECTION OF OPERATIVE SITE, TERMINAL ILEUM, AND PELVIC ORGANS

- Cecum and mesentery are first inspected for any injury.
- Terminal ileum is examined for Meckel's diverticulum up to 1 m in retrograde way starting at ileocecal junction.
- In females palpate the right uterine adnexa and uterus for any cyst or inflammation or growth.
- Inspect the invaginated area of cecum for any bleeding.
- Take out terminal ileum about 1 meter and look for Meckel's diverticulum, band adhesion, kinks, and Crohn's disease.
- The appendix and the contaminated knife, swab, forceps are placed in a kidney dish and taken away from operation site to avoid contamination.
- Peritoneal fluid should be sent for culture and sensitivity and gram staining.
- If the appendix cannot be totally released and distal part is difficult to retrieve then first the base of appendix, is dealt with, it is tied and divided, later on the whole appendix including apex is removed which was retrocecal or adhered with bowel.

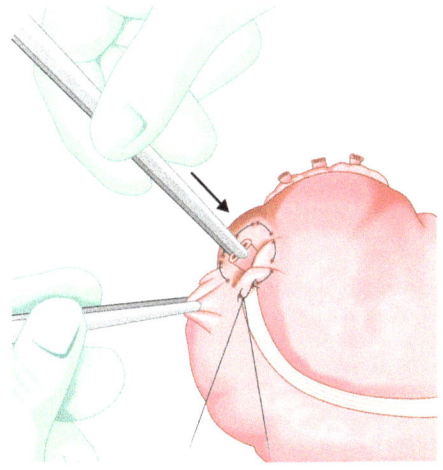

FIG. 11: Burying the base of appendix.

CLOSURE OF THE WOUND (FIG. 9E)

Wound is closed in layers. Staples are applied on skin.

> **Key Point**
>
> Do not try peritoneal lavage through gridiron incision, if required, close this incision and open through lower paramedian or midline incision.

Complicated situations during appendectomy:

The main purpose here is how to avoid injury to intestine and other organs while doing appendectomy in complicated situations.

- When the tip of the appendix is densely adherent then first do amputation of appendix at the base and then free the tip by careful dissection. It is easier than when both ends are fixed.
- If the whole appendix is fixed by dense adhesions then there is a risk of bleeding and injuring other structures by dissecting deep in adhesions. First free the base of the appendix then give traction by applying an artery forceps at this end of the appendix, cut the peritoneal covering over the appendix on its direction and appendix can be stripped.
- When omentum is adherent strongly with appendix then it is better to tie and excise the omentum with the appendix.
- When the appendix is totally concealed and cannot be identified then utilize various landmarks, especially cecum. Examine cecum minutely to find the base of appendix. If you directly attempt to enucleate the mass, you may land up with disaster.

- NP Dandridge reported a case with commendably frankness in order that others may profit by his experience ……. The appendix could not be found, a mass was found, thought to be exudate, …….. this exudate was freed with finger, a pulsating vessel of some size, which passed through it, was ligated. On removal, the parts proved to be a mass of enlarged glands…… the thickened and clubbed shaped appendix was found behind the cecum and was removed. The wound, which was completely closed, broke down after 8 days, fecal matter escaped, and afterward about 15 inches of small intestine and cecum sloughed away. This injury was repaired after four intestinal operations (Dandridge NP. Ann Surg. 1903;38:367).

LAPAROSCOPIC APPENDICECTOMY

'Incision heals from side-to-side, not from end-to-end, but length does matter.'
—**Moche Schein**

HISTORICAL BACKGROUND

- In 1982, Kurt Semm, German Gynecologist performed first successful laparoscopic appendicectomy, several years before laparoscopic cholecystectomy.
- For 10 years laparoscopic appendicectomy did not become popular. It became popular only after 1991 after success of laparoscopic cholecystectomy. It was also due to the fact that open appendicectomy through a small incision, is a minimal access surgery.[10]

INDICATIONS

Acute Appendicitis

- In suspected cases where diagnosis is not clear.
- In female of child-bearing age.
- In obese appendicitis patients, the laparoscopic technique proved to be superior to open technique in criteria such as perioperative-postoperative complications, operation time, etc.[11] In open appendectomy in obese patients sometimes incisions required to be enlarged, extra time is required and risk of wound complications is more.[12]
- In first trimester of pregnancy.
- Incidental appendicectomy when appendix is found inflamed during laparoscopy for other ailment.

Chronic or Subacute or Recurrent Appendicitis and Grumbling Appendix

Advantages of laparoscopic appendicectomy over open or conventional appendicectomy:
- A large meta-analysis comparing open to laparoscopic approach[13-17] showed that duration of surgery and operation costs are higher with laparoscopic appendicectomy.
- Faster convalescence, early mobility, shorter hospital stay, and early return to work.
- Less pain
- Better scar, so cosmetic
- Access to pelvic organ is better.
- Postoperative wound infection is less than open procedure.
- Exploration of peritoneal cavity is possible.
- Treatment of other causes of RIF pain is possible.
- Unnecessary laparotomy is avoided.
- Better in obese patients as there is less risk of wound infection in fat patients. Wound infections were about as likely (Peto or 0.47;95%–cl 0.36–0.62) after LA than after OA,....[18]
- Diagnostic laparoscopy before appendicectomy avoids negative appendicectomy.[19]

Disadvantages of laparoscopic appendicectomy over open approach:
- Procedure is costly
- Operation time is more
- Intra-abdominal abscesses are three times more common
- An experienced surgeon is required

Absolute contraindications:
- Inability to tolerate general anesthesia
- Refractory coagulopathy
- Diffused peritonitis with hemodynamic compromise
- Intestinal obstruction[20,21]

Two meta-analyses have confirmed the benefits of laparoscopic approach—this is at the expense of slightly longer operating time and a trend to higher incidence of intra-abdominal abscesses [Sauerland et al. Kargar, Basil, 1998:109-14. Golub R, Siddiqui F, Pohl D. J Am Coll Surg. 1998;186(5):545-53] **(Figs. 12 to 15)**.

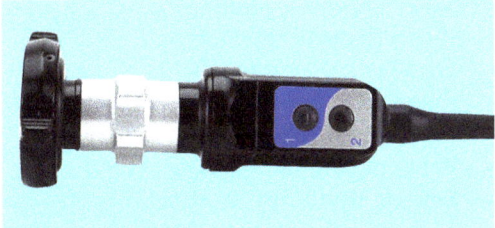

FIG. 12: Camera.

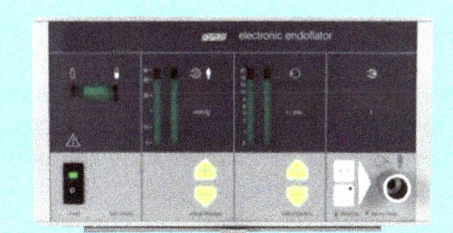

FIG. 13: Carbon dioxide insufflator.

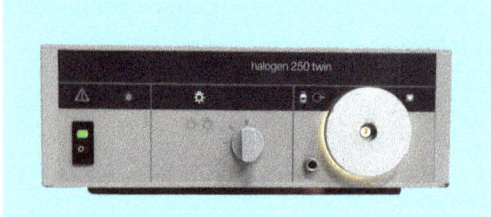

FIG. 14: Light source.

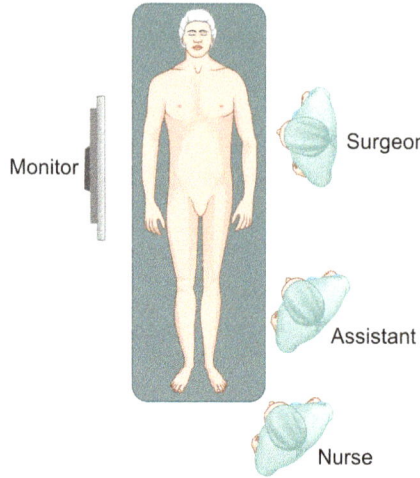

FIG. 15: Laparoscopic set up for appendectomy.

Relative contraindications:
- Inexperienced surgeon
- Suspicion of malignancy
- Pregnancy
- Previous lower abdominal surgery
- Pelvic inflammatory disease (PID)
- Severe systemic medical disease as congestive heart failure (CHF)

PREOPERATIVE PREPARATION

A Foley's catheter is passed to evacuate urinary bladder and monitor urinary output before sending the patient to OT which can be removed after operation in the operation theatre itself. A nasogastric tube should be passed to decompress stomach.

Anesthesia: General anesthesia.

Position: Supine in 15° Trendelenburg position with rotation of the table to left side. 15–20°, right side up.

Position of Surgical Team (Fig. 15)

- Surgeon stands on left side of the patient.
- First assistant also stands on left side of the patient next to surgeon.
- Second assistant stands between patients legs or on right side of the patient but sometimes it obstructs the vision of surgeon to monitor.
- The monitor is kept on right side of the patient.
- Anesthetist stands near the head of the patient.

Set up in Operation Theater

- Right arm of the patient is extended with IV cannula in it for drugs and IV fluids.
- Left arm is tucked under patient's side.
- Pulse oximeter is attached to thumb of right hand.
- Video monitor is at the eye level opposite the surgeon.
- Cables and CO_2 tubing are kept near the head end of the patient.
- Instrument tray is kept near foot end of the patient.

Instrument Tray

Following instruments are usually required for a laparoscopic appendicectomy other than a video camera, video monitor and carbon dioxide insufflator.
- One 10 mm trocar with a 5 mm reducer
- Two 5 mm trocars
- Two 5 mm atraumatic graspers
- One 5 mm bipolar diathermy forceps
- One 5 mm or 10 mm straight 0° endoscope
- Endoloops
- One linear stapler or clip applicator
- Specimen retrieval bag
- Harmonic scalpel

Steps of laparoscopic appendicectomy:
- Introduction of instruments by three ports
- Division of mesoappendix
- Extraction of appendix

Procedure

It is usually done with their ports. The fourth port is sometimes used in retrocecal appendix to mobilize it.

Pneumoperitoneum

- A stab wound is made at umbilicus with No. 11 blade and Veress needle is passed through it to produce pneumoperitoneum.
- Nowadays some surgeons use open technique by using Hasson's cannula than Veress needle to produce pneumoperitoneum.

Trocar Placement

- A 5 mm or 10 mm telescope is passed through umbilical port and peritoneal cavity is surveyed in all four quadrants **(Fig. 16)**.
- Safe access to peritoneal cavity is by Hasson's trocar, 3 cm incision is given infraumbilically in midline up to linea alba and Hasson trocar is bound to abdominal wall. It is fixed with 2-0 Vicryl with fascia.[22]
- Under vision of telescope the abdominal wall is transilluminated between umbilicus and pubic symphysis then another 1-cm incision is made in skin just above pubic symphysis without damaging any vessel which is visible in transillumination and a 10 mm port is introduced. Some surgeons prefer the port at the McBurney's point in LIF to avoid swording of instruments (collision of instruments).
- Another 10 mm post is introduced in LIF lateral to inferior epigastric artery.
- Intraperitoneal pressure is kept at 12 mm Hg and maximum to 14. In children the pressure equals the age.
- Trocars should be inserted in slightly oblique direction to prevent incisional hernia.
- Placement of trocars through rectus muscle is avoided to avoid injury to inferior epigastria vessels **(Figs. 17A and B)**.[23]
- The table is tilted in Trendelenburg position with right side up by 25°. By this maneuver the omentum and the coil of small bowel fall away from cecum and appendix.

Exploration

Sometimes as you introduce laparoscope in the peritoneal cavity, you find appendix lying in front. It is called 'handshake appendix' or 'how do you do appendix' **(Fig. 18)**. When the appendix is found shining and normal, it is called Lilly white appendix' **(Fig. 19)**.

- First the abdomen is thoroughly explored to exclude any other pathology.
- Now the search for appendix is started first identifying cecum by taenia coli. Follow the anterior taenia coli to find appendix.
- If the appendix is found normal then search for other causes of RIF pain, e.g., Meckel's diverticulitis, Crohn's ileitis, salpingitis, and tubo-ovarian pathology.

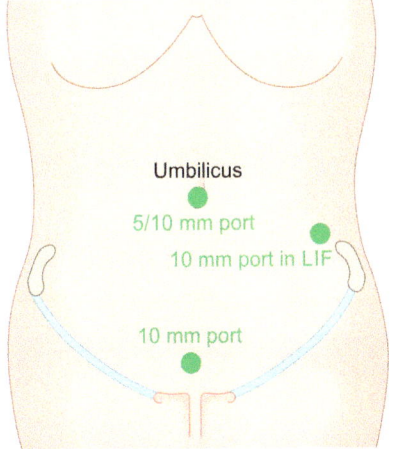

FIG. 16: Port placement in laparoscopic appendicectomy.

CHAPTER 7 Operative Surgery of Appendix

- If appendix cannot be found or cannot be exposed well then do not hesitate to convert the laparoscopy operation to open operation.
- Appendix is caught near the tip with Babcock's forceps, the mesoappendix is then visualized (**Figs. 20A and B**).

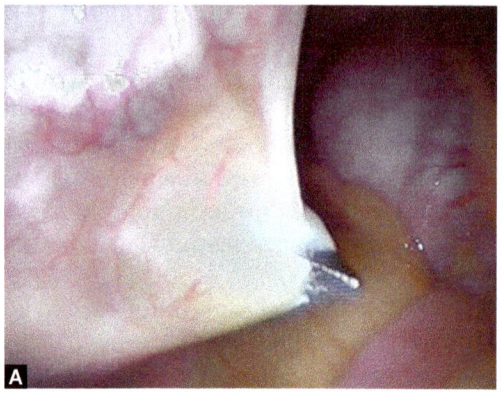 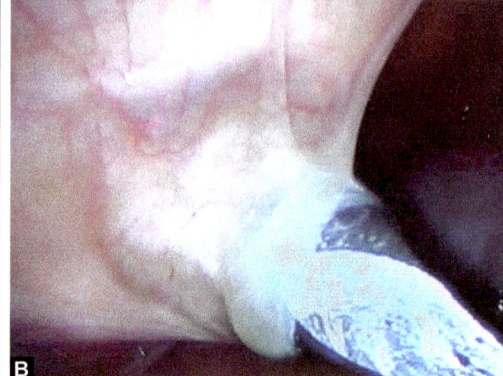

FIGS. 17A AND B: Insertion of trocar (**Video 9**).

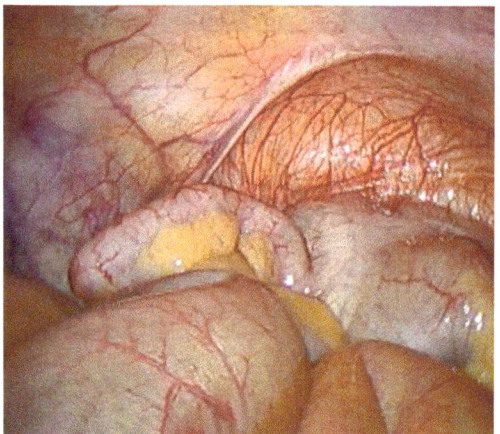 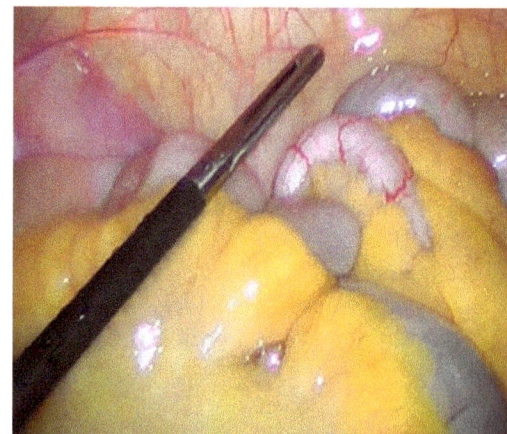

FIG. 18: Handshake appendix.

FIG. 19: Lilly white appendix (**Video 10**).

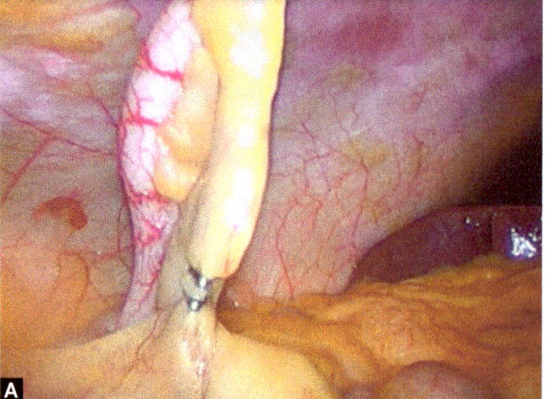 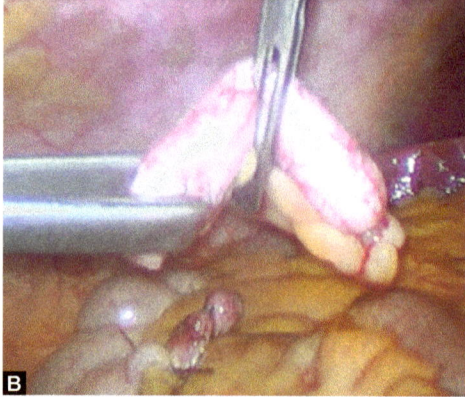

FIGS. 20A AND B: Appendix is held, and clips applied at mesoappendix (**Videos 11 to 14**).

- A window is created in mesoappendix near the base of the appendix, mesoappendix and base of appendix are dealt separately between clamps or staples.
- The mesoappendix is divided between two staples.

REMOVAL OF APPENDIX (FIGS. 21 TO 23)

- Two staples are applied at base of appendix then appendix is divided between two staples. Some surgeons prefer using endoloop at stump of appendix. If appendix appears gangrenous then catch it with Babcock's forceps to avoid perforation.
- The base of appendix is not inverted or buried.
- The appendix is put into endobag and the endobag is retrieved from 10 mm port.
- Area of appendix and cecum can be irrigated with saline if the site is soiled with pus or seropurulent fluid **(Figs. 21A and B)**.
- Inspect the stump of appendix and mesentery for any hemorrhage.
- Right lower quadrant (RLQ) may be irrigated if spillage is there **(Figs. 22A and B)**.

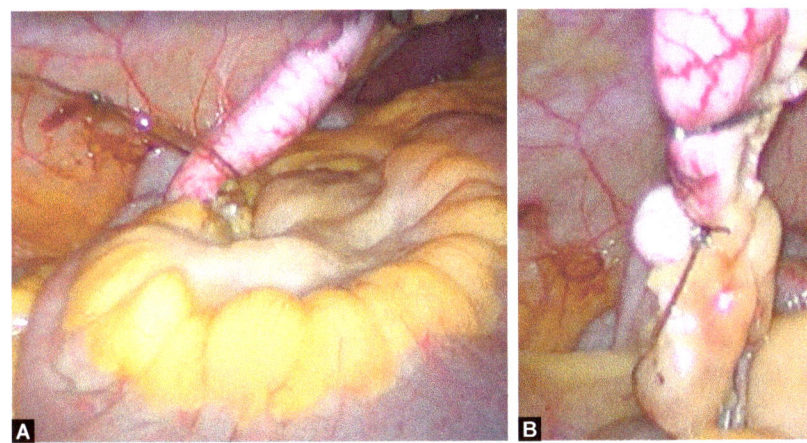
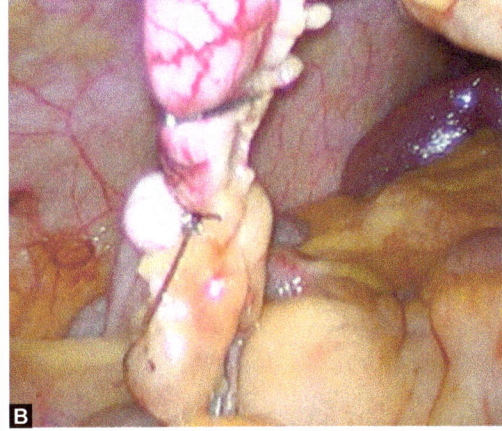

FIGS. 21A AND B: Endoloop applied on base of appendix **(Video 15)**.

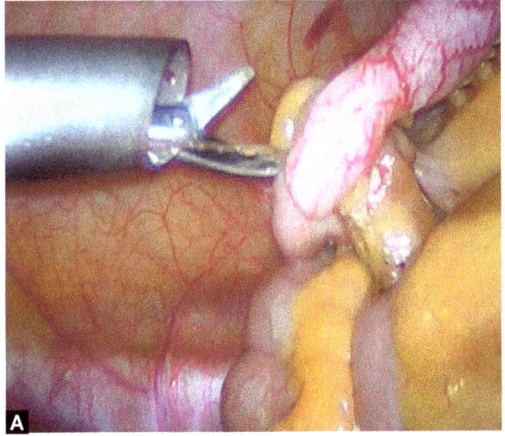
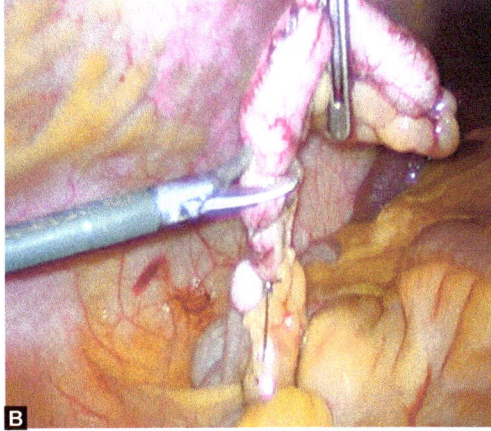

FIGS. 22A AND B: Cutting of base of appendix **(Video 16)**.

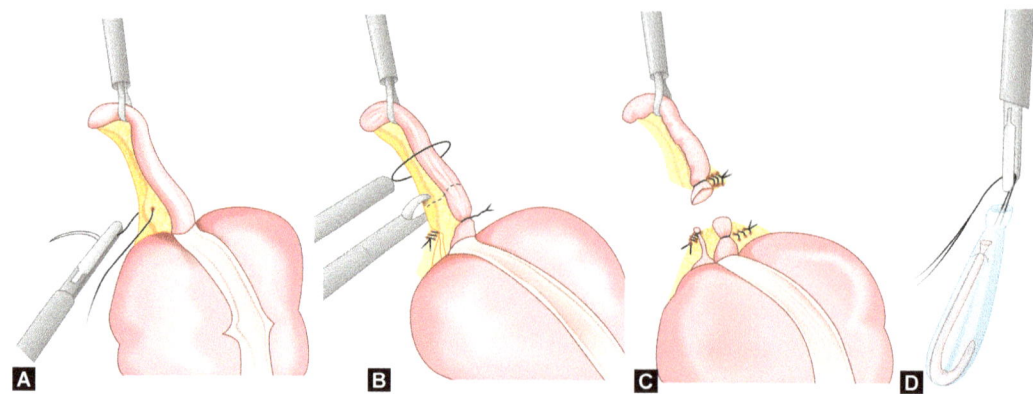

FIGS. 23A TO D: Various steps of laparoscopic appendicectomy **(Video 17).**

CLOSURE

- Remove all ports under vision so any bleeding from abdominal wall can be seen and stopped.[24,25]
- Skin staples are used at 10 mm port site.
- At the 5 mm post site adhesive band aid is applied.
- Drain is put if there was generalized peritonitis.
- It is advised to locally infiltrate long acting local anesthetic at three port sites for relief of postoperative pain.
- Some surgeons feel that in case of perforated appendix the CO_2 pneumoperitoneum enhances the bacteremia and toxemia though it is not confirmed.

Various inflammatory stages of appendix in appendicitis and how to deal:
- *If the appendix is normal:* Look for other sources of abdominal pain, if could not find then proceed for appendicectomy.
- *If the appendix is mildly inflamed without involvement of mesoappendix:* Appendix can be held with grasper gently and without fear of perforation, it can be removed by putting it in 10 mm trocar and removing trocar and appendix together protecting abdominal wall from contamination.
- *Highly inflamed appendix with thickened mesoappendix:* Be gentle and do not move the appendix too much unnecessarily. A 4th port, if required should be introduced to facilitate the dissection. The appendix must be removed on a retrieval bag to avoid spillage in peritoneal cavity. Adhesions can be relieved by gentle traction on appendix. A pretied ligature may be used to elevate grossly inflamed appendix with minimal trauma.[26]

Needlescopic Approach

- In laparoscopic approach two 10 mm port and one 5 mm port are used.
- In needlescopic approach one 10 mm and two 2 mm ports are used.

Postoperative Care

- Foley's catheter is removed in postoperative period.
- Rest of the care is same as in open procedure.
- Patient is discharged on second postoperative day.
- Two recent meta-analyses have confirmed the benefit of the laparoscopic approach in relation to less pain, faster recovery and a lower incidence of wound

infection.[27,28] But Cochrane database systemic review of over 4,000 patients suggested that there was a threefold increase in intra-abdominal abscesses and a longer operating time (16 minutes) in those patients undergoing laparoscopic procedure.[29]

> **Key Point**
> Use diathermy least and do not hesitate to convert to open procedure in difficulty.

INTERVAL APPENDICECTOMY

It is defined as 'an elective appendicectomy in the interval' between attacks of appendicitis.

It is the easiest appendicectomy. It is usually done 6–10 weeks after resolution of appendicular mass. Nowadays more and more surgeons are not following a strict regimens of advice of interval appendicectomy 6 weeks after appendicular mass, because it is seen that all cases do not get recurrence, only 20% patients will develop recurrence of appendicitis. Some surgeons advise interval appendicectomy after the inflammation has subsided.[30,31] While other consider subsequent appendicectomy unnecessary.[12] Some surgeons perform interval appendicectomy in children routinely after 8–10 weeks due to higher life time risk of recurrent appendicitis and the lower operative risk than in patients older than 30–40 years of age.[23]

So the interval appendicectomy is gradually fading out. Surgeons follow the dictum 'if require do it', appendicectomy is done only when recurrence develops. Some prefer to do it earlier than waiting 6–10 weeks as it is cost effective.[8]

Interval appendicectomy causes extra cost and hospitalization.[32]

INCIDENTAL APPENDICECTOMY

- It is an appendicectomy for normal appendix during laparotomy or laparoscopy for another condition.
- Centers for disease control using life table technique identified a lifetime risk of appendicitis of 86% in men and 67% in women as per this study 36 appendicectomy have to be performed to prevent one patient from developing appendicitis[33] in other words you have to spend 3.3 US dollar to save 1 dollar.[34] The incidental appendicectomy is neither clinically nor economically appropriate.

> Should normal appendix be removed as a prophylactic measure? This question was answered and seriously discussed by 88 American surgeons. It is sufficient to declare that the proposition was regarded almost unanimously as 'absurd', 'unjustifiable', 'unsurgical' or 'without excuse'. (St. Louis. Med Rev. March 17, 1900).

Indications of Incidental Appendicectomy[35-37]

- Children about to undergo chemotherapy
- Disabled, who cannot describe their symptoms
- Individuals who are about to travel to remote places where is no access to surgical care
- In patient of Crohn's disease whose cecum is free from macroscopic disease
- In Munchausen syndrome for psychological relief
- Along with Ladd's procedure for malrotation
- Doodley's lavage, during colonic lavage on operation table incidental appendicectomy does not significantly increase complications.[38]
- It appears that leaving a normal appearing appendix in fertile women with identifiable gynecological pathology is safe.[39]

Contraindications of Incidental Appendicectomy

- Immunosuppression
- Radiotherapy of cecum
- Crohn's disease involving cecum

In this condition the normal appendix is not removed due to following factors:
- Increased risk of infection.
- Increased chances of appendix stump leak.

RETROGRADE APPENDICECTOMY

When the appendix is found adherent to the posterior parietal peritoneum or even behind the peritoneum, it becomes difficult to do antegrade appendicectomy so we do retrograde appendicectomy. In retrograde appendicectomy, the base of appendix is dealt with first then we move toward tip of the appendix. The cecum is brought to the wound. The base of appendix is ligated and severed. The stump of appendix is invaginated in cecum and cecum is returned back in peritoneal cavity. Then the dissection is done gradually toward the tip of the appendix. Gradually by breaking adhesions we remove the appendix **(Video 17)**.

INVERSION APPENDICECTOMY

Indication

It is done when an incidental appendicectomy is performed.

Aim

- To avoid the risk of sepsis in otherwise clean laparotomy.
- In appendicectomy the bowel is opened and bacterial soiling of peritoneum may happen.

Steps

- Devascularize the appendix by ligating mesoappendix.
- Crush the base of appendix with an artery forceps.
- A probe is used to invert the appendix in cecum, leaving few millimeters not inverted.
- Tie the base of appendix with an absorbable ligature after removing the probe.
- This completely devascularizes the inverted appendix, which will slough out in the lumen of cecum.

HOW TO DEAL WITH SPECIAL CIRCUMSTANCES DURING APPENDICECTOMY?

'The art of medicine cannot be inherited, nor can it be copied from books.'
—**Paracelsus**

- If the wall of cecum is inflamed and edematous then either do not invaginate the stump of appendix or take sutures from healthier area away from stump of appendix due to fear of cut through.
- If base of appendix is edematous and highly inflamed then do not crush the base in fear of embolism and portal pyemia.
- If base of appendix is gangrenous then cut the appendix from base flushed with cecal wall and close the hole by two layers of seromuscular sutures.
- If the appendix is retrocecal and adhered and embedded in posterior cecal wall then you may do 'retrograde appendicectomy or base first appendicectomy'.
- If pus is in good quantity in pelvis and in peritoneal cavity it is better to introduce a rubber drain through a separate stab wound **(Fig. 24)**.

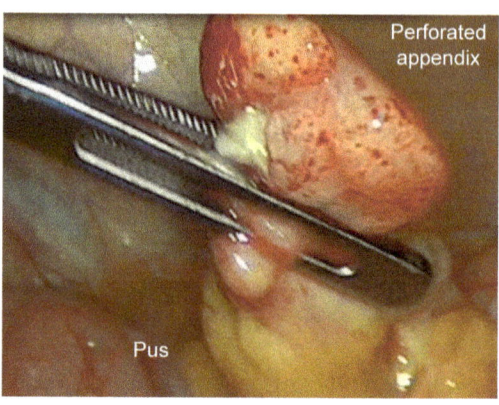

FIG. 24: Place a drain if pus in peritoneal cavity.

CHAPTER 7 Operative Surgery of Appendix

- If normal appendix is found on macroscopic examination. Appendix is then usually removed.
  - Search for other causes of RIF pain by exploring terminal ileum and pelvic organs.
  - Examine the tip of appendix for yellowish small, firm carcinoid tumor.
  - If you decide not to remove the normal looking appendix then explain it to the patient and relatives thoroughly so in future problem the surgeon will not assume that appendicectomy is already done.
  - Rates of negative appendicectomy are approximately 20% but it should be much lower with the present days advance facility for investigations such as ultrasound and computed tomography (CT) scan.
- If appendix is absent, search for retrocecal appendix by cutting peritoneum lateral to cecum along the line of Toldt.[40] Appendix can be at higher site may be subhepatic so extend the incision and search thoroughly by tracing taenia coli.
- If you find tumor of appendix then proceed as following plan:
  - If the tumor is <2 cm in size, appendicectomy is required.
  - If the tumor is >2 cm, right hemicolectomy is required.
  - If Crohn's disease is found with acute appendicitis treat conservatively with antibiotics. No appendicectomy. But if only tip of appendix is inflamed then appendicectomy is done.
- *If appendicular abscess is found*:
  - Drain the abscess
  - Do local peritoneal lavage. Put a drain.
- *If appendix gets burst while removing*:
  - Remove the fecalith from peritoneal cavity.
  - Lavage the local peritoneal cavity with normal saline.
  - Insert a drain.

- *If cecum is not seen*:
  - Follow with your right index finger the peritoneum reflecting from anterior abdominal wall to back.
  - Cecum may be higher up subhepatic, make a search.
- If the base of appendix and part of cecum is gangrenous. Remove all the gangrenous tissue with appendix, put a drainage tube and connect cecum wound edge with local wound skin edge. Remove the drain after few days.
- *Appendix is converted to a lump with abscess*:
  - Additional operating port is must
  - Blunt dissection is done gently
  - Pus is aspirated and collected for bacteriology
  - Cecum is carefully freed from adhesions and ileal loops
  - Resection is done with stapler
  - Appendix is removed with endobag
  - Suction of RIF done
  - A drain may be left in RIF
  - Port wounds are cleaned with 10% povidone—iodine solution
  - Metallic suction cannula can be used to separate appendix adhesions

> **Key Point**
> When doing appendicectomy, always keep in mind that you may find a normal appendix and decide beforehand whether you will remove or leave the appendix to save time during operation.

POSTOPERATIVE COMPLICATIONS OF OPEN APPENDICECTOMY

Age and perforation of appendix significantly increase the complications; one study showed the rate of complications 3% in nonperforated appendicitis and 47% in perforated cases **(Flowchart 1)**.

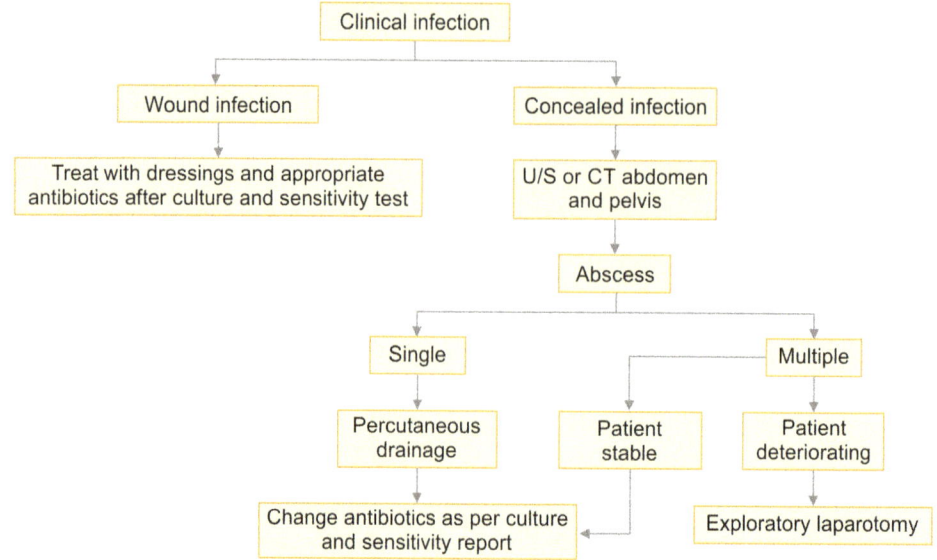

FLOWCHART 1: Algorithm of management of postappendectomy infection.

Complications of appendicectomy:
- Wound infection
- Hemorrhage
- Intraperitoneal abscesses
- Paralytic ileus
- Fecal fistula
- Portal pyemia (pylephlebitis)
- Postoperative adhesions
- Acute intestinal obstruction
- Right inguinal hernia
- Pelvic abscess

Postoperative sequelae after appendectomy are early, intermediate, and late. Early sequelae are due to anesthesia or operation such as hemorrhage, infection, and peritonitis continues. Intermediate sequelae develop within few days to few weeks such as abscess, ileus, phlebitis, embolus lodgment. Late sequelae arise after months or years such as hernia and intestinal obstruction.

Wound Infection

It is the most common postoperative complication. It occurs in <10% cases; it increases with perforated appendicitis to 15–20% and is highest with diffuse peritonitis (35%).[41] It is usually seen at home on 4th or 5th postoperative day. Infection is most commonly found in subcutaneous tissue.
- Wound infection is almost always confined to subcutaneous tissue and responds to simple drainage.
- Wound infection can cause dehiscence or burst abdomen in laparotomy wounds but not in gridiron incision.

Hemorrhage

Slipping of ligature of appendicular artery or accessory appendicular artery is usually the cause of reactionary hemorrhage. Take the patient to OT and open the wound and ligate the bleeding vessel.

Intraperitoneal Abscesses

The incidence of intraperitoneal abscesses has gone down due to preoperative and perioperative antibiotics. Locally increased pain, tenderness, and high fever suggest intra-abdominal abscess. CT scan of abdomen is diagnostic. The abscess can be in following forms:
- Appendix fossa abscess
- Right paracolic gutter abscess

- Pelvic abscess
- Pouch of Douglas abscess
- Subphrenic abscess
- Subhepatic abscess
- Inter small bowel loop abscess, usually multiple

Paralytic Ileus

It happens after every appendicectomy but usually stays longer in gangrenous, perforated appendix and generalized peritonitis.

Fecal Fistula

Nowadays fecal fistula is rare due to regular use of pre, peri, and postoperative antibiotics. It is an annoying but not a dangerous complication. The causes of development of fecal fistula after appendicectomy are:
- Cecal wall edema with inflammation and sloughing of part of cecum inside purse string suture.
- Attempted appendicectomy in appendicular mass.
- Leakage from appendicular stump due to slipping of ligature in noninvaginated stump.
- Appendicectomy in Crohn's disease, tuberculosis, actinomycosis and carcinoma of cecum.
- Tight and deep purse string suture sometimes causes necrosis and leakage.
- Erosion of cecum by drain.
- When carcinoma of appendix is the cause of appendicitis.
- By necrosis of cecum from an abscess. All fecal fistulae close spontaneously in few days unless there is distal obstruction.

> Fecal fistula formation is most common when the appendectomy is performed for gangrene or perforation of appendix.

- *Clinical features*:
  - Features of infection are present as fever, erythema over drain site or operation incision.
  - Foul smelling, feculent discharge from operation wound site or drain site.
  - The skin around fistula becomes excoriated.
- *Investigations*:
  - CT scan abdomen to look for other pathology.
  - CT fistulogram.
- *Treatment*: Conservative treatment are—antibiotic, IV fluids, dressing, protective cream on skin around fistula such as lacto calamine or zinc oxide cream. If the fistula does not close within 6 weeks then consider resection and anastomosis of ileocecal region.

Portal Pyemia (Pylephlebitis)

It is rare nowadays due to use of antibiotics. It is characterized by:
- High fever
- Chills and rigors
- Jaundice

It is due to spread of suppuration to portal vein via superior mesentery vein. It may lead to multiple liver abscesses.

Postoperative Adhesions

It is a late complication of appendicectomy. Diagnostic laparoscopy is required to diagnose. It causes:
- Persistent pain in RIF
- Intestinal obstruction

Acute Intestinal Obstruction

It can occur after appendicectomy due to adhesions. Initially may be paralytic but later on may become mechanical. Obstruction may occur due to band development but it is much less common than adhesions. It is seen in some studies occurring within 6 months and in 1% cases.[42]

Right Inguinal Hernia

It is direct inguinal hernia. The incidence of hernia is three times greater than in a normal person. It occurs more in lower right paramedian incision.[43,44] It can be caused by injury to iliohypogastric nerve, ilioinguinal nerve specially in Rutherford Morison incision.

> Professor Howard A Kelly taught that hernia is best avoided by operating early, before the advent of such symptoms and complications as necessitate drainage of the wound, that is to say, by a very early operation or by one in the interval.

Prophylaxis is, which is the best safeguard against hernia, the small incision whenever it can be employed with equal safety and in the separation of the muscular layers without cutting them (McBurney).

Pelvic Abscess

Nowadays it is reducing due to antibiotic cover. It is characterized by:
- High spiking pyrexia.
- Tenesmus or discomfort at defecation
- Loose stools
- Tender mass on digital rectal examination (DRE).
- Ultrasound and CT scan are diagnostic.

Treatment

- If untreated leads to generalized peritonitis.
- Transrectal drainage of pelvic abscess—DRE is done and then push the closed sinus forceps in pelvic abscess and abscess is drained.

Mortality

In a survey of 8,651 appendectomies done in England and Wales in 1992, the mortality rate was 0.24% and morbidity was 8%.[45-47]

> A patient with an acute appendicitis refused operation, later in the day the pain increased and when seen next morning ……. He was found with a peritonitis characterized by dissociation between pulse and temperature—the operation was then planned for 5 o'clock in the afternoon, but when the hour arrived, the patient was dead (Tuffier. Rev de Chir. 1895;705).

> Delay in operation for appendectomy may prove fatal. Delay may be either by two reasons, either by surgeon or by the patient, not giving consent. Professor Howard A Kelly used to say, 'the question of personal convenience ought not to be considered, and the night should be regarded as the day'…… it may be positively stated that no case of appendicitis where an operation was necessary was ever operated upon too soon, and when the decision to operate is made, no consideration, however, plausible, should be admitted as a reason for unnecessarily delay. Another source of fatal delay may be the desire of the patient or the relatives to await the arrival of members of the family from a distance. If the surgeon is convinced that an operation is imperative, he must not sacrifice the advantages of time to sentiment, but must assume the added responsibility of urging, and even insisting upon instant action.

POSTOPERATIVE COMPLICATIONS AFTER LAPAROSCOPIC APPENDICECTOMY

Anatomic Hazards

- Major vascular injuries during the initiation of a pneumoperitoneum is a much feared complication of laparoscopic procedures.[48]
- There are 2 main vessels in danger of injury while passing trocars and these are:
  - Inferior epigastric vessels
  - Ascending branch of deep circumflex iliac artery.

Inferior Epigastric Artery

It begins as a branch of external iliac artery and ascends medially along medial margin of deep inguinal ring, pierces fascia transversalis and crosses arcuate line entering rectus sheath and runs upward between rectus abdominis muscle and posterior rectus sheath. To avoid injuring to these vessels the trocars should be either in mid line or lateral to left rectus muscle.

Ascending Branch of Deep Circumflex Iliac Artery

Deep circumflex iliac artery arises as a branch of external ileac artery opposite origin of inferior epigastric artery. It runs up and laterally near ASIS it gives ascending branch which runs upward between internal oblique and transversus muscles to avoid its injury the trocar should be 1 finger breadth above ASIS.[49]

Bleeding

Aggressive dissection of mesoappendix is usually responsible for bleeding. Careful and minimal dissection prevents the bleeding. An additional trocar may be required to identify and grasp the bleeding vessel.

Leakage of Pus or Fecolith

It occurs when appendix is distended with pus and inflamed, careful dissection and removal in endobag prevents it. Remove the fecolith or pus immediately and irrigate and suck the field after removal of appendix.

Big Stump is Left or Appendix is Incompletely Removed

It can cause recurrent appendicitis so remove it.

Postoperative Abdominal Abscesses

Intra-abdominal abscess formation is three times more common after laparoscopic appendicectomy than after open appendicectomy.

> Electrocautery injury to bowel—most of the dissection should be done by blunt and sharp dissection and electrocautery is used least.

Key Point
If an appendicular mass fails to respond with antibiotics then it is converting to an abscess.

POSTOPERATIVE CARE

'I am dying from the treatment of too many physicians.'
—**Alexander the Great**

The in-charge of the case should give instructions and these should be followed. Not many persons of unit treat the patient.

The postoperative care instructions should be written clearly. Any change in treatment should also be written and not be verbal. Nurse on-duty must be explained by surgeon everything in detail.

- Nil orally for 24 hours but sips of water can be given from the same evening.
- IV fluids for 24 hours.
- Oral fluid intake allowed by next morning if no complication develops.
- Patient is allowed to be out of bed same evening so as not to get deep vein thrombosis **(Fig. 25)**.
- Gastric suction is not advised in uncomplicated cases of acute appendicitis after smooth appendicectomy.
- Soft diet is started from second postoperative day.
- In case of perforated appendicitis with generalized peritonitis oral intake takes more time so nasogastric suction is done till bowel sounds appear.
- *Antibiotic*:
  - In case of nonperforated acute appendicitis antibiotic coverage is given for 36–48 hours after appendicectomy
  - In perforated appendicitis with or without generalized peritonitis

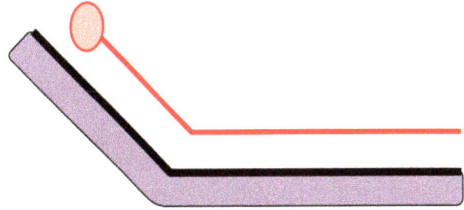

FIG. 25: Patient's position in postoperative period in bed.

antibiotic coverage is given for 7–10 days. IV antibiotics are given until:
- Patient becomes afebrile for 24 hours
- While blood count becomes normal
  - Peritoneal culture is not of much use as by the time the culture reports come, the patient recovers. Peritoneal culture is of use in following conditions:[45,50-54]
    - In immune suppressed patient
    - A patient who develops abscess

FOLLOW-UP OF APPENDICECTOMY PATIENT

- Patient is discharged on 2nd or 3rd day in uncomplicated appendicectomy and later in complicated cases.
- Oral antibiotics, NSAIDs (nonsteroid anti-inflammatory drugs), and PPI (proton pump inhibitor) are given for 5 days at home.
- On 8th postoperative day patient is called in surgical outpatient department (SOPD) for removal of sutures or clips.
- He is advised that he can drive car 10th postoperative day or so.
- He can join his work from 14th post-operative day approximately, depending upon his job.
- He can start his normal activity after 3 weeks of operation.

Postappendectomy checklist if patient is unwell:
- Examine the wound for infection or abscess
- Per-rectal examination to rule out pelvic abscess
- Examine lungs to rule out lobar pneumonia
- Rule out pylephlebitis, liver abscess, subphrenic abscess, and pyelonephritis.

Key Point

In postoperative pyrexia examine chest for atelectasis, dressing for wound infection, and calves for deep vein thrombosis (DVT).

THINGS TO REMEMBER ABOUT APPENDICITIS

- Appendicitis is most common in young males, 20–30 years of age.
- It is common in white race than Asian and Africans.
- It is common in low fiber diet eating individuals.
- It is common during May–August months, due to seasonal variations and viral infections.
- 30% of cases of appendicitis show family history in first degree relatives.
- The commonest position of appendix is retrocecal appendix. Pelvic position is second most common.
- Obstructive appendicitis is more common than catarrhal appendicitis.
- Purgatives are contraindicated in acute abdomen as may cause perforation.
- Fecolith is the most common cause of obstruction in appendicitis.
- Perforation of appendix with gangrene and peritonitis is more common in obstructive appendicitis than in catarrhal appendicitis.
- Pneumoperitoneum and gas under diaphragm on X-ray abdomen are not common findings in perforation of appendix.
- Retrocecal appendicitis does not cause muscular rigidity.
- Appendicular artery is an end artery and its thrombosis leads to early perforation of the tip of the appendix.
- In pregnancy, acute appendicitis is the most common cause of acute abdomen, it is advisable to remove appendix if required during pregnancy.
- In uncomplicated cases of acute appendicitis during pregnancy, the fetal mortality is 5% which becomes 20% in perforated appendix.
- In preileal, postileal and pelvic appendicitis diarrhea is common and it makes the diagnosis doubtful.

- In elderly patients, perforation and gangrene of appendix are common but picture resembles subacute obstruction due to low muscle tone and absence of muscular rigidity which leads to delayed intervention, leads to increased morbidity and mortality **(Fig. 26)**.
- Acute appendicitis is rare before 2 years, but perforation and generalized peritonitis are common due to ill developed omentum at this age. Omentum is bib in a child, but it is an apron in an adult. Rate of perforation in infancy is 80% and the rate of mortality is 50%.
- In children appendectomy should be performed early and conservative treatment should be avoided as peritonitis is common due to delay in diagnosis and poor localization.
- High risk factors in perforation of appendix, in acute appendicitis are:
  - Laxative abuse
  - Diabetes mellitus
  - Immunosuppression
  - Fecolith
  - Old age
  - Childhood
- In pelvic appendicitis, clinical picture may mimic ureteric colic if appendix is touching right ureter and causing its inflammation.
- Negative appendectomy rate is 20–30%.

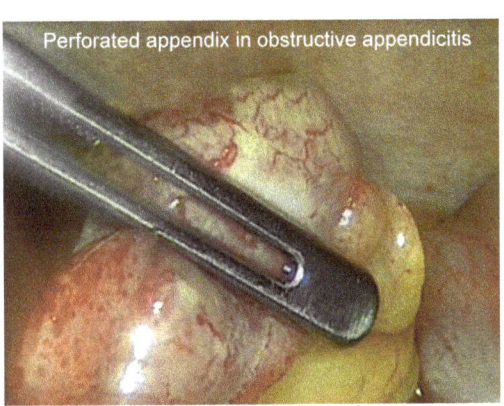

FIG. 26: Perforation of appendix in a patient of 76 years age.

VIDEOS

Video 9: Insertion of Trocar
Video 10: Cautery of Mesoappendix
Video 11: Exploration of Acutely Inflamed Appendix
Video 12: Cutting of Mesoappendix
Video 13: Extraction of Appendix
Video 14: Application of Clips on Mesoappendix
Video 15: Ligation of Base of Appendix
Video 16: Cutting of Base of Appendix
Video 17: Adhesiolysis

REFERENCES

1. Maizels G. Duplication of the vermiform appendix. S Afr Med J. 1966;40:1123-5.
2. Ang CW, Karandikar S. Surgical anatomy of the appendix. In: Nagral S, Nandy S (Eds). The Appendix-ECAB-E-BOOK. Elsevier; 2012.
3. Terasawa T, Blackmore CC, Bent S, Kohlwes RJ. Systematic review: computed tomography and ultrasonography to detect acute appendicitis in adults and adolescents. Ann Intern Med. 2004;141:537-46.
4. Adams ML. The medical management of acute appendicitis in a nonsurgical environment: A retrospective case review. Mil Med. 1990;155:345-7.
5. Serour F, Efrati Y, Klin B, Barr J, Gorenstein A, Vinograd I. Subcuticular skin closure as a standard approach to emergency appendectomy in children: Prospective clinical trail. World J Surg. 1996;20:38-42.
6. Brasel KJ, Burgstrom DC, Weigelt JA. Cost-utility analysis of contaminated appendectomy wounds. J Am Coll Surg. 1997;184:23-30.
7. Orgega JM, Ricardo AE. Surgery of the appendix and colon. In: Moody FG (Ed). Atlas of Ambulatory surgery. Philadelphia: WB Saunders; 1999.
8. Waters DA, Walker MA, Abernethy BC. The appendix stump: should it be invaginated? Ann R Coll Surg Eng. 1984;66:92-3.
9. Engstrom L, Fenyo G. Appendicectomy: assessment of stump invagination versus simple ligation: a prospective, randomized trial. Br J Surg. 1985;72:971-2.

10. Street D, Bodai Bl, Owens LJ, Moore DB, Walton CB, Holcroft JW. Simple ligation vs stump inversion in appendectomy. Ann Surg. 1988;123:689-90.
11. Ozozan OV, Guldogan CE, Gundogdu E, Ozmen MM. Obesity and appendicitis: Laparoscopic vs open technique. Turk J Surg. 2020;36(1):105-9.
12. Flum DR, Steinberg SD, Sarkis AY, Wallack MK. Appendicitis in patients with acquired immunodeficiency syndrome. J Am Coll Surg. 1997;184:481-6.
13. Fischer JE. Appendicitis and appendiceal abscess, Editors comment, mastery of surgery, 5th edition. Philadelphia: Lippincott Williams and Wilkins; 2007. p. 1439.
14. Dellinger EPI. Appendectomy, Commentary, controversies in laparoscopic surgery. Berlin/Heidelberg: Springer International Edition; 2006. p. 383.
15. Panton ON, Samson C, Segal J, Panton R. A four-year experience with laparoscopy in the management of appendicitis. Am J Surg. 1996;171:538-41.
16. Vallina VL, Velasco JM, McCulloocn CS. Laparoscopic versus conventional appendectomy. Ann Surg. 1993;218(5):685-92.
17. Garbutt JM, Soper NJ, Shannon WD, Botero A, Littenberg B. Meta-analysis of randomized controlled trials comparing laparoscopic and open appendectomy. Surg Laparosc Endosc. 1999;9:17-26.
18. Sauerland S, Lefering R, Neugebauer EA. Laparoscopic vs Open surgery for suspected appendicitis. Cochrane Database Syst Rev. 2002;(1):ID001546.
19. Lowy AM, Barie PS. Laparotomy in patients infected with human immunodeficiency virus: Indications and outcome. Br J Surg. 1994;81:942.
20. Arnbjornsson E. Invagination of the appendiceal stump for the reduction of peritoneal bacterial contamination. Curr Surg. 1985;42:184.
21. Golub R, Siddiqui F, Pohl D. Laparoscopic versus open appendectomy: A meta-analysis. J Am Coll Surg. 1988;186:545-53.
22. Hozman MD, Purut CM, Reintgen K, Eubanks S, Pappas TS. Laparoscopic ventral and incisional hernioplasty. Surg Endosc. 1997;11:32-5.
23. Andersen BR, Kallehave FL, Andersen HK. Antibiotics versus placebo for prevention of postoperative infection after appendectomy. Cochrane Database Syst Rev. 2003;(2):CD001439. Update in: Cochrane Database Syst Rev. 2005;(3):CD001439.
24. Hasson HM. Open laparoscopy: a report of 150 cases. J Reprod Med. 1974;12:234-8.
25. Apelgren KN. Laparoscopic Appendectomy, The SAGES Manual fundamental of laparoscopy, Thoracoscopy, and endoscopy, 2nd edition. Berlin/Heidelberg: Springer; 2006. p. 351.
26. Mueller GP, Williams RA. Surgical infections in Aids patients. Am J Surg. 1995;169(5A Suppl):34S.
27. Bova R, Meagher A. Appendicitis in HIV—Positive patients. Aust NZ J Sirg. 1998;68:337.
28. Dulucal JL. Tips and Techniques in Laparoscopic Surgery. Berlin/Heidelberg: Springer; 2005. p. 113-8.
29. Attard AR, Corlett MJ, Kidner NJ, Lestie AL, Fraser IA. Safety of early pain relief for acute abdominal pain. B Med J. 1992;30:554-6.
30. Thomas AH, Chema F, Reisner A, Aman S, Goldstein JN, Kumar AM, et al. Effects of morphine analgesia on diagnostic accuracy in emergency department patients with abdominal pain a prospective randomized trial. J Am Coll Surg. 2003;196(1):18-31.
31. Engstrom L, Renvo G. Appendicectomy: assessment of stump invagination: a prospective, randomized trial. Br J Surg. 1985;72:971-2.
32. Lally KP. Appendix. Sabiston Textbook of Surgery, volume 2, 17th edition. Amsterdam: Elsevier; 2004. p. 1392.
33. Marya SK, Garg P, Singh M, Gupta AK, Singh Y. Is long delay necessary before appendectomy after appendiceal formation? Can J Surg. 1993;36:268-70.
34. Samuel M, Holmes K: Prospective evaluation of nonsurgical versus surgical management of appendiceal mass. J Pediatr Surg. 2002;37:882.
35. Yamini D, Vargas H, Bongard F, Klein S, Stamos MJ. Perforated appendicitis: Is it truly a surgical urgency? Am Surg. 1998;64:970.
36. Jaffe BM, Berger DH. Schwartz's Principles of surgery, 8th edition. New York: McGraw Hill; 2005. p. 1133.
37. Cooperman M. Complications of appendectomy. Surg Clin North Am. 1983;63:1233.
38. Sugimoto T, Edwards D. Incidence and costs of incidental appendectomy as a preventive measure. Am J Public Health. 1987;77:471-5.
39. Wang HT, Sax HC. Incidental appendectomy in the era of managed care and laparoscopy. J Am Coll Surg. 2001;192:182-8.
40. Ritchey ML, Haase GM, Shochat SJ, Kelalis PP. Incidental appendectomy during nephrectomy for Wilms tumor. Surg Gynecol Obstet. 1993;176:423-6.
41. Hunter JG. Advanced laparoscopic surgery. Am J Surg. 1997;173:14.
42. Zollenger RM. Zollenger's Atlas of Surgical Operation, 8th edition. New York: McGraw Hill; 2006. p. 120.
43. Lemieur TP, Rodriguez JL, Jacobs DM, Bennett ME, West MA. Wound management in perforated appendicitis. Am Surg. 1999;65:339-443.

44. Andersson RE. Small bowel obstruction after appendicectomy. Br J Surg. 2001;88:1387-91.
45. Miranda R, Johnston AD, O' Leary JP. Incidental appendectomy: Frequency of pathologic abnormalities. Am Surg. 1980;46:355-7.
46. McGreevy JM, Finlayson SR, Alvarado R, Laycock WS, Birkmeyer CM, Birkmeyer JD. Laparoscopy may be lowering the threshold to operate on patients with suspected appendicitis. Surg Endosc. 2002;16:1046-9.
47. Flum DR, Koepsell T. The clinical and economic correlates of misdiagnosed appendicitis: nationwide analysis. Arch Surg. 2002;137:799-804.
48. Krishankumar S, Tambe P. Entry complications in laparoscopic surgery. J Gynecol Endose Surg. 2009;1(1):4-11.
49. Brooks DC. (1998), Laparoscopic Appendectomy current view of minimally Invasive surgery, Springer. p. 56.
50. Veress J. Neves instrument zur ausfuhrung von brustoder bachqunktionen and pneumothorax behandlung. Dtsch Med Wochenschr. 1938;64: 1480-1.
51. Brooks DC. Laparoscopic Appendectomy current view of minimally invasive surgery. Berlin/Heidelberg: Springer; 1998. p. 57.
52. Burkitt DP. The aetiology of appendicitis. Br J Surg. 1971;58:695.
53. Butler C. Surgical pathology of acute appendicitis. Hum Pathol. 1981;12(10):870-8.
54. Rautio M, Saxen H, Siitonen A, Nikku R, Jousimies-Somer H. Bacteriology of histopathologically defined appendicitis in children. Pediatr Infect Dis J. 2000;19(11):1078-83.

CHAPTER 8
Recent Advancements and Modern Trends

'If you are too fond of new remedies;
First, you will not cure your patient;
Secondly, you will have no patient to cure.'

—Astley Paston Cooper (1768-1841)

INTRODUCTION

Appendicitis is one of the most common emergency conditions faced by a general surgeon. Acute appendicitis if not diagnosed early or neglected leads to complications like gangrene of the appendix, perforation of the appendix and general peritonitis. The complications may prove fatal if not managed properly and early. Advancements in the field of diagnosis, investigations and treatment are continuously evolving. Imaging techniques of today can diagnose acute appendicitis earlier. Scoring systems indicate the severity of the inflammation quickly and help to avoid complications. The surgical technique advancements have made the operation less invasive and more fruitful with less complications.

IMMUNITY AND APPENDIX

Appendix is part of MALT (mucosa associated lymphoid tissue).
- The mucosa contains M-cells which transport antigen.
- The follicular and parafollicular zones of lymphoid follicles contain B and T- lymphocytes.

> It is proved recently that lymphoid follicle act as a local defense mechanism. The bacteria are trapped here while crossing the wall of appendix from lumen of appendix.

- The role of appendix in body's immunological competences is argued against by recent experimental studies. So removal of appendix does not compromise the body's defense mechanism.
- These experiments also argue against appendix being a vestigial organ rather than a specialized organ.
- Appendix secretes immunoglobulins especially IgA.

Dietary Fiber and Appendicitis

Recent studies have doubted the role of high-fiber diet in preventing acute appendicitis. It requires further research. The Cleveland Clinic Department of Gastroenterology says that 'There is no way to prevent appendicitis. However, appendicitis is less common in people who eat foods high in fiber, such as fresh fruits and vegetables.' A study about role of dietary fiber in the cause of acute appendicitis was done by the department of surgery, University of Lund, Sweden.

The results support the hypothesis that diet, in particular lack of fiber may be an important factor in the pathogenesis of acute appendicitis.[1]

Endoscopic Ultrasound

This new technology of doing ultrasound through endoscope (colonoscope) in appendicitis gives more accurate results. It prevents more negative appendicectomies and also prevents complications.

Scarless surgery (NOTES) is still an experimental surgery and requires a good and long follow-up **(Box 1)**.

Needlescopic Appendicectomy

Here we use one 10-mm port and two 2-mm ports.
- 10-mm port entry is dealt with Steri-strips.
- 2-mm port does not require any suture or Steri-strip.

SILS (Single Incision Laparoscopic Surgery)

Laparoscopic appendicectomy can be done through a single incision which if hidden in the umbilicus can make the surgery almost scarless.

Telesurgery

Telesurgery is a new surgical tool that uses robotic surgery by a surgeon on patients at distant location.

Robotic Appendicectomy

Appendicectomy using robot has an advantage of better visualization and may be helpful in complex cases.

Genetic Configuration

Getting appendicitis in several members of a family is not clear and it is thought provoking as far as the familial tendency is concerned. Genes are responsible or not requires more research.

DIMINISHING INCIDENCE OF APPENDICITIS

'What matters is not to add years to your life but to add life to your years.'
—**Alexis Carrel**

The incidence of acute appendicitis is diminishing in western countries. The factors observed as the probable cause of diminishing incidence of appendicitis and its complications are:
- *The increasing use of high fiber vegetarian diet with more use of fruits and green leafy vegetables.
- *Use of antibiotics*: Early operative intervention in case of perforated appendicitis may be associated with more postoperative complications compared to antibiotic therapy followed by interval appendicectomy.[2-4]
- Improved lifestyle changes and personal hygiene due to more awareness are also helpful.
  - In Europe and USA mortality rate of acute appendicitis has come down from 8.1 per 100,000 to 1 per 100,000.
  - Incidence of acute appendicitis fell 50% between 1960 and 1980 and is continuously falling.

BOX 1 Scarless surgery—NOTES.

NOTES:
- *Natural Orifice Transluminal Endoscopic Surgery (NOTES):*
  - Surgeons are trying to remove diseased abdominal organs through natural orifices
  - Flexible endoscope is used to remove the organ from natural orifice. Transvaginal removal of the normal appendix has been done recently[2]

Advantages of NOTES:
- Reduction of postoperative pain
- Shorter convalescence so less man-hour loss
- No wound infection
- No scar
- No abdominal wall hernia

APPENDICOSTOMY (MALONE PROCEDURE)

'I have noticed that doctors who fail in the practice of medicine have a tendency to seek one another's company and consultation. A doctor who cannot take out your appendix properly will recommend you to a doctor who will be unable to remove your tonsils with success.'

—**Ernest Hemingway**
(A Farewell to Arms)

Nowadays appendix is used for antegrade colonic enema via appendicostomy. Antegrade colonic enema via appendicostomy was started by Padraig Seamus Malone, Pediatric Urologist, Southampton General Hospital, Southampton, England. Appendix is connected to the umbilicus and a valve is created here which allows appendix to be catheterized and enema is done. It is done in children suffering with:

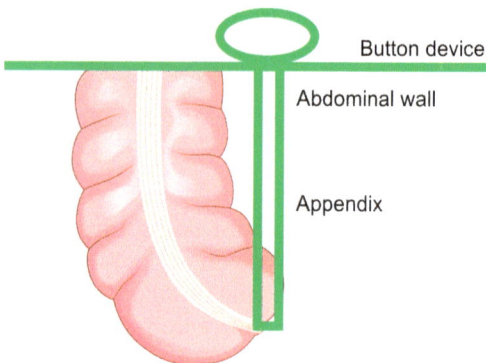

FIG. 1: Appendicostomy (Malone procedure).

- Anorectal malformation
- Neuropathic rectum
- *Appendicovesicostomy (Mitrofanoff procedure)*: It is done as patients with chronic catheterization.
- *Hepatoporto-appendicostomy*: Appendix is put between biliary tree and duodenum after resection of choledochal cyst **(Fig. 1)**.

Key Point

Modern equipment and techniques should be used by experienced surgeons, knowing his/her limitations and without compromising the outcome.

REFERENCES

1. Einar Arnbjornsson. Acute Appendicitis and Dietary Fiber. Arch Surg. 1983;118(7):868-70.
2. Oliak D, Yamin D, Udani VM, Lewis RJ, Vargas H, Arnell T, et al. Nonoperative management of perforated appendicitis without periappendicial mass. Am J Surg. 2000;179(3):177-81.
3. So JBY, Chiong EC, Chiong E, Cheah WK, Lomanto D, Goh P, et al. Laparoscopic appendectomy for perforated appendicitis. World J Surg. 2002;26(12):1485-8.
4. Hortwitz JR, Custer MD, May BH, Mehall JR, Lally KP. Should laparoscopic appendectomy be avoided for complicated appendicitis in children? J Pediatr Surg. 1997;32(11):1601-3.

CHAPTER 9

Some Rituals and Thoughts that are Becoming Obsolete

'In the carriages of the past you can't go anywhere.'
—**Maxim Gorky**

INTRODUCTION

Acute appendicitis is the routinely performed surgery by a general surgeon. Earlier the appendicitis was diagnosed by physical examination and Total Leucocyte Count (TLC), in a way it was diagnosed by surgeon's hands. Still the physical signs are reliable sources for diagnosis of appendicitis, but to increase the accuracy of the diagnosis now we take help from advance techniques such as CT scan and scoring systems. Sometimes, in confusing cases we have to take help of diagnostic laparoscopy also. As clinical diagnosis is not absolute, therefore, scoring systems combining with clinical signs and serum markers of inflammation are widely advocated. In laparoscopic appendicectomy the stump closure can be done either by stapler or endoloop, which is better is still debatable.

T Rasmussen et al. indicated that 'appendectomy had a low percentage of long term surgical complications'[1], but we have to drop obsolete practices and adopt new helpful advance techniques.

1. Appendix is a specialized organ but its removal does not cause any problem.
2. No one sign is diagnostic of acute appendicitis. It must be full clinical and investigative picture consideration for accurate diagnosis.
3. '1-2 hour urgent appendicectomy' can be extended to '3-4 hours appendicectomy with IV antibiotic'.
4. 'Long triple regimen' of antibiotics has become obsolete, in uncomplicated or simple cases 24 hours antibiotics cover is enough, in complicated cases (i.e., perforation) 3-5 days cover is sufficient.
5. Incision should be small 2.5-3 cm and then if required can be increased. The dictum 'Big surgeons make big incision' is obsolete.
6. Chemical cautery or electric cautery to free end of appendix stump is not a must. Although Povidone-iodine is frequently applied on appendicular stump, but in review of literatures, no definitive guidelines favoring its use on appendix stump could be retrieved.[2]
7. Burial of stump of appendix with purse string suture is not required. Some surgeons routinely burry the stum in the cecum, but it has not been proven to reduce leaks.[3]

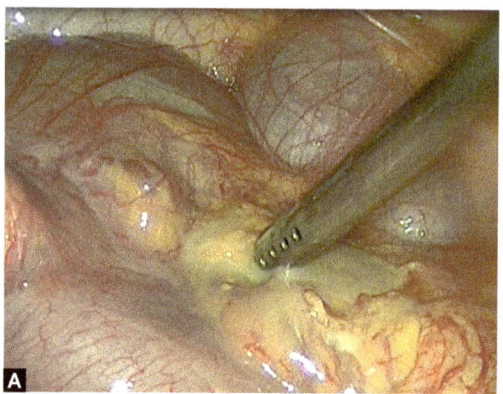 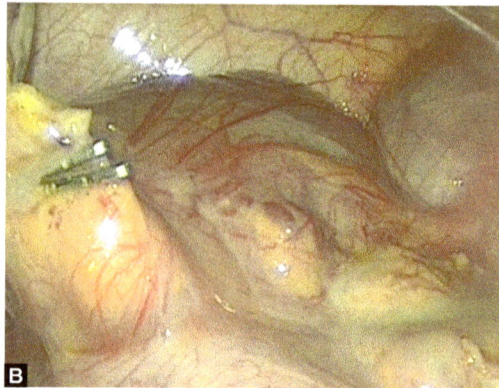

FIGS. 1A AND B: Suction of pus from peritoneal cavity.

8. Drain is not introduced unless abscess is present.
9. Suck the pus if present. Do not do peritoneal toilette **(Figs. 1A and B)**. Some authors have found that peritoneal irrigation seems to increase risk of developing postoperative intra-abdominal abscess (IAA) after appendectomy, independently from a laparoscopic or open approach.[4,5] Gloria Burini et al. indicated in their study that this meta-analysis suggest the use of an only-suction approach of purulent liquid in cases of localized peritonitis during appendectomy. In the presence of diffuse purulent peritonitis, a prolonged lavage until the abdomen is completed cleansed may still be preferable.[6]
10. Some surgeons stopped suturing peritoneal opening if small.
11. Muscles are not stitched together unless cut.

Key Point

It is an individual discretion based on personal experience to use staple or endoloop in stump closure.

REFERENCES

1. Rasmussen T, Fonnes S, Rosenberg J. Long Term Complications of Appendectomy: A Systematic Review. Scand J Surg. 2018;107(3):189-96.
2. Ahmad OA, Sarwar MZ, Muneera MJ, Latif W, Chatha A, Waheed K. Appendicular Stump Disinfection Using Povidone-Iodine Swab Compared With Electrocautery; which one is more effective? JFJMC. 2017;11(1):25-9.
3. Humes MD, Speake MWJ, Simpson MJ. Appendicitis. BMJ Clin Evid. 2007;2007:0408.
4. Cho J, Park I, Lee D, Sung K, Back J, Lee J. Risk factors for post operative intra-abdominal abscess after laparoscopy appendectomy: analysis for consecutive 1817 experiences. Dig Surg. 2015; 32(5):375-81.
5. Noore CB, Smith RS, Herbertson R, Toves C. Does use of intraoperative irrigation with open or laparoscopic appendectomy reduce post-operative intra-abdominal abscess? Am Surg. 2011;77(1):78-80.
6. Burini G, Cinanci MC, Cocetta M, Spizzirri A, Saverio SD, Coletta R, et al. aspiration versus peritoneal lavage in appendicitis: a meta-analysis. World J Emerg Surg. 2021;16(1):44.

CHAPTER 10

Questions Patients may ask

'I remember burying a girl fourteen years of age who had died with a ruptured appendix.'
—Tommy Douglas

INTRODUCTION

It is always good to part the knowledge and information about a sickness so that people can know what to do. By answering questions asked by people and patients we the surgeons, make them aware of seriousness of appendicitis, its complications and risk factors. The importance of early diagnosis and quick management can be explained this way. Q&A and discussions can help in avoiding serious complications of delayed and neglected treatment which may prove serious and even fatal sometimes. Bursting or rupture of inflamed appendix leading to general peritonitis can be prevented. Though it is not possible to prevent appendicitis, but healthy, balanced, plant based and fiber rich diet can reduce chances of developing appendicitis can be well explained. Atypical presentations such as back pain, diarrhea and burning sensation during micturition can be explained stressing for early medical consultation.

Question: What is appendix?
Answer: It is a small tube-like structure attached with intestine. It is situated in right lower part of the abdomen.

Question: What is the function of appendix in our body?
Answer: It is unknown, not clear. Some researchers feel it is a vestigial structure that has lost all or most of its functions. Others believe that it is designed to protect good bacteria in the intestine.

Question: What is the problem in appendicitis?
Answer: Appendicitis is the inflammation of appendix which is mostly due to blockage and appendix gets filled with pus. It causes pain in lower right side of abdomen.

Question: Why operation is necessary?
Answer: Operation is required to relieve symptoms of inflammation of appendix which are very painful and to prevent bursting of appendix leading to dangerous condition called peritonitis.

Question: What are the symptoms of appendicitis?
Answer: Common symptoms of appendicitis are:
- Pain in right lower part of abdomen
- Nausea and vomiting
- Fever
- Anorexia
- Right lower part of abdomen is tender to touch

Question: How is postoperative period?
Answer: In uncomplicated case you are allowed liquid orally in first 24 hours and then semisolid soft diet. Movement is encouraged.

Question: When can I be discharged from hospital?
Answer: You are discharged from hospital in 2–3 days, when you can walk and tolerate orally.

Question: When stitches are removed?
Answer: It usually takes 7–8 days for removal of stitches.

Question: What are the long-term effects of appendicectomy?
Answer: Usually there is no long-term effects of appendicectomy.

Question: Why appendix is so prone to infection?
Answer: Appendix is a tubular structure and is connected with lumen of intestine so it gets blocked by hard stool pieces called fecalith.

Question: Why the operation for appendicitis is urgent?
Answer: Delay in operation may lead to dangerous and life-threatening complications such as bursting of inflamed appendix and releasing infected material in whole of the abdomen cavity leading to very dangerous condition (**Fig. 1**).

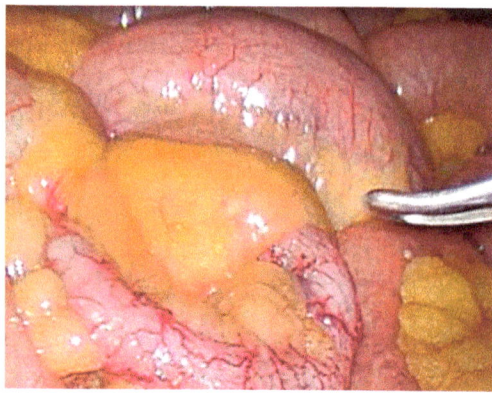

FIG. 1: Acute appendicitis.

In the United States, mortality following appendectomy is 0.1%, Worldwide it is estimated 0.3%.[1,2]

Question: How the operation is done?
Answer: Operation is commonly done under general or spinal anesthesia. A 3–4 inches cut is made in right lower part of abdomen. Abdominal cavity is opened and appendix is removed. It can also be performed by laparoscopic method.

Question: After how many days of appendix operation I can exercise?
Answer: Two weeks after laparoscopic operation and 4 weeks after open appendicectomy.

Question: How is the operation of appendix is done?
Answer:
By two ways:
1. Laparoscopic or keyhole operation
2. Open operation

Question: How much time does full recovery take after appendix operation?
Answer: 2–4 weeks.

Question: A child who is operated for appendix, when can join school?
Answer: 2 weeks.

Question: What are the complications of appendicitis?
Answer:
1. Bursting of appendix.
2. Abscess formation.

Question: How long does appendix surgery last?
Answer: Half an hour to 45 minutes depending upon its condition.

Question: How long do you stay in hospital for appendix operation?
Answer: 2–3 days.

Question: When you can fly after appendix surgery?
Answer: After 1 week.

CHAPTER 10 Questions Patients may ask

Question: When you can start your gym?
Answer: 6–8 weeks but do not lift heavy weight before 3 months.

Question: When I can drive my car after appendix operation?
Answer: After 10 days.

Question: How can I prevent appendicitis?
Answer: You cannot prevent appendicitis but increase fiber in your diet as it is seen that people who eat a plant-based diet of fresh fruits and vegetables have less incidence of appendicitis than nonvegetarians.

Question: Why do we require an appendix?
Answer: Scientists have discovered that appendix harbors beneficial gut bacteria and when one suffers from an attack of diarrhea and the beneficial bacteria are flushed out of body, appendix helps to recover the growth of these beneficial bacteria. That is why appendix is not considered a useless structure now.

Question: Is appendix in anyway related with body's immunity?
Answer: Appendix has some immune system cells which protect the beneficial bacteria residing in its lumen.

Question: Can I avoid operation for appendix and take medicines only?
Answer: The operative management of appendicitis is standard, but certain clinical situations are controversial. The conservative management of appendicitis with antibiotics is not durable in the short to medium term with high rates of complications eventually needing surgical management.[3,4]

Key Point

Appendix is not a useless structure, but it is an important organ acting as a reservoir for body friendly bacteria.

REFERENCES

1. Alove EA, Ward JL, Todd SR, Wilson CT, Gordy SD, Hoffman MK, et al. Population-level outcomes of early versus delayed appendectomy for acute appendicitis using the American College of Surgeons National Surgical Quality Improvement Program. J Surg Res. 2018;229:234-42.
2. Sartelli M, Baiocchi GL, Di Saverio, Ferrara F, Labricciosa FM, Ansaloni L, et al. Prospective Observational Study on acute Appendicitis Worldwide (POSAW). World J Emerg Surg. 2018; 13:19.
3. Ansaloni L, Catena F, Coccolini F, Ercolani G, Gazzotti F, Pasqualini E, et al. Surgery versus conservative antibiotic treatment in acute appendicitis: a systematic review and meta-analysis of randomized controlled trials. Dig Surg. 2011;28(3):210-21.
4. Fitzmaurice GJ, McWilliams B, Hurreiz H, Epanomeritakis E. Antibiotics versus appendectomy in the management of acute appendicitis: a review of the current evidence. Can J Surg. 2011;377:1545-6.

CHAPTER 11

Difficulties and Problems in Appendicectomy

'Open appendicectomy is the gold standard for appendicitis specially in complicated and difficult cases. Conversion of laparoscopic appendectomy to open appendectomy must not be delayed.'

—**Vinod Kumar Nigam**

INTRODUCTION

Laparoscopic appendicectomy is gradually increasing, but still the open appendicectomy is considered as gold standard for appendicitis, more so in difficult and complicated cases. In difficult cases where surgeon is facing problem going ahead, the laparoscopic surgery should be converted to open surgery to avoid injury to intestine and other structures and to reduce postoperative complications. In open surgery if difficulty is faced by the surgeon, the incision should be extended.

Carlos Augusto Gomes et al. defined and divided the complicated appendicitis in five grades, i.e., Grade 0- Normal looking appendix, Grade 1- Hyperemia and edema, Grade 2- Fibrinous exudate, Grade 3A- Segmental necrosis, Grade 3B- Base necrosis, Grade 4A- Abscess, Grade 4B- Regional peritonitis, Grade 5- Diffuse peritonitis.[1]

IF THE CECUM CANNOT BE FOUND?

It is due to two reasons:
1. Cecum is not descended to right iliac fossa (RIF)
2. Cecum is somewhere else in abdomen due to malrotation of gut.

What to do:
- Extend the incision in upward direction
- If you are convinced that cecum is elsewhere then close this incision and make a midline incision and search for cecum and appendix

IF CECUM IS FOUND BUT CANNOT BE DELIVERED IN WOUND?

It is due to diminished mobility of cecum due to tight peritoneal reflection.

What to do: The peritoneal fold is divided near lower pole of cecum on lateral side. Avoid injury to:
- Gonadal vessels
- Right ureter

IF APPENDIX CANNOT BE FOUND?

Follow one of the taeniae coli especially anterior taenia coli, this will lead to the base of appendix. If still not found then:
- Enlarge the incision
- Appendix may be buried in posterior wall of cecum. Cecum is pulled to left so the parietal peritoneum reflection on lateral side of cecum is made tense and visible. A vertical incision is made which is curved at the lower end of cecum. Blunt dissection is done with a pledget on artery forceps and cecum further retracted to left, gradually the posterior surface of cecum and buried appendix will be visible. Take care of following two structures:
  i. Right ureter
  ii. Right gonadal vessels
- Appendix may be intussuscepted and you will find a dimple or umbilication in cecum.
- Appendix has sloughed off and appendix is not present at all

CECUM MAY NOT BE CECUM BUT IT IS SIGMOID COLON OR TRANSVERSE COLON

- Sigmoid colon is recognized by:
  - Mesentery
  - Appendices epiploicae
- Transverse colon has:
  - Omentum attached to it
  - Appendices epiploicae

What to do:
- Pack the sigmoid colon toward pelvis and transverse colon medially and up
- Bring the appendix to wound

Experienced surgeon will put his index finger and will hook out the appendix. Hooking of appendix is not for a beginner as it is a dangerous procedure. A beginner should enlarge the incision.

WHEN WHOLE APPENDIX IS NOT REMOVED?

Always examine the appendix after its removal and see that it is completely removed with its intact tip. If a piece of appendix is left in, then it will liquefy and cause infection and may form intraperitoneal abscess. Sometime the proximal end of the appendix is not removed as it is buried in cecal wall.

What to do: A piece of appendix must not be left behind. It must be removed. You may need to extend the incision for better access.

WHEN IN GANGRENOUS APPENDIX THE DISCOLORATION HAS REACHED UP TO CECUM?

The appendix base is removed with cuff of cecum and the cecal hole is closed with few interrupted sutures. Sutures are applied before removal of appendix **(Fig. 1)**.

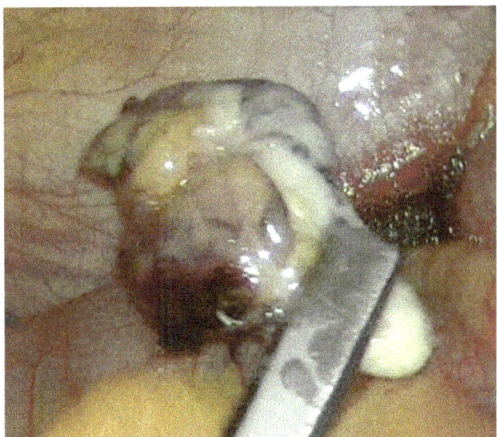

FIG. 1: Gangrenous appendix, gangrene reaching to the cecum.

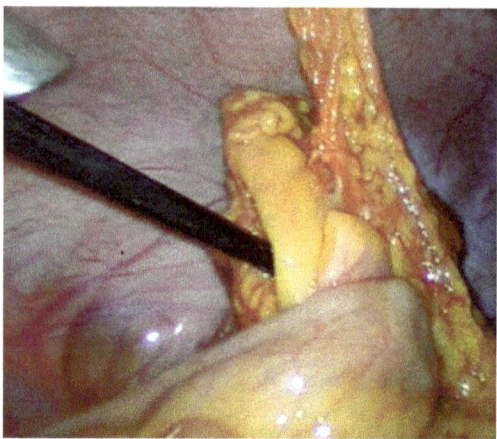

FIG. 2: Appendix engulfed by omentum due to adhesions. Therefore omentum is called 'abdominal policeman'.

WHEN THE OMENTUM IS ADHERENT TO THE APPENDIX?

Sometime it is difficult to separate appendix and omentum. A piece of omentum is also removed between hemostats with appendicectomy **(Fig. 2)**.

WHAT IF A TUMOR IS FOUND?

Relationship of carcinoma of cecum and appendicitis is studied widely and is found that rarely appendicitis may be due to carcinoma.
- Carcinoma of cecum may obstruct the orifice of appendix and can cause acute obstructive appendicitis.
- Sometimes the doubt of a carcinoma of cecum is created when an already drained appendicular abscess does not heal and further exploration reveals a carcinoma.

What to do: Right hemicolectomy.

WHEN A STUMP AFTER APPENDICECTOMY LEAKS?

Furthermore, appendiceal stump leakage secondary to inadequate stump closure is a recognized complication following laparoscopic appendectomy.[2,3]

It happens rarely but when happens may cause local collection or even generalized peritonitis.

What to do:
- Normal saline peritoneal lavage
- Cecostomy:
  - Deflate the cecum and decompress it by squeezing it or with a low pressure suction.
  - A no 20 Foleys catheter is introduced in cecum and taken out from abdominal wall and fixed. Or a Blowhole cecostomy is done by suturing the cecum to abdominal wall and a colostomy bag is applied.

WHEN HEMORRHAGE OCCURS FROM APPENDICULAR MESENTERY?

It is not a common event, it occurs rarely. There is pain in RIF and tachycardia. There may be localized or generalized peritoneal irritation.

What to be done:
- Reopen the abdomen
- Do suction for collected blood
- Identify the bleeding site. Ligate the bleeding vessel:
  - Tissue becomes friable in infection so be gentle
  - Be careful about ileocecal vein ligation as it may cause bleeding and congestion and semi-infarct to cecum.

A patient with multiple comorbidities or with severe sepsis will require intensive care admission for support. Apart from resuscitation, adequate analgesia is essential and the appropriate antibiotics should be given to obviously unwell patients. Urgent surgery is required as delay increases the morbidity and mortality.[4,5]

CHAPTER 11 Difficulties and Problems in Appendicectomy

> **Key Point**
> First step in appendectomy is finding the cecum and then searching for the attachment of appendix on it.

REFERENCES

1. Gomes CA, Sartelli M, Gomes CC, Ansaloni L, Catena F, Coccolini F, et al. Acute appendicitis: proposal of a new comprehensive grading system based on clinical, imaging and laparoscopic findings. World J Emerg Surg. 2015; 10:60.
2. Makram N, Knight SR, Ibrahim A, Patil P, Wilson MSJ. Closure of appendiceal stump in laparoscopic appendectomy: A systematic reviewed of the literature. Ann Med Surg. 2020;57:228-35.
3. Rickert A, Krieger CM, Runkel N, Kuthe A, Köninger J, Jansen-Winkeln B,. The TICAP-Study (titanium clips for appendicular stump closure): a prospective multicentric observational study on appendicular stump closure with an innovative titanium clip. BMC Surg. 2015;15:85.
4. Ditillo MF, Dziura JD, Rabinovici R. Is it safe to delay appendectomy in adults with acute appendicitis? Ann Surg. 2006;244:656-60.
5. Nundi S, Nagral S. The Appendix. In: Chandra R, Wong A, Keck JO (Eds). Acute Appendicitis. Elsevier; 2014.

CHAPTER 12

Arguments, Controversies, and Discussions in Diseases of Appendix

'The human appendix, formerly thought to be vestigial, is now known to be a functioning component of the immune system.'
—**William A Dembski**

INTRODUCTION

Acute appendicitis is one of the most common diseases for which a surgeon is called. The diagnosis and management of appendicitis though straightforward but sometimes even the experienced and senior surgeon gets baffled. Delay in diagnosis and management leads to complications which can prove serious and even fatal. In spite of this, more than 1/4 patients of acute appendicitis come to the hospital after 48 hours.

In uncomplicated cases of acute appendicitis, generally it is believed that the laparoscopic appendicectomy has advantages over open appendicectomy such as cosmetic, less pain, short hospital stay, low incidence of wound infection and good for obese patients, but the chances of postoperative intra-abdominal abscesses in case of perforated appendix increase in laparoscopic appendicectomy.

Controversy persists regarding the use of imaging studies for diagnosis, laparoscopic versus open surgical methods, nonoperative management of uncomplicated appendicitis, delayed management of the patient with phlegmon from severe appendicitis, the necessity for interval appendectomy, and the merits of deferral of off-hour appendectomy until following morning.[1]

There are many areas of controversies in diseases of appendix. The main topics are following:
- Appendicectomy—open or laparoscopic.
- Perforated appendix—open or laparoscopic appendicectomy.
- Appendicectomy—ligation of base or stapling.
- Normal looking appendix—remove or leave it.
- Pregnancy—open or laparoscopic appendicectomy.

> Acute appendicitis is one of the most common surgical problems in general surgery. Diagnostic accuracy of acute appendicitis has not much improved in spite of increased use of diagnostic modalities such as ultrasound and CT scan.[2-4]

WHETHER APPENDIX IS VESTIGIAL ORGAN OR NOT

Earlier researches could not link the appendix to any of the purposeful function and that is why the appendix was called as a vestigial organ.

Now the appendix is found having link with immunological status.
- Lymphoid follicles of the wall of appendix help in maturation of lymphocytes.

- Gut-associated lymphoid tissue (GALT) forms globulin and appendix is a part of GALT due to its abundant lymphoid follicles.

The appendix is now considered as a specialized organ.

So it is not taken as a vestigial organ any more now.

OPEN OR CONVENTIONAL VERSUS LAPAROSCOPIC APPENDICECTOMY

In fact the most important determinant factor whether an open or a laparoscopic appendicectomy is done appears to be the preference of the surgeon who treats the patient.[5]

Laparoscopic appendicectomy has not gained as much popularity as laparoscopic cholecystectomy. The reasons behind this are:

- Open appendicectomy is an easy and small procedure and not like an open cholecystectomy. It requires less time also so its popularity is not being dented by laparoscopic appendicectomy.
- In suppurative or perforated appendicitis the probable risk of spread of infection due to pneumoperitoneum restricts some surgeons to go for laparoscopic appendicectomy.

Two big studies confirmed that laparoscopic appendicitis has advantage over conventional appendicectomy but with laparoscopic appendicectomy intraabdominal abscess increase up to three fold in presence of perforation, in such cases open approach should be preferred due to increased chances of residual intraabdominal abscesses.

David C Brooks, Professor of Clinical Surgery, Harvard Medical School Brigham and Women's Hospital, follows a standard policy to use laparoscopy in all women of child-bearing age who have a negative pregnancy test. If there is an obvious appendicitis, appendectomy is performed, in absence of gross sign of appendicular pathology, prophylactic appendectomy is not done; however, in any equivocal case, a laparoscopic appendectomy is performed to avoid future ambiguity between the diagnosis of an acute appendicitis and a gynecologic condition.[6]

Advantages of Laparoscopic Appendicectomy

- Less pain on 1st postoperative day
- Shorter hospital stay
- Faster recovery and early return to normal activity
- Low incidence of wound infection
- Almost no scar
- Good for obese patients
- Good for females of child-bearing age as it excludes the gynecological cause of right iliac fossa (RIF) pain.

The Cochrane library published randomized controlled trials comparing laparoscopic with open appendectomy in 2003 and found laparoscopic appendectomy superior to open appendectomy as regards to postoperative recovery, short length of hospital stay, and reduced time to return to normal activity.

In the morbidly obese patients, laparoscopic appendicectomy performed for acute and perforated appendicitis is associated with a short length of stay and lower morbidity and costs. Laparoscopic appendicectomy should be the procedure of choice for the treatment of acute appendicitis in the morbidly obese population.

DISADVANTAGES OF LAPAROSCOPIC APPENDICECTOMY

- Longer operation time
- More incidence of intra-abdominal abscesses
- More expensive
- Requires experienced surgeon

The laparoscopic appendicectomy is to be encouraged. The disadvantages are reduced to only being more expensive procedure in hands of experienced surgeons and then there is always a chance to convert to open if problems arise.

Does Laparoscopic Appendectomy Influence Risk of Infection?

- One of the principal advantages of laparoscopy over open surgery is the decreased incidence of wound complications including surgery site infection.
- In contrast the use of pneumoperitoneum, dependent positioning and increased duration of surgery in laparoscopic appendectomy may increase the risk of developing intra-abdominal infection as compared with that of open surgery.

Laparoscopic appendicectomy has replaced open appendicectomy in most of the countries, but still the open appendicectomy is important in complicated cases of appendicitis such as perforated or gangrenous appendicitis and other complicated cases. It has been observed that the incidence of intra-abdominal abscess formation is more in laparoscopic appendicectomy than open appendicectomy. Wound infection in open appendicectomy is more common than laparoscopic appendicectomy especially in case of perforated appendicitis.

DEBATE I: PERFORATED APPENDIX —OPEN OR LAPAROSCOPIC APPENDICECTOMY

Laparoscopic appendicectomy has less incidence of wound infection than open appendicectomy.[7]

Pneumoperitoneum, dependent positioning and increased duration of surgery with laparoscopic appendectomy may increase the risk of developing intra-abdominal infection as compared with that of open surgery.[8] The modern management of intra-abdominal infection has substantially reduced the morbidity **(Fig. 1)**.[9]

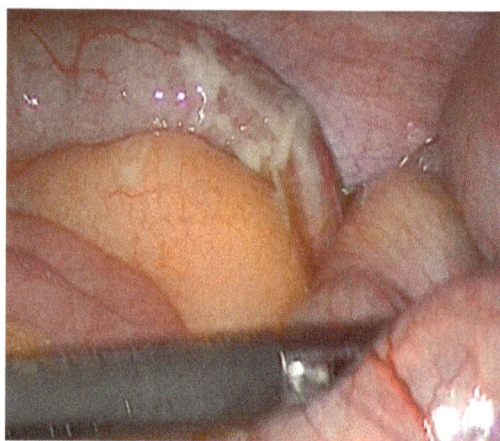

FIG. 1: Perforated appendix with localized peritonitis.

In presence of gross perforation with generalized peritonitis, peritoneal toilette may be more effective with open surgery than with laparoscopic surgery. If perforation is discovered during laparoscopic appendicectomy, if feasible 'not to convert' to open surgery.[10]

DEBATE II: APPENDICECTOMY— LIGATION OR STAPLING OF BASE OF APPENDIX

Endoloop ligation of the base of appendix does not take care of mesoappendix but stapler can deal with the base of appendix and mesoappendix at the same time **(Figs. 2 and 3)**.

The base of appendix can be divided after treating with endoloop or divided by a linear stapler. Linear stapler is having advantages over ligature. These are:
- Appendix base and mesoappendix can be divided in single maneuver even in presence of inflamed mesoappendix, though the time of procedure remains almost same.[10]
- When appendix is grossly inflamed with mesoappendix the linear stapler is of great help without causing much manipulation.
- A randomized comparative study by Orlege[11,12] showed that ligation was asso-

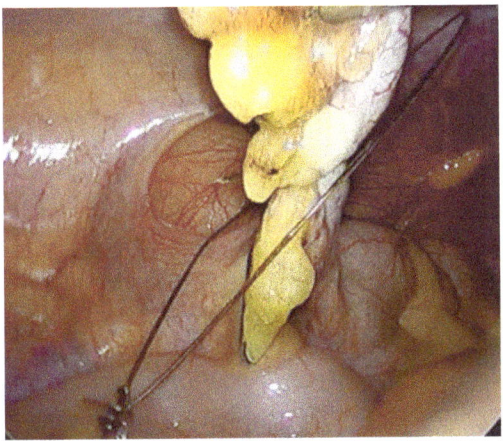

FIG. 2: Application of endoloop.

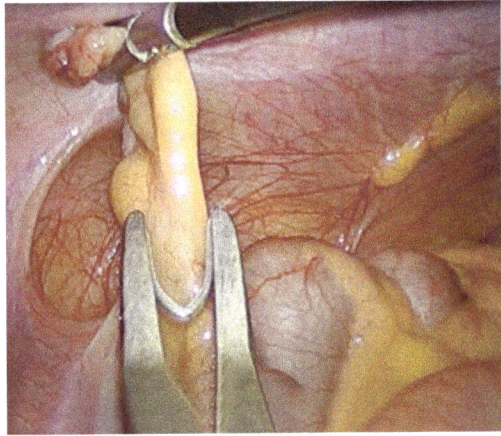

FIG. 3: Application of clip.

ciated with higher incidence of vomiting than laparoscopic linear stapler on appendectomy.

DEBATE III: NORMAL LOOKING APPENDIX—REMOVE OR LEAVE IT?

Approximately 20% appendices on histopathology are found normal. If the percentage of normal appendix is high then it means that we are removing unnecessary appendices and if the figure is much less then we are waiting too long.

- When you find a normal appendix on operation. Explore the abdomen for possible causes of such pain such as Meckel's diverticulitis, amoebic typhlitis, terminal ileitis, salpingitis, and other tubo-ovarian diseases then remove the appendix if every other cause is excluded to avoid future RIF pain and future diagnostic dilemma send the appendix for histopathology.
- The infection and inflammation starts in the mucosa of the appendix and then spreads out to the serosa, so in spite of inflammation in mucosa, the outside macroscopic findings may be normal as 25–30% of appendices on appendicectomy are macroscopically normal. If you cut open the appendix some of these will be found having inflamed mucosa. The inflammation may later be confirmed by histopathology.
- Before taking a decision for removal of an appendix which is normal consider the RIF pain cause in that particular case including any previous history of RIF pain. Weight the merits and demerits of appendicectomy in this particular case and then take the decision.
- Removal of noninflamed appendix does less harm than the nonremoval of inflamed appendix.
- Some surgeons feel that removal of normal appendix on exploration or on laparoscopy is to be done for following reasons:[13]
  - If pain occurs in future then the diagnosis of appendicitis will not be considered.
  - Normal looking appendix may be inflamed and can be shown on pathological examination.
- Up to 45% normal appearing appendices are found in young females. There may be pathological inflammation in normal looking appendix it can be confirmed by exploring the appendix macroscopically.[14] A study showed that 16%

normal appendix not removed returned to emergency department because of recurrent abdominal pain after a median time of 8 month.[15] Appendicectomy for a normal looking appendix is a quick and uncomplicated operation.[16]

DEBATE IV: PREGNANCY— OPEN OR LAPAROSCOPIC APPENDICECTOMY?

There is always danger of spontaneous abortion in first trimester and of premature labor in third trimester.[17] Acute appendicitis is an emergency and delay can cause perforation and disaster. Laparoscopy during pregnancy carries risks due to following factors:

- Untoward effects of pneumoperitoneum
- Increased intrauterine pressure over uterine blood flow
- Fetal acidosis
- Risk of surgery to uterus and fetus
- Uterine and fetal injury can occur from Veress needle and trocars.

Various studies have shown that laparoscopic appendectomy can be done with low incidence of fetal loss but it must be done with caution. Open approach should be used after first trimester.

Key Point
Abdominal surgery in a pregnant patient should be deferred till pregnancy is over except emergency requiring urgent surgical intervention due to risk of premature labor and loss of fetus and mother.

REFERENCES

1. Meeks DW, Kao LS. Controversies in Appendicitis, Surg Infect (Larchmt). 2008;9(6):553-8.
2. Addiss DG, Shaffer N, Fowlers BS, Tauxe RV. The epidemiology of appendicitis and appendectomy in the United States. Am J Epidemiol. 1990;132: 910-25.
3. Wen SW, Naytor CD. Diagnostic accuracy and short term surgical out comes in cases of suspected acute appendicitis. CMAJ. 1995;152:1617-26.
4. Flum DR, Movris A, Koepsell T, Dellinger EP. Has misdiagnosis of appendicitis decreased over time? A population based analysis. JAMA. 2001;286:1748-53.
5. Grvini P, Smith LC, Urbach DR. The surgeon on call is a strong factor determining the use of a laparoscopic approach for appendectomy. Surg Endosc. 2002;16:1774-7.
6. Assalia A, Gagner M, Schein M. Is laparoscopic appendectomy "Bitter" than open appendectomy? In: Controversies in Laparoscopic Surgery. Springer, Berlin, Heidelberg; 2006. p. 376.
7. Holzman MD, Lurut CM, Rientgen K, Eubarks S, Pappers TS. Laparoscopic ventral and incisional hernioplasty. Surg Endosc. 1997;11:32-5.
8. Balague Ponz C, Tnas M. Laparoscopic surgery and surgical infection. J Chemother. 2001;13 Spec No 1(1):17-22.
9. Pedersen AG, Petersen OB, Wara P, Rønning H, Qvist N, Laurberg S. Randomized controlled trial of laparoscopic versus open appendectomy. Br J Surg. 2001;88:200-5.
10. Ortega AE, Hunter JG, Peters JH, Swanstorm LL, Schirmer B. Laparoscopic appendectomy, study group: A perspective randomized comparison of laparoscopic appendectomy with open appendectomy. Am J Surg. 1995;169:208-12.
11. Grunewald B, Keating J. Should the normal appendix be removed at operation for appendicitis? JR Coll Surg Edinb. 1993;38:158-60.
12. van den Broek WT, Bijnen AB, de Ruiter P, Gouma DJ. A normal appendix found during laparoscopic appendectomy should not be removed. Br J Surg. 2001;88:251-4.
13. Greeson KL, Pappold JF, Liberman MA. Incidental laparoscopic for acute right lower quadrant abdominal pain. Its time has come. Surg Endosc. 1998;12:223-5.
14. Buser KB. Laparoscopic surgery in the pregnant patient—one surgeon's experience in a small rural hospital. J Soc Laparoendosc Surg. 2002;6:121-4.
15. Lyass S, Pikarsky A, Eisenberg VH, Elchalal U, Schenker JG, Reissman P. Is laparoscopy safe in pregnant woman? Surg Endosc. 2001;15(4):377-9.
16. de Perrot M, Jenny A, Morales M, Kohlik M, Movel P. Laparoscopic appendectomy during pregnancy. Surg Laparosc Endosc Percutan Tech. 2000;10:368-71.
17. Friedman JD, Ramsey PS, Ramin KD, Berry C. Pneumonia and pregnancy loss after second— trimester laparoscopic surgery. Obstet Gynacol. 2003;99:512-3.

CHAPTER 13

Pharmacology of Drugs Used in Diseases of Appendix

*'If you can control the patient by dietary means,
do not turn to drugs.'*
—**Hebrew**

INTRODUCTION

Appendicitis is one of the commonest causes of acute abdomen. The treatment of appendicitis is appendicectomy. Inspite of the surgery as a treatment of appendicitis some drugs are also used in appendicitis and even after appendicectomy. The drugs used commonly are antibiotics to control infection and analgesics to relieve pain. Analgesics are used to relieve pain of the disease and the operation also. The role of antibiotics in the management of appendicitis is increasing as in certain situations the antibiotics are used in place of appendicectomy. Antibiotic treatment alone is not suggested for children, older adults or patients who are pregnant, or for patients with sepsis or who are immunocompromised.[1-4]

Following are the common drugs used in diseases of appendix:
- Antibiotics
- Analgesics
- Antispasmodic
- Antiemetics
- H$_2$ receptor antagonists
- Proton pump inhibitors (PPI)

ANTIBIOTICS

The appendicitis is an infection with mixed bacterial flora, i.e., aerobic and anaerobic. So the antibiotics are given to cover all organisms.

In uncomplicated cases of acute appendicitis 1–2 days antibiotics are given, but in perforation and peritonitis 5–7 days of antibiotics are must depending upon the organisms responsible and nutritional and general condition of patient and until, the patient is afebrile with a normal WBC count.[5]

Antibiotics commonly used in appendicitis are:
- Penicillin:
  - Ampicillin with cloxacillin
  - Amoxicillin with clavulanic acid
  - Cephalosporin – 1st, 2nd, 3rd, and 4th generation.
- Aminoglycosides
- Metronidazole
- Ampicillin with Cloxacillin:
  - *Dosage:* 1–4 g daily in divided dose
  - *Contraindication:* Hypersensitivity to penicillin
  - *Precaution:* Renal and hepatic impairment

- *Safety:* Usually safe with pediatric patient, pregnancy, lactation, and old age.
- *Side effects:* Skin rash, pruritus, urticaria, GI upset, and pseudomembranous colitis.
- *Drug interaction:* Simultaneous use with oral contraceptives may lead to break through bleeding. Effect reduced by bacteriostatic agent. Synergy with clavulanic acid. Food interferes with absorption.
- Amoxicillin with clavulanic acid:
  - *Dosages:* IV 500 mg to 1.2 g, 8 hourly.
  - *Contraindication:* A history of an allergic reaction to the penicillin and pregnancy.
  - *Precaution:* Assessment of renal, hepatic, and hematopoietic functions.
  - *Interaction:* Reduces absorption of oral contraceptives.
  - *Side effects:* Nausea, vomiting and diarrhea. Urticaria, skin rashes, and serum sickness. Rise in SGOT, anemia, thrombocytopenic purpura, eosinophilia, leucopenia, and agranulocytosis
- *Cephalosporins*: Four generations of cephalosporins are in use nowadays. These are:
  - *First generation:* Have high activity against gram positive but weaker against gram-negative bacteria. These are cefazolin, cefalexin, cephradine, and cefadroxil.
  - *Second generation:* More active against gram-negative organisms, active against anaerobes, these are cefuroxime, cefuroxime, and cefaclor.
  - *Third generation:* Active against gram negative, enterobacteriaceae, inhibits pseudomonas as well. Less active on gram-positive cocci. These are cefotaxime, cefpodoxime proxetil, cefdinir, and ceftibuten.
  - *Fourth generation:* Similar to that of 3rd generation compounds is highly resistant to beta lactamases, hence active against many bacteria resistant to the earlier drugs. These are cefpirome:
    - *Dosage:* Different doses. Mostly given by IV route.
    - *Contraindication:* Hypersensitivity to penicillin or cephalosporin.
    - *Side effects:* GI disturbances, pseudo membranous colitis.
- *Interaction with aminoglycoside:* Increase in nephrotoxicity, oral contraceptives—decrease effectiveness of oral contraceptives; anticoagulants—increase hypoprothrombinemic effect.
- *Aminoglycosides*: Active against anaerobic and gram-negative bacilli. Commonly used aminoglycosides are amikacin, gentamycin, and netilmicin.
  - Amikacin:
    - *Dosage:* 15 g/kg body weight/day in two or three divided doses. Maximum of 1.5 g/day.
    - *Side effects:* Ototoxicity, nephrotoxicity, neuromuscular blockage, skin rash, tremors, eosinophilia, headache, nausea, and vomiting.
    - *Contraindication:* Known hypersensitive to aminoglycoside.
    - *Precautions:* Impaired renal function, use with caution.
    - *Drug interaction:* Increased ototoxic or nephrotoxic effects with ethacrynic acid and neuromuscular blocking drugs potentiates actions of penicillin, cephalosporin **(Fig. 1)**.
- *Metronidazole*: Metronidazole is active against a wide range of bacteria including bacteroides.
  - *Dosage:* Orally 400 mg, 8 hourly, by rectum 1 g, 8 hourly for 3 days followed by 1 g, 12 hourly. IV 500 mg, 8 hourly all up to 7 days.
  - *Side effects:* Anorexia, nausea, metallic taste, abdominal cramps. Thrombophlebitis of injected vein.
  - *Contraindication:* First trimester of pregnancy.

CHAPTER 13 Pharmacology of Drugs Used in Diseases of Appendix

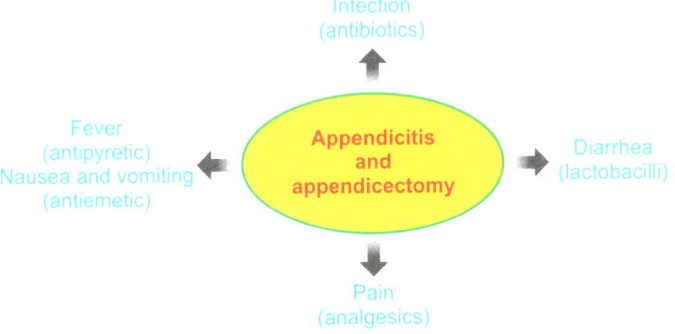

FIG. 1: Drugs used in appendicitis and appendicectomy.

- *Precautions:* Disulfiram like intolerance to alcohol.
- *Drug interaction:* Enhances action of coumarin anticoagulants.

ANALGESICS

- Opioid analgesics: Tramadol hydrochloride—it is commonly used.
  - Advantages:
    - No respiratory depression in therapeutic doses or other side effects of opioid analgesics.
    - No drug dependencies.
  - *Dosage:* 50–100 mg, 12 hourly or 8 hourly
  - *Side effects:* Nausea, vomiting
  - *Contraindication:*
    - Hypersensitivity.
    - Do not use in children below 16 years of age, pregnancy, and lactation.
  - *Special precautions:* Alcohol intake
  - Drug interaction:
    - Potentiates, sedative effects of tranquilizers
    - Fatal interaction with MAOIs.
- Nonopioid analgesics

  These are nonsteroidal anti-inflammatory drugs (NSAIDS). Commonly used NSAIDS are:
- Ibuprofen
- Ketoprofen

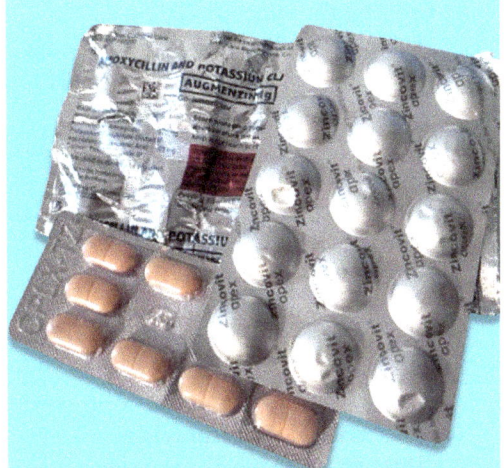

FIG. 2: Various drugs used in appendicitis.

- Etoricoxib
- Mefenamic acid
- Diclofenac sodium
- Aceclofenac

Diclofenac sodium: It is most commonly used NSAID. It has powerful analgesic, antipyretic and anti-inflammatory **(Fig. 2)** actions.

Dosage: 50 mg, two-three times a day
- **Contraindications:**
  - Hypersensitivity
  - Peptic ulcers
- *Side effects:* Epigastric pain, nausea, and retention of fluids.

CHAPTER 13 Pharmacology of Drugs Used in Diseases of Appendix

ANTISPASMODICS

There are many chemical used as antispasmodics.

- **Dicyclomine:** It is a smooth muscle relaxant and weak anticholinergic agent.
  - *Dosages:* 20 mg, three times a day.
  - *Contraindication:* Glaucoma
  - *Special precautions:* BPH
  - *Side effects:* Dry mouth, dizziness, and atonic constipation
  - *Drug interaction:* Increase adverse effects of anticholinergic drugs.
- **Hyoscine butylbromide:** Especially antispasmodic effect on GIT.
  - *Dosages:* 10–20 mg, three times a day.
  - *Contraindication:* Glaucoma, BPH
  - *Special precautions:* Driving
  - *Side effects:* Tachycardia, vision disturbances
  - *Drug interaction:* Potentiates effect of other anticholinergic drugs.

ANTIEMETICS

- **Domperidone:** It increases LES pressure, causes antral and duodenal contraction and increases gastric emptying.
  - *Dosage:* 20–40 mg, three times a day.
  - *Contraindication:* Pregnancy
  - *Drug interaction:*
    - Reduces absorption of oral digoxin.
    - Increase absorption of aspirin, paracetamol, and diazepam.
- **Ondansetrons:** It is a highly potent antiemetic so used in vomiting due to anticancer drugs and radiotherapy also. It can cause atonia and extrapyramidal effects like metoclopramide.
  - *Dosage:* 8 mg IV slowly. 8 mg orally 12 hourly.
  - *Contraindication:* Hypersensitivity
  - *Special precautions:* Liver diseases
  - *Side effects:* Headache, face flushing, constipation
- **Metoclopramide:** It is an effective antiemetic.
  - *Dosage:* 10 mg, three times a day.
  - *Contraindications:* Hypersensitivity, GI symptoms, extrapyramidal syndrome, and GIT atony.
  - *Special precautions:* Fast IV injection causes restlessness and anxiety. Renal and hepatic insufficiency.
  - *Side effects:* Restlessness, GIT atony and extrapyramidal effect.

H$_2$ RECEPTOR ANTAGONISTS

- Cimetidine
- Ranitidine
- Famotidine

These are potent acid reducing agents:
- *Dosage:* 150 mg twice a day (Ranitidine). 40 mg, two times a day (Famotidine) lafutidine (10 mg before going to bed).
- *Contraindication:* Hypersensitivity
- *Special precaution:* Gastric malignancy
- *Side effects:* Skin rashes, blurred vision, leucopenia, and thrombocytopenia

PROTON PUMP INHIBITORS

- Omeprazole
- Rabeprazole
- Lansoprazole
- Pantoprazole
- *Esomeprazole:*
  - *Dosage:* 20 mg once or twice a day on empty stomach (Omeprazole).
  - *Contraindication:* Hypersensitivity
  - *Special precautions:* Gastric malignancy
  - *Side effects:* Headache, diarrhea, nausea, and backache.

Key Point

Remember: A good operative technique cannot be replaced or substituted by a substandard technique and postoperative heavy antibiotics.

REFERENCES

1. Farooq A, Fournier FR, Brown C. Antibiotics alone in the treatment of appendicitis. CMAJ. 2021;193(21):E769.
2. Al-Omran M, Mamdani MM, McLeod RS. Epidemiologic features of acute appendicitis in Ontario, Canada. Can J Surg. 2003;46:263-8.
3. Salminen P, Tuominen R, Paajanen H, Rautio T, Nordström P, Aarnio M, et al. Five-year follow-up of antibiotic therapy for uncomplicated acute appendicitis in the APPAC randomized clinical trail. JAMA. 2018;320:1259-65.
4. Huang L, Yin Y, Yang L, Wang C, Li Y, Zhou Z. Comparison of antibiotic therapy and appendectomy for acute uncomplicated appendicitis in children: a meta-analysis. JAMA Pediatr. 2017; 171:426-34.
5. Keller MS, McBride WJ, Vane DW. Management of complicated appendicitis: A rational approach based on clinical course. Arch Surg. 1996;131: 261-4.

CHAPTER 14

Statistics about Appendix and its Diseases

'Statistics is the grammar of science.'
—Carl Pearson

INTRODUCTION

Statistics in medicine is of utmost importance as it reveals the various aspects of a disease such as its behavior, common features, risk factors, morbidity and mortality. In appendicitis the statistics have been proved very helpful in assessing value of different investigations and imaging techniques and best possible treatment in different situations. Statistics has proved that the gold standard for treatment of appendicitis is appendicectomy and antibiotics help in lowering the rate of postoperative complications. Statistics help in improving the accuracy of diagnosis of appendicitis by scoring systems.

- The appendix was first described in 1521 and inflammation of the appendix has been known to be a clinical problem since 1759.[1,2]
- Incidence of acute appendicitis is 8–10% in Western countries. In India, it is much less probably due to high fiber vegetarian diet.
- Maximum incidence of acute appendicitis occurs between 20 and 30 years.
- Male to female ratio of acute appendicitis is 2:1 before 30 years and then gradually comes to 1.7:1.
- Above 90% patients suffering with acute appendicitis suffer with anorexia, 70% with nausea and vomiting, and <10% have diarrhea especially children.
- Appendicitis occurs one in 1,500–2,000 pregnancies.
- Mortality rate of fetus is 1.5–3% with uncomplicated acute appendicitis whereas 30–35% in perforated appendix with peritonitis.
- 5–20% negative appendicitis are usually seen. Recently, there has been a consistent decline in negative appendicectomy rate (NAR) in United States because of better diagnostic imaging tools.[3,4]
- 15–40% of appendicitis removed during emergency appendectomy are found normal on histopathology.
- Negative appendicitis with laparotomy in pregnant patient carries fetal death up to 3%.
- 50% acute appendicitis patients with perforation are either below 10 years or above 50 years of age.
- Post appendectomy wound infection occurs in 3% operations in non-perforation cases and 4.7% in perforated appendices.

CHAPTER 14 Statistics about Appendix and its Diseases

- Appendicitis is rare before 2 years of age, but if occurs, the rate of perforation is 80% and of mortality is 50%.
- 30% cases of acute appendicitis in children have family history of appendicitis in first degree of relatives.
- 60% patients of obstructive acute appendicitis developed perforation.

- One in five cases of appendicitis is misdiagnosed.
- 60% of obstructed appendicitis have lymphoid follicular hyperplasia especially most common between 20 and 30 years.
- Fecalith is the commonest cause of obstruction (35%) in adult and children.
- Perforation of appendix with generalized peritonitis causes 10-20% mortality. However, the incidence of perforation (perforation rate) in acute appendicitis varies widely: a perforation rate between 4 and 39% has been reported in the West African Subregion.[5-9]
- 37–45% patients of acute appendicitis do not present a classic clinical picture.
- Barium enema cannot visualize normal appendix in 50% healthy persons.
- Conservative nonoperative management of appendicitis with high doses of antibiotics is reported to be effective in 60% patients.
- There have also been several studies promoting the treatment of uncomplicated appendicitis solely with antibiotics and avoiding surgery altogether.[10,11]
- *In carcinoid tumor of appendix:*
  ○ If tumor is <1 cm—never metastasizes.
  ○ If tumor is 1-2 cm—1% metastasizes.
  ○ If tumor is >2 cm—30% metastasize **(Fig. 1)**.

6% Lifetime risk of appendicitis

5–20% Negative appendicitis usually seen

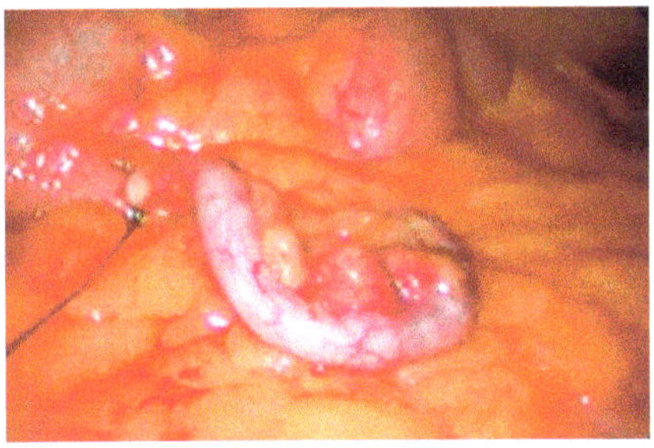

Appendicitis before 2 years of age rare, if occurs 80% perforation chances and 50% mortality

Post appendicectomy wound infection in 3% in uncomplicated cases and 4.7% in perforated appendices

FIG. 1: Role of statistics in appendicitis.

Key Point
Statistics show that incidence of acute appendicitis is decreasing, diagnostic accuracy is increasing, number of appendicectomies increasing but percentage of perforation remains almost same.

REFERENCES

1. Rendle S. The causation of appendicitis. Br J Surg.1920;8:171-88.
2. Deaver J (Ed). Appendicitis, 3rd edition. Philadelphia: P Blackston's Son and Co.; 1905.
3. Alhamdain YF, Rizk HA, Algethami MR, Algarawi AM, Albadawi RH, Faqih SN, et al. Negative Appendectomy Rate and Risk Factors That Influence Improper Diagnosis at King Abdul Aziz University, Hospital. Mater Sociomed. 2018;30(3):215-20.
4. Seetahal SA, Bolorunduro OB, Sookoleo TC, Oyetunji TA, Greene WR, Frederick W,et al. Negative appendectomy: a 10-year review of a nationally representative sample. Am J Surg. 2011;201(4):433-7.
5. NjoKu TA, Okobio MN. Perforated appendicitis: Risk factors and outcomes of management. Niger J Surg Sci. 2006;16:76-7.
6. Adeyanju MA, Adebiyi A. An audit of appendicitis at a tertiary Centre in Lagos, Nigeria. J Sci Res Stud Nigerian. 2015;2:126-34.
7. Edinos ST, Mohammed AZ, Ochichia O, Anumah M. Appendicitis in Kano, Nigeria: A 5 year review of pattern, morbidity and mortality. Ann Afr Med. 2004;3:38-41.
8. Ohene-Yeboah M, Togbe B. An audit of appendicitis and appendectomy in Kumasi, Ghana. West Afr J Med. 2006;25(2):138-43.
9. Balogun OS, Osiowo A, Afolayan M, Olajide T, Lawal A, Adesanya A. Acute perforated Appendicitis in Adults: Management and Complications in Lagos, Nigeria. Ann Afr Med. 2019;18(1):36-41.
10. Vaos G, Dimonpoulou A, Gkioka E, Zavras N. Immediate surgery or conservative treatment for complicated acute appendicitis in Children? A meta-analysis. J Pediatr Surg. 2019;54(7): 1365-72.
11. Zani A, Hall NJ, Rahman A, Morini F, Pini Prato A, Friedmacher F, et al. European Pediatric Surgeon's Association Survey on the Management of Pediatric Appendicitis. Eur J Pediatr Surg. 2019;29(1):53-61.

CHAPTER 15

Surgical Audit

'Surgery without audit is like playing cricket without keeping the score.'
—HB Devin

INTRODUCTION

Appendicitis is a common disease, but sometimes it is misdiagnosed and leads to postoperative complications. We cannot improve the outcome of the treatment of appendicitis unless we understand the importance of effective surgical audit. The record of patient's history, physical examination, hematological investigations and imaging results must be properly preserved, documented, studied and compared with other standard works to show the trend of the disease. What to be done in doubtful, but not clear cut cases of appendicitis has to be treated on a locally prepared policy. Operative findings both in open and laparoscopic appendicectomy should be properly and elaborately recorded. What was done in different difficult situations should also be observed and the results and postoperative complications to be compared with international standards. All these points will help to make a successful policy to deal with different situations in appendicitis to reduce the postoperative complications.

Clinical audits are the best source of feedback. So far, in India the clinical audit for appendicitis is not a common thing. If we wish to improve upon the incidence of misdiagnosis, postoperative discomforts and complications, and negative appendicectomies, we have to streamline the postoperative feedback in the name of clinical audit and registers.

AUDIT

Audit is fundamental part of surgical practice in UK.[1] Local audit can be improved by applying the guidelines given by national audit and projects,[2] etc.

Clinically-led initiative which seeks to improve the quality and outcome of patient care through structured peer reviews, whereby clinicians examine their practice where indicated.[3]

REGISTER

It is the prospective recording of information concerning diagnosis and operations of individual follow-up over time beyond the mere coding according to official classifications.

AIMS

- To increase the postoperative care of patients.
- To increase the QOL (quality of life) after surgery.
- To reduce the cost of operation with better care.
- New operative techniques can be studied and assessed for surgery.
- A plan and policy can be made for appendix surgery.

> Surgical audit keeps a control on operation standards. If they are falling then they are improved or sometimes even the policy is changed.

The main areas of help are:
- Postoperative discomforts
- Postoperative complications
- Morbidity
- Mortality
- Postoperative QOL
- Return to work and man-hour loss
- Recurrence rate

Whether the surgery procedure was correct and effective can be judged by the outcome. The outcome of surgery depends upon:
- Selection of patients
- Quality of surgical procedure
- Postoperative procedure
- Postoperative treatment, antibiotic policy, and follow-up program.

An audit cycle if properly completed only then the outcome of appendix surgery will improve.

Outcome: Analyze outcome goal or target
- Achieving, not achieving, why not achieving?
- Where is the fault?
- How it can be improved?
- Do the changes?

There are five stages of surgical audit:
1. Preparation for audit
2. Selection of criteria
3. Assessment of performance
4. Making changes to improve performance
5. Continuous and sustained improvement

In India some audit projects are doing a good job.[4,5]

Given the pressure, our healthcare system's economic evaluations are crucial if we are to allocate scarce resources efficiently.[6]

- Ask yourself that your line of surgical treatment is giving desired results or not.
- Can you justify yourself to your patients and to your peers?
- Do not hesitate to ask for help or opinion from senior colleagues **(Fig. 1)**.

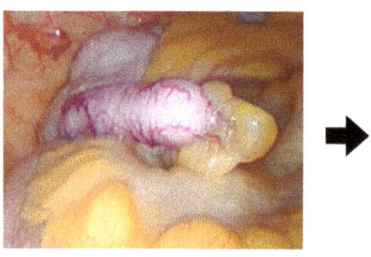 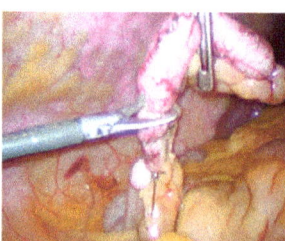

Record postoperative pain, discomfort, wound, infection, fever, vomiting, diarrhea, morbidity, and other postoperative complications. Analyze for improving the procedure

FIG. 1: Role of surgical audit in appendicitis.

Key Point
If results fall short of the criteria chosen, some changes in the care must be proposed.

REFERENCES

1. Brown CJ, Emberton M. Surgical audit and the evaluation of surgery. Surg Int. 2006;43:276.
2. Thomas K, Emberton M. Modern surgical audit. Surgery. 2000;18(10):250-2.
3. O'Riordan DC, Kingsnorth AN. Audit of patients outcomes after herniorrhaphy. Surg Clin North Am. 1998;78(6):1129-39.
4. Surgical Audit 2000. Department of Surgery, ESI Hospital, Basaidarapur, New Delhi, India.
5. Surgical Audit 2000. Department of General Surgery. Christian Medical College, Vellore, Tamil Nadu, India.
6. Campbell HE. Health economics and surgical care. Surg Int. 2006;43:271.

CHAPTER 16

Medicolegal Aspects: Legal Eagle

'Laws sometimes sleep, but never die.'
—**Law Maxim**

INTRODUCTION

The role of medicolegal factor is very important now a days, it is more relevant than yesteryears. Proper record keeping and maintaining documents help surgeons to avoid medicolegal proceedings against them. Opinions and suggestions given by a surgeon to the patient and relatives about surgery or conservative treatment in appendicitis are to be properly recorded. Detailed recording of history, physical examination and investigations in case sheet is valuable as it may be required later on. Whenever a medicolegal proceeding comes up in case of appendicitis the medical records are reviewed and analysed to decide negligence, delay in diagnosis, delay in operation, mistakes during operation and improper management of postoperative complications.

Gradually as economy is opening in India, law suits against doctors especially surgeons are increasing. The emergency surgery is the main area where surgeon is always on trial both medically as well as legally. To avoid legal entangles take in considerations the following points:

- Register yourself with some law firms of repute which deal with medical cases.
- Always sit in a comfortable room with relatives of the patient and politely discuss the matter of operation.
- Be nice to patient and his relatives but do not overdo.
- Try to be honest and sincere.
- Explain the sickness, need of operation, and explain the indication of operation in simple language.

> Get the detailed informed consent signed. The consent should be clear in that what is the condition of patient; when operation was advised; why the operation is required urgently; and what the consequences of not getting operated now are. The consent must also be signed by a witness. The consent if signed in detail will be of help even years after operation, if required by court.

- Never guarantee a cure as there are many ifs and buts between surgery and full recovery.

- Write down the conversation during meeting with patient and relatives in case sheet or record in camera.
- Get your professional indemnity insurance.

Long back in 1898 this problem of medicolegal aspect of appendicitis was considered by surgeons. WB Small of Lewiston, Maine, writing upon the relation of trauma of appendicitis (NY Med Rec, 1898, Volume 54, p. 364), says: 'I believe the true cause of the greater percentage of appendicitis in young men is found in the more frequent exposure to accidental injuries and strains, and to the strong contractions of the abdominal muscles necessary in their work. This explanation brings the subject into prominence from a medicolegal point of view. Some cases show plainly the direct results of external violence, and I believe accident insurance companies or corporations and individuals responsible for the occurrence of accidents, are as plainly liable as for a broken limb'.

A retrocecal appendicitis may not produce local signs of peritonitis since the inflamed area is covered by the overlying bowel.[1] This confusing feature of acute appendicitis should not make surgeon to do wrong diagnosis as it may involve legal issues **(Fig. 1)**.

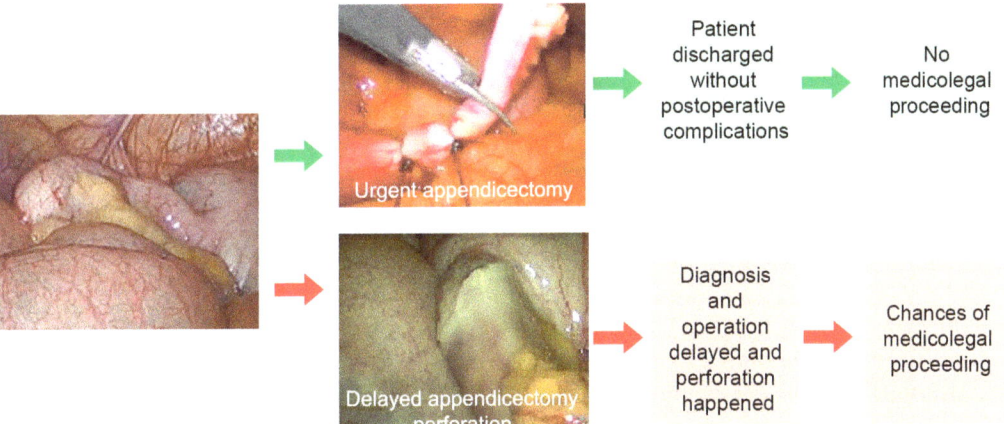

FIG. 1: Medicolegal proceeding chances in management of appendicitis.

Key Point

Ask yourself, would you recommend the treatment you are offering to the patient to your father or mother. You will not make mistake.

REFERENCE

1. Guidry SP, Poole GV. The anatomy of appendicitis. Am Surg. 1994;60(1):68-71.

CHAPTER 17

Mnemonics

'Memory is the mother of all wisdom.'
—Aeschylus

INTRODUCTION

The word 'Mnemonic' is derived from the ancient Greek word, 'Mnemonikos', meaning 'of memory' or 'relating to memory'. It is also related to Greek goddess of memory, 'Mnemosyne'. Mnemonic word was discovered by a Greek poet, Simonides in 447 BC. According to Oxford dictionary mnemonic can be defined as a word, sentence or poem used to help remember a rule, name, etc. Mnemonics help our memory to retain information and make it easy to remember.

Mnemonics are used in medicine as instrument to remember medical knowledge for long term. Various medical terms and facts which are difficult to remember can be remembered for long with the help of mnemonics. A mnemonic couplet to help students learn the names of cranial nerves has been in use in the United States since the mid-ninteenth century.[1]

- *Murphy's triad*:
  - Mnemonic (Mn): PVP
    - P = Pain in abdomen
    - V = Vomiting
    - P = Pyrexia

- *Etiology of appendicitis (common causes)*:
  - Mn: DR SODA
    - D = Diet
    - R = Racial familial and geographical factor
    - S = Socioeconomical level
    - O = Obstruction of appendix by fecalith and worms
    - D = Diseases of cecum; cancer, Crohn's disease, and tuberculosis
    - A = Abuse of purgative

- *Alvarado scoring*:[2]
  - M = Migrating right iliac fossa (RIF) pain
  - A = Anorexia
  - N = Nausea, vomiting
  - T = Tenderness RIF
  - R = Rebound tenderness
  - E = Elevated temperature (>37.3°C)
  - L = Leukocytosis (>10 × 1037.3 cells)
  - S = Shift to left (segmental neutrophils) (>75%)

- *Ochsner-Sherren regimen*:
  - A = Aspiration—Ryle's tube
  - B = Bowel care—no purgatives

- C = Charts for pulse/temperature/BP/size of mass
- D = Drugs, antibiotics
- E = Exploration is avoided in appendicular mass
- F = Fluids, IV

- Common differential diagnosis of acute appendicitis:
  - Mn: PUNAM TRIPS MRCP
    - P = Perforated peptic ulcer
    - U = Ureteric colic
    - N = Nonspecific mesenteric lymphadenitis
    - A = Acute gastroenteritis
    - M = Mittelschmerz
    - T = Torsion of ovarian cyst
    - R = Regional ileitis
    - I = Intestinal obstruction
    - P = Pancreatitis
    - S = Salpingitis
    - M = Meckel's diverticulitis
    - R = Ruptured ectopic gestation
    - C = Cholecystitis, acute
    - P = Pyelonephritis, acute

- Clinical features of carcinoid syndrome:
  - Mn: DABAR
    - D = Diarrhea
    - A = Attack of bronchial asthma due to histamine
    - B = Increased borborygmi
    - A = Attack of flushing of face, induced by alcohol
    - R = Reddish blue hue (cyanosis) due to histamine

- Differential diagnosis of appendicular mass:
  - Mn: TIC-T-TAC
    - T = TB (Ileocecal TB)
    - I = Ilial lymphadenitis
    - C = Crohn's disease
    - T = Tumor, carcinoma of cecum
    - T = Tumor, carcinoma of ovary
    - A = Amoebic typhlitis, actinomycosis
    - C = Twisted ovarian cyst

- Important signs of acute appendicitis:
  - Mn: Remember Best Teachers Certify MCH
    2   2   2   2
    - R = Rebound tenderness
    - R = Rovsing sign
    - B = Bed shaking test of Bapat
    - B = Baldwin's test
    - T = Tenderness in RIF
    - T = Tenderness in digital rectal examination (DRE)
    - C = Cope's psoas test
    - C = Cope's obturator test
    - M = Muscle guarding
    - C = Cough sign
    - H = Hyperesthesia in Sherren's triangle

- Complications of acute appendicitis:
  - Mn: GAPSAP
    - G = Generalized peritonitis
    - A = Appendicular abscess
    - P = Perforated appendix
    - S = Septicemia
    - A = Appendicular lump
    - P = Portal pyemia

- Important tumors of appendix:
  - Mn: CAP
    - C = Carcinoid tumor
    - A = Adenocarcinoma
    - P = Pseudomyxoma peritonei (PMP)

- Complications of appendicectomy:
  - Mn: 2 PACIF
    - P = Portal pyemia
    - P = Paralytic ileus
    - A = Abscess, pelvic and intra-peritoneal
    - A = Adhesions, postoperative
    - C = Complication of any operation, wound infection
    - C = Complication of any operation, hemorrhage
    - I = Intestinal obstruction, acute
    - I = Inguinal hernia, right
    - F = Fecal fistula

CHAPTER 17 Mnemonics

- *Two layers of subcutaneous tissue in RIF:*
  - Mn: CS (C comes before S as alphabet)
    - C = Camper's superficial fatty layer
    - S = Scarpa's deep membranous layer

- *Names of three taenia coli:*
  - Mn: MOL
    - M = Taenia mesocolica
    - O = Taenia omentalis
    - L = Taenia libera

> **Key Point**
> Remember MAO Mnemonics Murphy's triad, Alvarado scoring, and Ochsner–Sherren regimen.

REFERENCES

1. Lanska DJ. On old olympus? Oliver Wendell Holmes and origin and evolution of a mnemonic couplet for the cranial nerves. J Hist Neurosci. 2022;31(1):20-9.
2. Alvarado A. A practical score for the early diagnosis of acute appendicitis. Ann Emerg Med.1986;15:557-64.

CHAPTER 18

Frequently Asked Questions

'Ignorance is like knowledge; there is no end to it.'
—**Anonymous**

INTRODUCTION

FAQs is a method to improve the knowledge of the readers. This format provides quick answers to the common questions about the article or topic. It gives a chance to ask about the clinical features, presentation and management of acute appendicitis. Generally people wish to know about the treatment of appendicitis, removal of appendix is a must or can be delayed or treated conservatively? What happens when the appendix is removed? Can I delay the operation for appendicitis as I am alone here and wish to wait for my family members for few days? What are the complications and side effects of appendicectomy? What foods are allowed after appedicectomy operation? How long I will be in the hospital? Can I get operated by keyhole or laparoscopic method?

Appendicitis, the inflammation of the vermiform appendix, is a common problem. Appendix is a worm like tubular structure attached to part of large intestine called cecum. When the appendix is inflamed it cases pain in RLQ of the abdomen with loss of appetite, nausea, vomiting and fever. Usually the appendicitis is caused by blockage of the lumen of appendix. The best way to treat appendicitis is by removing it (appendicectomy). You cannot prevent appendicitis, but definitely you can reduce chances of its occurrence by eating plant based fiber rich diet.

Question 1: What is the difference between the terms "appendectomy" and "appendicectomy"?

Answer: Both terms mean "operation for removal of appendix"; "appendectomy" term is used in North America and "appendicectomy" in rest of the world.

Question 2: If on exposure during appendicectomy an appendix is macroscopically found normal, it should be removed or not?

Answer:
- Explore the abdomen for possible causes of such pain such as Meckel's diverticulitis, amoebic typhlitis, terminal ileitis, salpingitis and other tubo-ovarian diseases then remove the appendix if every other cause is excluded to avoid future right iliac fossa (RIF) pain and future diagnostic dilemma.
- The infection and inflammations start in the mucosa of the appendix and then spread out to the serosa so the outside macroscopic findings may be normal, 25-30% of appendixes on appendicectomy are macroscopically normal. If you cut open the appendix some of these will

be found having inflamed mucosa. The inflammation may later be confirmed by histopathology.
- Before taking a decision for removal of a macroscopically normal appendix consider the RIF pain cause in that particular case. Appendicectomy should be considered in any previous history of RIF pain.

Question 3: Can appendicectomy cause inguinal hernia?

Answer: The ilioinguinal and iliohypogastric nerves run between internal oblique muscle and transversus abdominis muscle down to the inguinal canal. Injury to these nerves causes paralysis of conjoint tendon which results in inguinal hernia.

Question 4: What are the names of three taenia coli?

Answer:
- Taenia libera—on anterior surface of cecum
- Taenia mesocolica—on poster medial surface of cecum
- Taenia omentalis—on posterolateral surface of cecum

Question 5: What is a carcinoid tumor of appendix and what is its most common site?

Answer: Carcinoid tumor of appendix arises from Kulchitsky cells or Argentaffin cells found at the base of crypts of appendix. The most common site of carcinoid tumor is appendix.

Question 6: What is a vestigial organ?

Answer: Vestigial organ is an undeveloped organ that in the embryo or in some more or less remote ancestor was well developed and functional.

Question 7: Why Appendix is prone to get infected?

Answer:
- It is a long, narrow, blind ended tube (cul-de-sac), it encourages stasis of its contents which gives chance to bacteria to multiply.
- The lumen of appendix has a tendency to become obstructed by dried and hard fecal mass (enterolith or fecalith), which leads to further stasis.
- The wall of appendix has large number of lymphoid tissue masses, which trap the bacteria going from appendix wall and get enlarged and enhance the narrowing of lumen and accelerate obstruction.

Question 8: Why appendix is prone to perforate?

Answer:
- The appendicular artery is an end artery. The inflammatory edema of the wall of the appendix compresses the appendicular artery near the tip of the appendix where it lies directly on the wall of the appendix causing thrombosis in the artery leading to perforation and gangrene of appendix.
- The muscular layer in the wall of the appendix is not well developed that is why it cannot withstand the high intraluminal pressure and gets ruptured early at "Hiatus Muscularis".
- It is a cul-de-sac and can be easily blocked.
- Lumen of appendix is very narrow so can be easily blocked.

Question 9: How to locate the appendix during surgery?

Answer:
- First find out the ileocecal junction. Identify the terminal ileal loop, follow it, it leads to cecum, appendix is attached to cecum.
- Follow the three taenia coli. All three taenia coli meet at the base of appendix.
- Sweep from lateral abdominal wall and find cecum.

Question 10: Why appendicitis is generally uncommon in infants and elderly?

Answer:
- The obstruction of the lumen of appendix is the usual precipitating factor in most of cases of acute appendicitis. The lumen of appendix is usually wide in infants so the fecal material cannot be retained

due to wide lumen so obstruction cannot happen.
- In old age the infected fecal matter cannot enter the lumen as it gets narrowed so appendicitis is not common in old age.

Question 11: What are the risk factors for perforation of appendix in acute appendicitis?
Answer:
- Extreme of age
- Obstructive appendicitis
- Diabetes mellitus
- Immunosuppression
- Pelvic appendix

Question 12: Recurrent appendicular artery is a branch of?
Answer: Posterior cecal artery.

Question 13: Appendicular artery is branch of?
Answer: Ileocolic artery.

Question 14: Most common position of appendix.
Answer: Retrocecal.

Question 15: What do you mean by left side appendicitis?
Answer:
- Diverticulitis of descending colon or pelvic colon. Symptoms resemble those of appendicitis.
- Appendicitis in situs inversus.

Question 16: What is "appendicitis obliterans" or "protective appendicitis"?
Answer: It is a rarely encountered—logical diagnosis after an appendicectomy. Fibrous obliteration of appendix is considered as a part of the ageing process. Mucosa and submucosa are replaced by fibrous tissues. It mimics acute appendicular due to obliteration of its lumen. In the appendicitis the submucous tissue shrinks and sclerosis develops which obliterates the lumen so protects against perforation.

Question 17: What is "appendicolithiasis"?
Answer: In the lumen of appendix become obliterated with calculi. It runs in families.

Question 18: What is "How do you do appendix"?
Answer: When you open the peritoneum and find inflamed appendix lying there and no search is required as if appendix is asking surgeon "How do you do".

Question 19: What is "Lilly white appendix"?
Answer: On exploration if a normal appendix is found. It is called "Lilly white appendix" as it is not inflamed so it is white and not reddish.

Question 20: What is "Chandelier Sign"?
Answer: In pelvic inflammatory disease (PID), on pelvic examination a touch on cervix moves the inflamed uterine adnexal suddenly makes the patient to jump-like hitting chandelier. The positive "chandelier" sign differentiates PID from acute appendicitis.

Question 21: What is "white worm"?
Answer: A normal appendix found on exploration for removal of appendix. 10–20% are white worms on appendicectomy.

Question 22: If Crohn's disease is found in appendix then what to do?
Answer: If only tip of appendix is involved—do appendicectomy. If the base of appendix is involved—conservative treatment.

Question 23: Can acute cholecystitis mimic acute appendicitis?
Answer: Yes especially retrocecal appendicitis, when its tip is inflamed it resembles acute cholecystitis. Both are acute abdomen problems. Laparoscopy is diagnostic as well as therapeutic.

Question 24: Why does tip of appendix get commonly perforated?
Answer:
- It is most distal part of appendix so it is least vascular especially in long appendix.

- It is devoid of mesentery so no protective cover.
- Appendicular artery is here lying directly on the wall of appendix so it gets easily thrombosed due to inflammation and necrosis happens in the distal part of appendix.

Question 25: What is MALT and GALT?

Answer: MALT means mucosa-associated lymphoid tissue. GALT means gut-associated lymphoid tissue. MALT is also called as "epithelia-lymphoid tissue". MALT are encapsulated collection of lymphoid nodules located in alimentary tract near epithelium, when MALT become active, they migrate deeper in submucosa. MALT associated with alimentary tract are called GALT.

Question 26: What are 6Fs of acute appendicitis?

Answer:
Which are:
F – Foetor
F – Fever
F – Flushed appearance
F – Furred tongue
F – RIF pain
F – Fast pulse

Question 27: If you find normal appendix on exploration, what you will do?

Answer: Exclude other causes of RIF pain and then do appendicectomy.

Question 28: In acute appendicitis can the microscopic picture of urine resemble that of UTI?

Answer: Yes, urine shows pus cells and RBCs if the inflamed appendix touches ureter or urinary bladder.

Question 29: What is "CT – appendix"?

Answer: When a patient of right lower quadrant (RLQ) pain comes to hospital emergency room and urgent CT scan of abdomen done, patient is kept on conservative treatment till diagnosis is made. By the time CT report comes patient improves but radiologist now diagnoses it as acute appendicitis.

Question 30: What is "Appendicitis epiploica"?

Answer: It develops due to torsion of appendix epiploica (fat pockets attached to taenia coli).

Pain disappears when epiploica sloughs out. If operation is done appendix epiploica is excised.

Question 31: What is "Valentino appendix"?

Answer: Appendix can mimic acute appendicitis even if it is not inflamed. Due to any intraperitoneal pathology surface of appendix becomes red due to contact with inflammatory exudates and looks like acute appendicitis. Famous actor Rudolf Valentino in 1926 in New York was operated for appendicectomy while he was having perforated peptic ulcer. He died in postoperative period. The autopsy revealed the real cause.

Question 32: What factors encourage inflammation in acute appendicitis?

Answer:
- Age—common between 20 and 30 years
- Use of steroids
- Free lying preileal or postileal appendix
- Fecolith in lumen, causing obstruction
- Purgation—use of purgative to open bowel in constipation
- Impaired blood supply

Question 33: What is the role of plain X-ray abdomen in acute appendicitis?

Answer: To rule out ureteric stone.

Question 34: Why the base of appendix is crushed in appendicectomy?

Answer:
- It blocks the lumen to avoid spread of infection by spillage.
- Ligature can easily be tied here and does not slip on this narrow area.

CHAPTER 18 Frequently Asked Questions

Question 35: Why stump of appendix is buried?
Answer:
- It is an infected area so avoids soiling of peritoneal cavity.
- It avoids adhesions formation.

Question 36: What are the causes of nonresolving appendicular mass?
Answer:
- Appendicular abscess
- Carcinoma of cecum

Question 37: What are the disadvantages of burying of stump of appendix in appendicectomy?
Answer:
- May cause cecal wall abscess
- Later on in life a barium enema for some other disease may show it as a filling defect and will cause diagnostic problem.

Question 38: What are the atypical presentations of acute appendicitis?
Answer:
- Pelvic appendicitis—loose motions—acute gastroenteritis
- Retrocecal appendicitis—psoas muscle spasm
- Subhepatic appendicitis—pain in right hypochondrium mimicking acute cholecystitis
- Acute appendicitis in pregnancy—high and lateral location of pain

Question 39: What is "good morning appendix"?
Answer: As soon as the abdomen is opened, the appendix pops out and surgeon has not to search for it.

Question 40: Why complications are common in infants and elderly persons?
Answer:
- *In infants*:
  ○ Early diagnosis is sometimes difficult so delay happens in treatment
  ○ Omentum is small like a bib and so it cannot control infection by sealing it at original site
- *In elderly patients*:
  ○ Poor immunity
  ○ Lax muscles cause delay in diagnosis due to absence of muscle guarding
  ○ Use of purgative is common at this age

Question 41: In which position appendicitis is dangerous?
Answer: Ileal at 2 o'clock position, as its tip is free in general peritoneal cavity and perforation can cause general peritonitis directly and easily.

Question 42: What is appendicular artery of Seshachalam?
Answer: It is an accessory appendicular artery arises from posterior appendicular artery and supplies the base of appendix. It was described by Seshachalam anatomist from Madras Medical College, Chennai, Tamil Nadu, India.

Question 43: What is the conversion rate of laparoscopic to open appendectomy?
Answer: 5-25% depending upon the degree of inflammation, adhesions, and perforation of appendix.[1,2]

Question 44: What are the important clinical features of retrocecal appendicitis?
Answer:
- Shifting pain from periumbilical area to RIF may be absent
- Pain is in loin
- Tenderness is in loin and not in RIF
- Psoas sign is present

Question 45: What are the important clinical features of pelvic appendicitis?
Answer:
- Pain and tenderness may be in hypogastrium instead in RIF.
- Digital rectal examination (DRE) reveals tenderness in right side of pouch of Douglas.
- May be associated with diarrhea due to contact of inflamed appendix with rectum.
- May be associated with burning during micturition due to contact of inflamed appendix with urinary bladder.

CHAPTER 18 Frequently Asked Questions

Question 46: What are the important clinical features of postileal appendicitis?
Answer:
- RIF pain may be more medial.
- Diarrhea is present due to contact of inflamed appendix with ileum.

Question 47: What is appendix?
Answer: It is a diverticulum-like structure from cecum of large intestine or colon.

Question 48: What is the function of appendix?
Answer:
- It is thought to be a vestigial organ.
- Its function is not definitely known, except immunological link.

Question 49: Why appendicectomy is required?
Answer: Appendicectomy is usually an emergency operation. It is performed for:
- To relieve symptoms of acute appendicitis.
- From preventing appendix to burst and cause serious complications like peritonitis.
- It prevents more complex and serious operation.

Question 50: What is done in appendicectomy?
Answer: This operation is usually done under general anesthesia but can also be done under spinal anesthesia. Appendix is excised and removed.

A small incision is given in lower part of right side of abdomen or can be done by laparoscopy (keyhole surgery), the inflamed appendix is removed. The stump of appendix base is closed. The abdominal wound is closed.

Question 51: When patient is allowed orally after appendicectomy?
Answer:
- Oral liquids are allowed from 2nd postoperative day.
- Soft diet is given from 3rd postoperative day.

Question 52: When sutures are removed?
Answer: 7th or 8th postoperative day.

Question 53: What about patient mobility after appendicectomy?
Answer: Patient is allowed and encouraged to move from 2nd postoperative day. Patient is allowed freely to move from 7th postoperative day.

Question 54: What is the classic presentation of acute appendicitis?
Answer: Periumbilical pain that migrates to RLQ in a patient who is anorexic.

Question 55: What is McBurney's point?
Answer: The point of maximum tenderness in RLQ.

Question 56: Who coined the term appendicitis?
Answer: McBurney, Surgeon from New York, USA and Fitz, Physician from Boston, USA, coined the term appendicitis in 1886.[1]

Question 57: Who were Rockey–Davis?
Answer: Rockey–Davis were a pair of surgeons, AE Rockey and GG Davis, who developed RLQ transverse, muscle splitting incision that extends into rectus sheath.[2]

Question 58: What is the mortality risk involved with appendicitis?
Answer:
- Nonperforated appendicitis <0.1%
- Perforated appendicitis ≤5%

Question 59: What is "Line of Toldt" and what is its importance in appendicectomy?
Answer: This is an imaginary line also called "White line of Toldt". It is the line on lateral peritoneal fold from anterior surface of cecum and ascending colon to abdominal wall.

Incision on this line is bloodless and it is used to mobilize the cecum to find out retrocecal appendix.

CHAPTER 18 Frequently Asked Questions

> **Key Point**
>
> In postoperative period if fever appears and does not subside, ask questions to yourself about the cause of this pyrexia, think fast and reach to a diagnosis, delay may harm your patient.

REFERENCES

1. Meakin JL. Appendectomy and appendicitis. Can J Surg. 1999;42(2):90.
2. Rockey AE. Transverse incisions in abdominal operations. Med Rec. 1905;68:779.

CHAPTER 19

Multiple Choice Questions

'They know enough, who know how to learn.'
—Henry Brooks Adams

INTRODUCTION

Multiple choice questions (MCQs) are essential tool for a student to prepare for examination. In medicine, the value of MCQs is unparalleled as the examination are very tough and require a lot of preparation. MCQs in medicine are helpful in measuring the preparation for examination as they self assess the preparedness. MCQs are helpful in motivating the students and developing self-esteem. They can be used as pre-test assessing method to test the self knowledge by the student. MCQs can help in preparation for objective tests and also to improve the understanding of the subject. MCQs are prompt and quick way of feedback. MCQs are also a way to keep concentration, attention and stimulation of the student for preparation for an examination.

The following multiple choice questions (MCQs) were asked in various examinations of postgraduate entrance tests of various universities such as PGI, AIIMS, JIPMER, AP, AMU, AI, LB, etc.

1. Recurrent appendicular artery is a branch of:
   a. Ileocolic artery
   b. Right colic artery
   c. Middle colic artery
   d. Posterior cecal artery

2. Appendicular artery is branch of:
   a. Ileocolic artery
   b. Right colic artery
   c. Middle colic artery
   d. Posterior cecal artery

3. Most common site of appendix:
   a. Retrocecal
   b. Preileal
   c. Paracecal
   d. Postileal

4. Earliest symptom in acute appendicitis is:
   a. Pain
   b. Fever
   c. Vomiting
   d. Rise of pulse rate

5. McBurney's point:
   a. Lies in the middle of right spine umbilical line

b. At the junction of lateral 2/3 and medial 1/3 of line
c. At the junction of lateral 1/3 and medial 2/3 of line
d. Lies at the umbilicus-liver junction

6. The following signs are not seen in acute appendicitis, *except*:

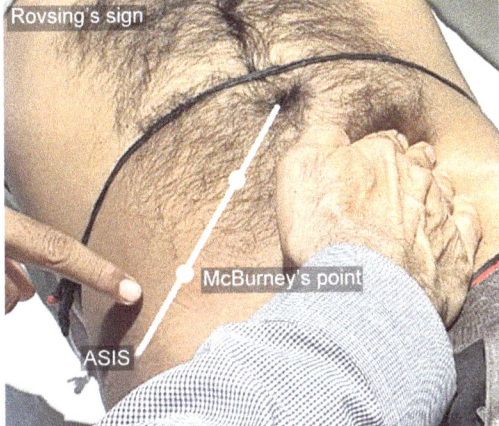

FIG. 1: McBurney's point.

   a. Rovsing's sign
   b. Murphy's sign
   c. Boa's sign
   d. Macewen's sign

7. Rovsing's sign is seen in:
   a. Acute appendicitis
   b. Acute cholecystitis
   c. Pancreatitis
   d. None of the above

8. Pointing index sign is seen in:
   a. Acute appendicitis
   b. Acute pancreatitis
   c. Perforated DU
   d. Acute cholecystitis

9. A gridiron incision becomes a Rutherford–Morrison incision when the incision is extended by:
   a. Splitting the muscle laterally
   b. Cutting the muscles laterally
   c. Cutting the muscles medially into the rectus sheath
   d. Incising vertically along the rectus muscle

10. Which of the following statements is not true of McBurney's incision?
    a. Most suitable if the diagnosis of appendicitis is definite
    b. If it is converted into a muscle cutting incision it is called Rutherford–Morrison incision
    c. Inguinal hernia is a sequelae of the incision
    d. The incision can be extended upward or downward

11. All are true about appendicular rupture, *except*:

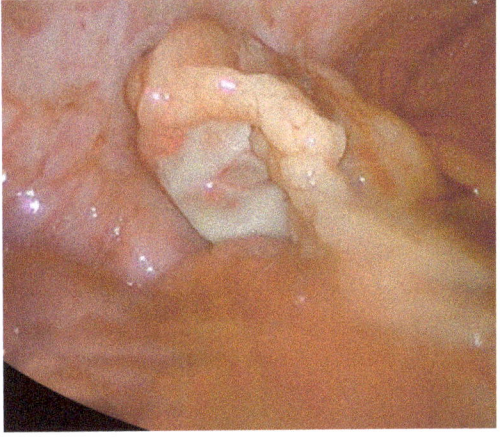

FIG. 2: Appendicular rupture.

    a. Common in low socioeconomic status people
    b. Common in extremes of age
    c. Early antibiotics prevent perforation
    d. Appendicectomy done even in presence of rupture

12. All of the following are early complications arising after appendicectomy for acute appendicitis, *except*:
    a. Ileus

b. Sterility
c. Intestinal obstruction
d. Pulmonary complications

13. Ochsner–Sherren regimen is used in management of:
   a. Appendicular abscess
   b. Chronic appendicitis
   c. Appendicular mass
   d. Acute appendicitis

14. Mucocele of the appendix is:
   a. Benign tumor
   b. Low grade malignancy
   c. Retention cyst
   d. Infective process

15. Most common site of carcinoid is:
   a. Ileum
   b. Liver
   c. Rectum
   d. Appendix

16. Carcinoid of which site is least likely to be malignant?
   a. Appendix
   b. Stomach
   c. Small intestine
   d. Lung

17. Most common tumor of appendix is:
   a. Argentaffinoma
   b. Lymphoma
   c. Leiomyosarcoma
   d. Adenocarcinoma

18. Surgery for carcinoid tumor of the appendix:
   a. Right hemicolectomy
   b. Appendicectomy
   c. Limited resection of the right colon
   d. Right hemicolectomy with removal of inches of the ileum also

19. What do you do for a 2.5-cm carcinoid in the appendix?
   a. Right hemicolectomy
   b. Appendicectomy with yearly CT scan
   c. Total colectomy with ileoanal pouch anastomosis
   d. Limited colonic resection with adjuvant chemotherapy

20. In an incidental diagnosis of carcinoid of appendix covering an area of 2.5 cm, the line of action will be:
   a. Appendicectomy
   b. Appendicectomy with yearly follow-up of 24 hours estimation of hydroxy-indoleacetic acid (HIAA)
   c. Appendicectomy along with right hemicolectomy
   d. Appendicectomy and annual CT scan

21. When rectum is inflated with air through a rectal tube, pain, and tenderness occur in RIF in case of appendicitis. This is known as:
   a. Aaron's sign
   b. Battle sign
   c. Bastede's sign
   d. McBurney's sign

22. All of the following are parts of prolonged antibiotic therapy in intra-abdominal sepsis, *except*:
   a. Masking of general signs
   b. Subacute intestinal obstruction
   c. Malignant change
   d. Frozen pelvis

23. Odorless peritoneal fluid is noticed in:
   a. Perforated peptic ulcer
   b. Perforated ileum
   c. Perforated appendix
   d. TB peritonitis

24. All are useful in acute appendicitis, *except*:

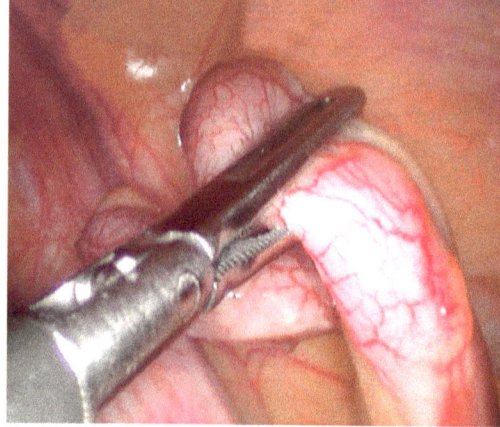

FIG. 3: Acute appendicitis.

a. Antibiotics
b. Analgesics
c. IV fluids
d. Purgative

25. What is "peritoneal mice"?
a. Pseudomyxoma peritonei
b. Appendices epiploicae
c. Peritoneal seedings of tumor
d. Endometriosis

26. Epidemic appendicitis is due to:
a. Fecalith
b. Worms of ileocecal region
c. Streptococcal infections
d. Abuse of purgatives
e. None of the above

27. The frequent mechanism in perforation of appendix is:
a. Impacted fecalith
b. Tension gangrene due to accumulated secretions
c. Necrosis of lymphoid tissue
d. Carcinoid tumor

Answers

1. (d)	2. (a)	3. (a)	4. (a)	5. (c)	6. (a)	7. (a)	8. (a)	9. (b)	10. (c)
11. (d)	12. (b)	13. (c)	14. (c)	15. (d)	16. (a)	17. (a)	18. (b)	19. (a)	20. (c)
21. (c)	22. (c)	23. (a)	24. (d)	25. (b)	26. (c)	27. (b)			

Key Point

Only advice "Learn surgery by doing".

REFERENCE

1. McBurney C. Experience with early operative interference in cases of disease of the vermiform appendix. NY State Med J. 1889;50:676.

Further Readings

1. Kelly HA, Hardon E. The Vermiform Appendix and its Diseases. Philadelphia: W.B. Saunders; 1905.
2. Ortega JM, Ricardo AE. Atlas of Ambulatory Surgery. Philadelphia: W.B. Saunders; 1999.
3. Hai A, Srivastava RB. Textbook of Surgery: The Association of Surgeons of Indian. New Delhi: Tata McGraw-Hill Publishing Company Limited; 2003. pp. 462-6.
4. Chaurasia BD. Human Anatomy, 4th edition, volume 2. New Delhi: CBS Publication; 2020. pp. 256-60.
5. Richard S. Snell Clinical Anatomy, 7th edition. Lippinoott William and Wilkins; 2004. pp. 246-51.
6. Decker GAG, Plessis DDu. Lee McGregor's Synopsis of surgical Anatomy: Indian Edition, 12th edition. K.M. Varghese Company; 1986. pp. 41-4.
7. Singh V. Clinical Anatomy. 1st edition. Elsevier; 2001. pp. 120-21.
8. Williams PL, Dyson M. Gray's Anatomy, 37th edition. 1989. pp. 1366-7.
9. Dorland. Dorland's Illustrated Medical Dictionary, 30th edition. W.B. Saunders Co. Ltd.; 2003. pp. 118-9.
10. Williams N, Bulstrode C, Russell RCG. Bailey and Love's Short Practice of Surgery, 24th edition. Hodder Arnold. 2004. pp. 1203-18.
11. Alvarado A. A practical score for the early diagnosis of acute appendicitis. Ann Emerg Med. 1986;15:557-64.
12. Burnand KG, Young AE, Lucas JD, Rowlands B, Scholefield J. The New AIRD's Companion in Surgical Studies. 3rd edition. Churchill Livingstone; 2005. pp. 579-84.

Index

Page numbers followed by *f* refer to figure and *fc* refer to flowchart.

A

Abdomen 66
  acute 52
  ultrasound of 65
Abdominal crisis 85
Abdominal pain, algorithm for acute 71*fc*
Abdominal policeman 150*f*
Abdominal surgery 156
Abdominal wall 110*f*
  anterior 108, 109
  muscles of 109*f*, 110*f*
Abscess 95
  appendicular 86, 89, 91
    causes of 89
    fate of appendicular 91
    indications of appendicular 89
  intra-abdominal 144
  intraperitoneal 87, 132
    residual 91
  locations of appendicular 90*f*
  paracolic 91, 92
  pelvic 91, 92, 132, 134
  periappendiceal 67
  postoperative abdominal 135
  pyemic 95
  rupture of appendicular 91
  site of appendicular 91
  small 88
  sub-diaphragmatic 91, 92
  sub-hepatic 91, 92
  sub-phrenic 89
Accessory appendicular artery 17, 17*f*
Actinomycosis 93
Acute appendicitis 28, 30, 31*f*, 33, 34*f*, 44, 48, 49, 49*f*, 52*f*, 55, 59, 64*f*, 65*f*, 67, 67*f*, 69*f*, 71, 71*fc*, 72, 72*f*, 74-76, 77*fc*, 84, 97, 123, 143, 146*f*, 152, 175-177, 182
  pain 52

Acute cholecystitis 70
  mimic acute appendicitis 175
Adenocarcinoma 100
Adhesions, postoperative 133
Alvarado scoring 170
  system 68
Amebic typhlitis 81, 85, 93
Amikacin 111, 158
Aminoglycoside 111, 157
  interaction with 158
Amoebic typhlitis 79
Amoxicillin 157, 158
Ampicillin 157
Amyand's hernia 4*f*, 14*f*
Analgesics 157
Anatomic hazards 134
Anesthesia 113
Angioma 100, 101
Anorectal malformation 142
Anorexia 51
Antibiotics 157
  role of 98
  use of 141
Antiemetics 157, 160
Aortic aneurysm, leaking 85
Appendectomy 82, 112, 173
  laparoscopic 150, 156
  set up for 124*f*
Appendical gland 19
Appendicectomy 4, 8, 48, 97, 108, 112, 136, 148, 173, 174, 178
  complications of 132
  conventional 113
  drugs in 159*f*
  incidental 113, 129
  incisions for 114*f*
  indications of 112*f*, 113
  interval 113, 129
  inversion 113, 130
  long-term effects of 146
  ondications of incidental 129
  open 131

  preoperative preparation for 111
  retrograde 113, 130
  role of interval 91
  steps of 114
    laparoscopic 128*f*
    open 114, 120*f*
  urgent 97
Appendices epiploicae 85
Appendicitis 2, 28, 30, 58, 76, 93, 112, 128, 136, 140, 157, 162, 165, 173
  acute 178
  catarrhal 34, 34*f*, 76*f*
  obstructive 46*fc*, 60
  case of 8
  chances of 38*f*
  chronic 22, 30, 31, 31*f*, 32*f*, 113
    recurrent 123
  classical acute 48
  clinical audit for 165
  complications of 86, 96, 146
    acute 96
  diagnosis of 66, 78
    acute 70, 72
  differential diagnosis of acute 78, 171
  diminishing incidence of 141
  distribution of 41*f*
  drugs in 159*f*
  early stages of acute 59
  epidemic of acute 42
  epiploica 176
  etiological factors of 37
  etiology of 170
    acute 37
  granulosa 30, 32
  incidence of acute 162, 163
  investigations for 62
  larvata 30, 32
  management of 169*f*
  migration of pain in 51*f*
  nonobstructive 42*f*, 45, 47*f*, 47*fc*, 60, 60*f*

Index

obliterans 175
obstructive 42f, 47f, 59, 60f
  acute 44
operation for 146
operative management of 147
pain in acute 50
pathology of acute 43
perforated 69f
perforative 36, 37f
position of 177
post-ileal 62
pre-ileal 62
prevent 147
problem in 145
prognosis of acute 97
protective 175
purulent 35, 35f
recurrent 30, 31, 86, 96, 113
residual 30, 32
retrocecal 13, 13f, 61, 61f, 169
role of
  statistics in 163f
  surgical audit in 166f
seasonal variation of acute 42
signs of acute 53, 171
stump 77
subacute 22, 30, 34f, 100, 113
symptoms of 145
  acute 50
treatment of acute 97
type of 30, 31, 59
  acute 44
valentino 82
Appendicolith, asymptomatic 77
Appendicolithiasis 175
Appendicostomy 142, 142f
Appendicovesicostomy 142
Appendicular artery 16, 17f, 175
  of Seshachalam 177
Appendix 12, 24, 88, 101, 118, 126f, 140, 145, 149
  absence of 28
  acts 26f
  acutely inflamed 48f
  adenocarcinoma of 101, 102
  agenesis of 11f, 28, 29f
  aiverticula of 100f
  and rectum 91
  and sigmoid colon 91
  and small bowel 91
  and urinary bladder 91
  anti-mesenteric border of 87
  arterial supply of 17, 18f
  base of 61f, 121, 121f, 127f, 154
  benign tumors of 101

burial of stump of 143, 177
carcinoid tumor of 163, 174
conditions of 99
congenital anomalies of 28, 29
cut section of 22f
cutting of base of 127f
cyst of 99
delays 27
development of 10, 11f
diseases of 28, 152, 157
diverticula of 29, 30f
diverticulum of 29, 99, 100, 113
drugs of 157
duplication of 29, 29f
emboli from 18f
empties 26f
empyema of 99, 113
endometriosis of 113
engulfed 150f
epiploicae, torsion of 79, 85
function of 25, 145, 178
highly inflamed 128
histology of 22, 22f
hyperaemia of 82
inflammatory stages of 128
into cecum, intussusception of 79f
intussusception of 99, 100
investment of 23
isolation of 118
location of 12f
lumen of 11, 15, 15f, 40
lymph drainage of 19f
lymphatic drainage of 18, 19f
malignant tumors of 101
mass effect around 64
mesentery of 16
mildly inflamed 23f
mucocele of 99, 99f, 113, 113f
nerve supply of 20
normal 65f
obliteration of 96
obstruction of lumen of 40
operation of 146
  recovery after 146
operative surgery of 108
perforation of 72f, 73, 86, 87f, 88f, 137f, 154f, 175
position of 12, 13f, 61
pyocele of 99
removal of 113, 119, 127
rupture of empyema of 99
size of 15
statistics about 162
stump of 120f, 177

sub-hepatic 13, 14f, 29, 30f
subserous 14, 14f
surface marking of 12
surgery, relation to 108
tip 87, 175
  gangrene of 37f
treatment of empyema of 99
tumors of 22, 100
Valentino 82, 82f, 176
venous drainage of 18, 18f
vermiform 1-3, 10, 11f, 10f, 12, 25, 26, 28
wall of 16f
Argentaffinoma 101
Artery
  of Seshachalam 17, 17f
  recurrent appendicular 175
Ascaris lumbricoides 41
Auscultation 53

B

Bacteria 40
  beneficial 147
  reservoir of 26f
  toxins of 36
Bacteroides
  fragilis 44
  species 44
Baldwin's test 57
Barium meal 65
Bastede sign 58
Battle's pararectal incision 118
Beneficial intestinal bacteria 2
Bleeding 135
Blood urea 64
Blowhole cecostomy 150
Blumberg's sign 55
Bowel
  abscess, interloop small 92
  sentinel loops of 64
Bradykinin 102
Broken limb 169

C

Caeco-appendical angle 19
Calcified fecaliths 64
Calcium 64
  phosphate 40
Camper's fascia superficial fatty layer 108
Carbon dioxide insufflator 123f
Carcinoid syndrome 101, 102
  clinical features of 171

Carcinoid tumor 100-102
Catarrhal appendicitis 34, 45
Cecum 11f, 148
   carcinoma of 86, 93, 150
   delivering 118
   vascular fold of 20f
Cephalosporin 111, 157, 158
Cervical lymph nodes 78
Chandelier sign 175
Charles Darwin's theory 1
Chemical cautery 143
Cimetidine 160
Cirrhosis 85
Clado's gland 19
Clavulanic acid 157, 158
Clip, application of 155f
Clostridium species 44
Cloxacillin 157
Colon, carcinoma of 79, 84
Complete blood count 63
Congenital anomalies 28
Congestion 46
Conjoint tendon 109
Constipation 52
Cope's psoas test 57
C-reactive protein 64
Crease incision 116
Creatinine 64
Crohn's disease 40, 70, 80, 93, 175
Crohn's ileitis 32
Crypts of Lieberkühn 101
Cutaneous arteries 109
Cutaneous nerves 109
Cutaneous veins 109
Cystadenocarcinoma 99
Cystadenoma 99
Cysts, appendicular 96
Cytomegalovirus 77

D

Deep circumflex iliac artery,
   ascending branch of 135
Dehydration 63
Diabetes mellitus 85
Diarrhea 52
Diclofenac sodium 159
Dicyclomine 160
Dietary fiber 140
Digestion, disorders of 41
Digital rectal examination 58, 91
Distal colonic obstruction 40
Diverticulitis 79, 84
Domperidone 160

Dunphy's sign 56
Duodenal ulcer, perforation 80, 81f
Dyspepsia
   appendicular 58
   cause of appendicular 58

E

Early appendicular perforation 74f
Echinococcus granulosus 41
Ectopic pregnancy 79, 83
Edema 46, 67
Electric cautery 143
Electrolytes 64
Eliciting muscle guarding,
   method of 56
Endoloop, application of 155f
Endometriosis 79, 83, 84, 101
Endoscopic ultrasound 141
Enema 65
Entamoeba histolytica 41
Enteritis, regional 80
Enterobius vermicularis 41
Enterococcus 43
   species 44
Epigastric artery, inferior 109f, 110, 110f, 111, 134
Epiploic appendicitis 85
Epithelial debris 40
Escherichia coli 44, 44f
Esomeprazole 160
Etoricoxib 159
External oblique
   aponeurosis, division of 115f
   muscle 109, 109f, 110, 110f

F

Famotidine 160
Fascia, superficial 108
Fate of appendicular lump 95
Fecal
   fistula 132, 133
   material 40
Fecalith 40
Femoral artery 110f
Femoral canal 110f
Femoral nerve 110f
Femoral vein 110f
Fever 51
Fibers, direction of 109, 110
Fibrinopurulent peritonitis, acute 88

Fibrinous peritonitis, acute 88
Fibroma 100, 101
Fibrosis 40
Fluid collection 67
Fold of Douglas 110
Follicular cyst rupture, mid-cycle 79
Foreign body 40
Fowler–Weir approach 117
Fusobacterium species 44

G

Gallbladder, rupture of 84
Gallstone colic 79, 84
Gangrene 149f
Gangrenous 33
   appendicitis 36
   appendix 149
Gastroenteritis, acute 70, 78, 79, 171
Genetic configuration 141
Good morning appendix 177
Gram-negative bacilli 44
Gram-positive
   bacilli 44
   cocci 44
Gridiron incision 115
   advantages of 115
   disadvantages of 115
   steps of 115
Grumbling appendix 30, 31, 123
Gut flora 25
Gut, malrotation of 13, 29f

H

H_2 receptor antagonists 157, 160
Handshake appendix 126f
Hasson's trocar 125
Hematuria 52
Hemicolectomy, right 150
Hemorrhage 132
Henoch–Schönlein purpura 79, 80
Hepatoporto-appendicostomy 142
Herbivorous animals 1
Hernial sac 14f
Histamine 102
Human immunodeficiency virus
   infection 76
Hyoscine butylbromide 160
Hypersensitivity 159

Index

I

Ibuprofen 159
Ileitis, regional 80, 171
Ileocecal fold
  inferior 20, 20f
  superior 20
Ileocecal hyperplastic
  tuberculosis 93
Ileocecal recess
  inferior 20, 20f
  superior 20, 20f
Ileocecal region 19f
Ileocecal valve 15f
Ileum 11f
Ilial lymphadenitis 93
Immune function 26
Immunity 140
Immunoglobulin A, secretion
  of 25
Immunosuppression 85
Incidental appendicectomy,
  contraindications of 129
Incision 114
  closure of 116
Infection 146, 155
Infertility 96
Inflammation 28, 155
  spreads 60
Inflammatory diseases 82
Inguinal hernia 174
  right 133
Inguinal ligament 109
Instrument tray 124
Internal oblique muscle,
  aponeurosis of 110
Intestinal flora 25
Intestinal obstruction 96, 171
  acute 70, 79, 84, 132, 133
Intestine, tuberculosis of 80
Intra-abdominal infection,
  management of 154

J

Jackson's membrane 20, 21f
Jar tenderness 58

K

Kallikrein 102
Kaposi's sarcoma 77
Ketoprofen 159
Klebsiella species 44
Kulchitsky cells 101

L

Lansoprazole 160
Lanz incision 116
  advantages of 116
  disadvantages of 116
Laparoscopic appendicectomy
  122, 134, 148, 153, 154
  disadvantages of 153
  port placement in 125f
Laparoscopic to open
  appendectomy, conversion
  rate of 177
Laparoscopy
  diagnostic 68
  principal advantages of 154
Laparotomy 162
Lawson tait 6f
Leannander 39
Left iliac fossa 29, 29f
Leukemic ileocecal syndrome
  79, 85
Light source 124f
Lilly white appendix 126f, 175
Limited respiratory movements
  54
Linea semilunaris 110
Lobar pneumonia 80
Local peritoneal irritation, signs
  of 77
Lower midline incision,
  advantages of 117
Lump
  appendicular 91, 92f, 94f
  constituents of appendicular
    92
Lymph follicles 24f
Lymph gland 19
  main 19f
Lymph node, enlarged
  appendicular 19f
Lymphoid follicles 16, 16f
  hyperplasia of 40
Lymphoma 100, 101

M

Malone procedure 142, 142f
Manson–Bahr point 82f
Markle sign 58
Mass
  appendicular 91, 92f
  causes of nonresolving
    appendicular 177
  differential diagnosis of
    appendicular 93, 171

Mayo's scissors 115
McBurney's gridiron incision
  115f
McBurney's incision 7f
McBurney's point 7f, 12, 12f, 15,
  82f, 115, 178, 181f
  tenderness at 54f
Meckel's diverticulitis 70, 78, 79,
  171
Meckel's diverticulum 78f
  rule of 2 of 79
Medicolegal factor, role of 168
Mefenamic acid 159
Memory, goddess of 170
Menstruation 43
Mesenteric infarction 79, 85
Mesenteric lymphadenitis 70
  acute 78
Mesoappendix 16, 16f, 20f, 126f
  arising 16f
  cutting of 119
  thickened 128
Metoclopramide 160
Metronidazole 111, 157, 158
Mitrofanoff procedure 142
Modern equipment and
  techniques 142
Mortality, causes of 93
Mucocele, malignant 99
Mucosa 23
Mucosal hyperplasia 99
Murphy's syndrome 50, 52
Murphy's triad 52, 52f, 170
Muscle 109
  coat 23
  guarding 55
Muscularis mucosa, neutrophilic
  infiltration of 46
Myoma 100, 101
Myxoma 100, 101

N

Nasogastric tube 111
Nausea 51
Needlescopic appendicectomy
  141
Needlescopic approach 128
Neoplasm 40
Nephrotic syndrome 85
Neuropathic rectum 142
Neurovascular bundle, location
  of 110f
Nigam's scoring system 68, 69f
Nonobstructive theory 41

Index

Nonopioid analgesics 159
Nuclear medicine investigations 70

O

Oblique muscle, internal 109, 109f, 110, 110f
Obstruction, causes of 40
Ochsner–Sherren regimen 89, 94, 95, 170
   contraindications of 94
   principle of 94
Omentum, size of 73f
Omeprazole 160
Ondansetrons 160
Operation
   site preparation 114
   theater, set up in 124
Operative site, inspection of 121
Opioid analgesics 159
Orifice, appendicular 15, 15f
Ovarian carcinoma 93
Ovarian cyst
   torsion of 70, 84, 171
   twisted 93
Ovarian follicle, ruptured 70

P

Pain 50, 52, 56
   cause of 2
   recurrent bouts of 31
Palpation 52
Pancreatitis, acute 70, 81
Pantoprazole 160
Paralytic ileus 132, 133
Parametritis 93
Parasite, presence of 41
Parietal peritoneum 75
Pelvic appendicitis 61, 62, 62f
   clinical features of 177
Pelvic inflammatory disease 79, 83
Pelvic organs 121
Pelvic position 13
Penicillin 8, 157
Peptic ulcers 159
Peptostreptococcus species 44
Percussion 53
Peritoneal cavity 130f
   safe access to 125
   suction of pus from 144f

Peritoneal fluid cultures 43
Peritonitis
   general 88
   localized 154f
   primary 85
   purulent 74f, 88f
Phlegmon 67, 91
Pneumoperitoneum 125, 154
Pointing test 54, 54f
Porphyromonas gingivalis 43
Portal pyemia 86, 95, 132, 133
Postappendectomy infection, management of 132fc
Post-appendicectomy pyrexia 92, 93f
Postileal appendicitis, clinical features of 178
Potassium 64
Pott's spine 85
Pregnancy test 63
Preherpetic pain 85
Proton pump inhibitors 157, 160
Pseudoappendicitis 30, 32, 82
Pseudomonas aeruginosa 44
Pseudomyxoma peritonei 100-102
Pulmonary tuberculosis, thoracoplasty for 8
Purgatives 41
Purse string suture 120f
Purulent peritonitis, acute 88, 89f
Pyelonephritis 79, 83
   acute 70
   right-sided acute 81
Pylephlebitis 133
   suppurative 95
Pyrexia 53

R

Rabeprazole 160
Ranitidine 160
Rebound tenderness 55
Recess 20f
Rectus abdominis muscle 109f, 110, 110f
Rectus sheath hematoma 81
Retention cyst 99
Retrocecal appendicitis, clinical features of 177
Retrocecal position 12
Right iliac fossa 56
   anatomy of 108
   pain 98

Right paramedian incision 117
   advantages of 117
Ripasa scoring system 68
Robotic appendicectomy 141
Rockey–Davis incision 118
Rovsing's sign 56f, 181
Rupture, appendicular 181f
Ruptured ectopic
   gestation 171
   pregnancy 70
Rutherford Morison's incision
   disadvantages of 117
   indications of 117
Rutherford Morison's muscle cutting incision 116
Ryle's tube 170

S

Salpingitis 83, 171
   acute 70
Scarless surgery 141
Scarpa's fascia deep membranous layer 108
Septic
   factor 63
   peritonitis 88
Septicemia 95
Serofibrinous peritonitis, acute 88
Serosa 23
Sherren's triangle 56, 57f
Sickness, diagnosis of 22
Sigmoid colon 149
Sigmoid diverticulitis 86
Single incision laparoscopic surgery 141
Skin 108
Sodium 64
Spinal conditions 85
Spine, tuberculosis of 85
Stitches 146
Streptococcus species 44
Stricture 40
Strongyloides stercoralis 41
Subcecal position 13
Submucosa 23
Subserous appendix, dissection for 14
Surgical anatomy 10
Surgical audit 165
Surgical team, position of 124
Sympathetic nerves 20

Index

T

Tabetic crisis 85
Tachycardia 53, 60
Telesurgery 141
Tenderness 60
Terminal ileum 121
Testis, torsion of 81
Thoracic nine 20
Thoracic ten segments 20
Tongue, dry 54
Total leucocyte count 143
Tramadol hydrochloride 159
Transverse colon 149
Transversus abdominis muscle 109f, 110, 110f
Trauma 42, 74
Trocar placement 125
Trocar, insertion of 126f
Tuberculosis 77
Tubo-ovarian sepsis 83
Tumor
  appendicular 113
  benign 100
  malignant 100
Typhoid 80

U

Ulcerative colitis 27
Ulcers 32
Ultrasound scan
  false negative 66
  false positive 66
Ureteric colic 80
  right 70
Urinary 5-hydroxyindoleacetic acid 70
Urinary tract infection 63
Urine examination 63
Uterine adnexa, right 82

V

Vaginal examination 70
Valentino syndrome 82
Valve of Gerlach 15
Vascular infections 96
Vascular occlusion 41
Veins draining 18
Vermiform appendix, surface of 26
Vestigial organ 174
Violent pain, sudden onset of 60
Viral infection 39
Visceral peritoneum 75
Vomiting 51, 88

W

Wallbridge classification 29
White worm 175
Worms 41
Wound
  closure of 122
  infection 132, 154

Y

Yersinia 32
  ileitis 82

EU GSPR Authorised Reprsentative
Logos Europe, 9 rue Nicolas Poussin
1700, La Rochelle, France
Phone: +33 (0) 6 67 93 73 78
E-mail: contact@logoseurope.eu

www.ingramcontent.com/pod-product-compliance
Ingram Content Group UK Ltd.
Pitfield, Milton Keynes, MK11 3LW, UK
UKHW050429150426
5217IPUK00019B/1300